the
A-Z Guide to Food
as Medicine

the
A-Z Guide to Food
as Medicine

Diane Kraft
Ara DerMarderosian

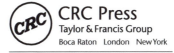

CRC Press
Taylor & Francis Group
Boca Raton   London   New York

CRC Press is an imprint of the
Taylor & Francis Group, an **informa** business

CRC Press
Taylor & Francis Group
6000 Broken Sound Parkway NW, Suite 300
Boca Raton, FL 33487-2742

© 2016 by Taylor & Francis Group, LLC
CRC Press is an imprint of Taylor & Francis Group, an Informa business

No claim to original U.S. Government works

Printed on acid-free paper
Version Date: 20150914

International Standard Book Number-13: 978-1-4987-3523-0 (Paperback)

Library of Congress Cataloging-in-Publication Data

Kraft, Diane, 1963-
    The A-Z guide to food as medicine / Diane Kraft and Ara DerMarderosian.
        pages cm
    Includes bibliographical references and index.
        ISBN 978-1-4987-3523-0 (alk. paper)
        1. Nutrition. 2. Medicine, Preventive. 3. Self-care, Health. I. DerMarderosian, Ara.
    II. Title.

    RA784.K67 2016
    613.2--dc23   2015029282

Visit the Taylor & Francis Web site at
http://www.taylorandfrancis.com

and the CRC Press Web site at
http://www.crcpress.com

The A-Z Guide to Food as Medicine is honored to have received a 2016 American Library Association/Choice Magazine Outstanding Academic Title award.

Contents

Foreword

There is a growing consumer interest in health and the role that nutrition can play in promoting health and preventing nutrition-related chronic diseases. This heightened interest in nutrition has been accompanied by many questions about what specifically can be done with nutrition to promote health and prevent disease. There is a growing interest in phytochemicals because of the ongoing research demonstrating their many health benefits. Phytochemicals are present in plant foods such as fruits, vegetables, beans, grains, nuts, seeds, soy products, as well as liquid vegetable oils. Thousands of phytochemicals have been identified; common classes include antioxidants, flavonoids, flavanols, flavanones, isoflavones, catechins, epicatechins, anthocyanins, anthocyanidins, proanthocyanidins, isothiocyanates, carotenoids, allyl sulfides, polyphenols, and phenolic acids, among others. The list of phytochemicals may be overwhelming to grasp. Given their plethora and their myriad biological actions, there is a need for an authoritative resource that provides important basic information about many individual foods and phytochemicals. Having all of this information compiled in *The A–Z Guide to Food as Medicine* will be of benefit to readers in understanding the current evidence base for individual phytochemicals. This guide is an important resource because it presents concise and key science-based information that can be quickly and easily accessed. It can also be used as a filter for "junk science," which clutters many information resources and causes a lot of confusion among the public. The guide is formatted to define the food, spice, bioactive compound, or topic of interest; its origin, including how it is used; a summary of the scientific findings, including references; the bioactive dose, when known; and safety information, when applicable. This guide presents germane information concisely in one place. This is of benefit to readers who wish to follow good nutrition practices that are based on sound science. Readers will find that the guide is "go to" resource when trying to sort fact from fiction in response to the burgeoning nutrition misinformation that is everywhere. Key topics of interest include nutrients, bioactive components, specific foods, spices, and other topics of interest. Readers will value the extensive list of topics covered and the concise information presented for each one. *The A–Z Guide to Food as Medicine* will serve as an expedient resource for quickly accessing fact-based information about foods and phytochemicals in a manner that obviates the need to spend unnecessary time hunting down reputable information in the literature and other sources. I highly recommend *The A–Z Guide to Food as Medicine* as a valuable, "quick-access" resource for obtaining sound, science-based information that can be used to implement dietary practices that benefit health.

Penny M. Kris-Etherton, PhD, RD
Distinguished Professor of Nutrition, Penn State University

Preface

Traditional use of foods as medicine has been practiced worldwide since ancient times. In the third century BC, Hippocrates said, "Let food be thy medicine." In the centuries that followed, records show that foods and plant materials were the basis of early medicines in practically every country. In contrast to folkloric use of foods as medicine, when an apple a day was recommended to keep the doctor away but for unknown reasons, modern science has isolated immune-enhancing constituents in apples and recommends the number of servings (a bioactive dose) of fruits one needs daily for health to prevent certain diseases[1] and makes practical recommendations to eat not only white-fleshed fruits but also to consume as many different colors of fruits as possible to ingest as wide an array as possible of nutrients and phytochemicals associated with health and disease prevention.

Phytochemicals, literally "plant chemicals," are produced by the plant for survivability, that is, as protection against pathogens and pests,[2] and they also provide health benefits when consumed.

For example, glucosinolates in brassica family vegetables are both plant-protective[3] and have been shown to exert anticancer properties when consumed.[4] Phytochemicals are also responsible for the characteristic colors, flavors, aromas, and textures of plant foods.

The beneficial pharmacological properties of foods, nutrients, and phytochemicals are highlighted in this guide.

Whole food, with few exceptions, is preferable as a source of nutrients and phytochemicals. Phytochemicals, similar to nutrients, are best utilized by the body when provided as part of the whole food matrix, rather than as individual entities. This is due to the numerous symbiotic elements contained within foods that work in concert with one another, both enhancing the beneficial elements and diluting the less desirable elements.[3]

The actions of phytochemicals in the diet are characterized by Dillard and German as follows:

1. Substrates (fuels) for biochemical reactions
2. Cofactors of enzymatic reactions

3. Inhibitors of enzymatic reactions
4. Absorbents/sequestrants that bind to and eliminate undesirable constituents in the intestine
5. Ligands (substances that bind to another molecule to form a complex) that agonize or antagonize cell surface or intracellular receptors
6. Scavengers of reactive or toxic chemicals
7. Compounds that enhance the absorption and/or stability of essential nutrients
8. Selective growth factors for beneficial gastrointestinal bacteria
9. Fermentation substrates for beneficial oral, gastric, or intestinal bacteria
10. Selective inhibitors of deleterious intestinal bacteria

This guide is a dictionary of foods and bioactive ingredients found in foods. The authors included fruits, vegetables, and other natural foods identified in the scientific literature as having been studied for a physiological effect. Individual entries (foods, nutrients, and phytochemicals) are organized alphabetically so information can be easily accessed. Only naturally occurring foods and food constituents are addressed while dietary supplements are not, because their physiological effects may be due to dose, whereas, our focus was on natural physiological effects of foods and food constituents. Only enteral, and not topical uses of foods, nutrients, and phytochemicals are addressed.

Each entry provides

- The food or food constituent name, definition, and common use.
- Scientific findings for its beneficial effects or lack thereof.
- A bioactive dose, if known, that is, if supported by scientific consensus; for example, the quantities of food groups that one should eat daily that are consistent with health are known and are presented as a "bioactive dose." Likewise, the quantities of nutrients that one should consume daily, in the foods they select, are known, and the recommended dietary allowance (RDA) or adequate intake (AI) of nutrients is presented as a "bioactive dose." In many cases, data about the physiological effects of a phytochemical are limited to laboratory research, suggesting the research on that particular food component is preliminary. The reader is aware that *in vitro* and animal studies do not prove *in vivo* biological activity. By including such preliminary data, the guide is informing the reader that a phytochemical is in its infancy in terms of research. Rarely have foods or their constituents been adequately tested in well-designed, adequately powered clinical trials. When a clinical trial's bioactive dose has been reported, the guide attempts to include it in the scientific findings section, but for the majority of foods and phytochemicals

presented herein, typically a bioactive dose is not known and "bioactive dose: not known" is stated.

- Safety data, such as the tolerable upper level of intake (UL), for nutrients are stated. Safety concerns for certain groups or individuals have been captured when they were identified in the scientific literature whether or not studies in scientific findings address these groups. For example, there may have been no studies conducted in pregnant women and no studies on pregnant women will appear in the scientific findings sections, but when pregnancy precautions have been published and could be identified in the scientific literature, the safety section will state that safe use has not been established during pregnancy.

All foods are generally recognized as safe (GRAS) by the U.S. Food and Drug Administration, and many food constituents, for example, limonene and vanillin, also have GRAS status. Generally, the statement "Presumed safe when consumed in normal dietary quantities by non-allergic individuals" is stated in the safety section for the majority of foods, nutrients, and phytochemicals, followed by safety concerns for certain groups or individuals.

Important advice and notes

With regard to using information in this guide, it is important to keep the caveats of good science and common sense in mind:

1. Most common foods are known to be safe when properly prepared and consumed in normal amounts. However, some can interact with prescription drugs and some should not be consumed when certain diseases or conditions exist. Some foods must also be avoided in cases of food intolerance, sensitivity, or allergy.
2. Phytochemicals and food constitutents that are medicinal in nature in small quantities may be deleterious to health in large quantities.
3. All data provided in this guide are intended for reference and to enhance knowledge of foods and food constituents.

Diane Kraft and Ara DerMarderosian

References

1. National Cancer Institute. Cancer Progress Trends Report. http://progress-report.cancer.gov/prevention/fruit_vegetable. Accessed February 06, 2015.
2. Joseph JA, Shukitt-Hale B, Willis LM. Grape juice, berries, and walnuts affect brain aging and behavior. *J Nutr.* 2009;139:1813S–1817S.

3. Björkman M, Klingen I, Birch AN, Bones AM, Bruce TJ, Johansen TJ, Meadow R et al. Phytochemicals of Brassicaceae in plant protection and human health—Influences of climate, environment and agronomic practice. *Phytochemistry* 2011;72(7):538–556.
4. Kumar G, Tuli HS, Mittal S, Shandilya JK, Tiwari A, Sandhu SS. Isothiocyanates: A class of bioactive metabolites with chemopreventive potential. *Tumour Biol.* 2015 Apr 3. [Epub ahead of print].

Acknowledgments

The authors thank Katharine Yuengling for her considerable work and intellectual contribution to this book over many years; their families, Kevin and Noah Kraft and Evelyn DerMarderosian, for their support and sacrifice throughout the long process of developing this manuscript; our CRC Press/Taylor and Francis Group editor Randy Brehm for her can-do attitude and professionalism that made every phase of work on this book enjoyable; project coordinators Ashley Weinstein and Kat Evans, cover designer John Gandour, project editor Marsha Hecht, and project manager Karthick Parthasarathy from Techset Composition.

Thanks also to the following individuals whose knowledge or assistance enhanced the content of this work or furthered the manuscript toward publication: Rachel Ackerman, Bruce Auerbach, Joseph M. Betz, Bill Bowman, Kevin Burns, Evelyn DerMarderosian, Melissa Fellenbaum, Elizabeth Gardner, Kathleen Gardocki, Monica Henson, Susan Kane, Ned Kraft, Joseph Kremer, Penny M. Kris-Etherton, Robert C. Langan, Evelyn J. Little, Miroslaw Liwosz, Melissa G. Marko, Krisan Matthews, David Meharg, Sharon Neal, Michael Nerino, Justin Padinske, M.A. Tomasz Pazdro, Joel Pearce, Laura Pelehach, David Pompilio, Ralph Porrazzo, Bobbie Rohrbach, T.C. Smith, Karen Thacker, Becky Thornburg, Laura Torcomian, Kathy Webb, and Shirley Williams.

Authors

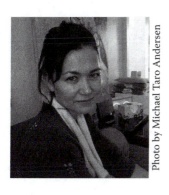

Photo by Michael Taro Andersen

Diane Woznicki Kraft, MS, RD, LDN, holds a Master of Science degree in clinical nutrition from New York University and a Bachelor of Science degree in human nutrition from Penn State University. She and her coauthor created this handbook as a reference for healthcare professionals to access scientific findings on the health aspects of foods, food groups, nutrients, and phytochemicals to assist clients educationally on diet and nutrition. Woznicki Kraft teaches nutrition at Alvernia University, Reading, Pennsylvania. She has authored consumer and professional articles on nutrition for The American Council on Science and Health and The American Academy of Nutrition and Dietetics and has edited chapters in science text books and manuals, including the dietary supplements chapter of *The Merck Manual*. This is her first book.

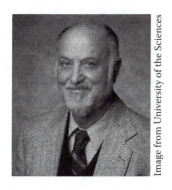

Image from University of the Sciences

Ara DerMarderosian, PhD, Emeritus Professor of Pharmacognosy and Medicinal Chemistry, University of the Sciences, Philadelphia, Pennsylvania. He has authored several books on pharmacognosy topics, chapters in *Remington's Pharmaceutical Sciences*, and numerous scientific articles, and has served as editor and/or coeditor of *The Review of Natural Products*, a reference book on natural products addressing the botanical, historical, clinical, chemical, pharmacological, and toxicological aspects of natural products, through the eighth (2015) edition. He is the herbal and dietary supplement chapter author for several editions of *The Merck Manual*, and has spoken on nutrition and pharmacognosy topics to medical professionals for several decades.

A

Açaí berry (Euterpe oleracea)

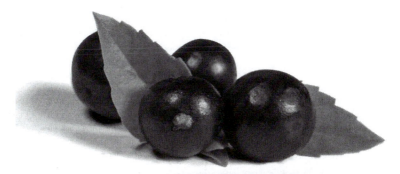

Acai fruit. (Image from diogoppr/Shutterstock.)

definition

Dark purple fruit of the açaí palm native to South America. Commonly sold as juice or juice drink.

scientific findings

An *in vitro* study found that acai juice polyphenols exhibited antioxidant properties and inhibited LDL (low-density lipoprotein) oxidation but found "no consistent clinical evidence of antioxidant potency" of acai compared to other beverages, such as red wine.[1] In rats fed a hypercholesterolemic diet, acai supplementation improved antioxidant status and reduced non–high-density lipoprotein (HDL) cholesterol.[2] In a small crossover clinical trial of healthy human volunteers (n = 12), acai juice and pulp, dosed at 7 mL/kg of body weight, raised plasma antioxidant capacity but did not affect other markers of antioxidant activity such as antioxidant capacity of urine.[3] A small nonblinded, non–placebo-controlled trial of healthy overweight adults (n = 10) showed that consuming 100 g of acai pulp for 1 month improved insulin, total cholesterol, and postprandial plasma glucose.[4]

1

bioactive dose

Not known.

safety

Presumed safe when consumed in normal dietary quantities by non-allergic individuals. There is insufficient safety data available to evaluate the use of acai during pregnancy or lactation.[5]

Alfalfa (Medicago sativa)

definition

Herb which is made into tea and used medicinally; the seeds and sprouts are also consumed.[6] Alfalfa sprouts are used fresh in salads, on sandwiches, or juiced. *M. sativa* contains saponins, flavonoids, phytoestrogens, alkaloids, phytosterols, and terpenes.[7] In traditional medicine, *M. sativa* has been used to treat atherosclerosis, heart disease, stroke, cancer, diabetes, and menopausal symptoms.[7]

scientific findings

In laboratory research, the *M. sativa* plant has exhibited neuroprotective, hypocholesterolemic, antioxidant, antiulcer, antimicrobial, hypolipidemic, and estrogenic properties.[7] In a clinical trial (n = 15 hypercholesterolemic subjects), eating 40 g of alfalfa seeds three times daily with meals for 8 weeks reduced elevated total and LDL cholesterol,[8] due to saponins' inhibition of the absorption of cholesterol or bile in the gut,[8] an effect that also was demonstrated in two laboratory studies.[9,10]

bioactive dose

For high cholesterol, a typical oral dose of 5–10 g of the alfalfa herb steeped, strained, and drunk as tea three times daily has been used.[6]

safety

Presumed safe when consumed in normal dietary quantities by non-allergic individuals. Alfalfa seeds and sprouts have the potential for bacterial contamination and should be avoided by children, older adults, and immune-compromised individuals.[11] Chronic ingestion of alfalfa seeds has been associated with pancytopenia and drug-induced lupus-like effects.[5] Alfalfa constituents may exert estrogenic effects and therefore may be unsafe during pregnancy and lactation when used in amounts greater than those found in foods.[5] When the alfalfa herb is prepared and used as a tea as described in Bioactive Dose, it is considered to be possibly safe for use by adults, but excessive or long-term use is not recommended.[5]

Allium vegetables

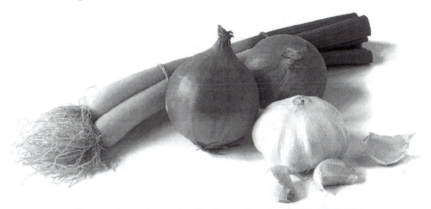

Spring onion, onion, and garlic. (Image from jopelka/Shutterstock.)

definition

Bulbous culinary herbs of the Alliaceae family that include approximately 500 species such as onion (*Allium cepa*), shallot (*Allium ascalonicum*), garlic (*Allium sativum*), green onion (*Allium macrostemon*), leek (*Allium porrum*), scallion (*Allium tartaricum*), and others. Commonly used raw or cooked for their flavor and pungent odor due to organosulfur compounds such as allyl derivatives.[12] Allium vegetables are rich in flavonoids.[13] They have been used for medicinal purposes throughout recorded history.

scientific findings

In laboratory studies, allyl derivatives inhibited carcinogenesis in the stomach, esophagus, colon, mammary gland, and lung of experimental animals[14] and improved immune function, reduced blood glucose, and conferred radioprotection and protection against microbial infection.[15] Clinical trials to investigate anticancer effects of allium vegetables and their constituents are lacking,[15] but epidemiological studies have provided preliminary evidence of allium vegetables' anticancer effects in certain types of cancer. For example, a population-based case–control study (n = 238 case subjects with confirmed prostate cancer and 471 control subjects) found that men who consumed the highest amount of allium

A

vegetables (>10.0 g/day which is approximately one tablespoon[16]) had a statistically significant lower risk of prostate cancer than those who consumed the least.[17] Allium vegetable intake of ≥1 portion per week compared with low or no consumption was associated with a reduced risk of myocardial infarction in a case–control study (n = 760 patients with a first episode of nonfatal acute myocardial infarction and 682 controls).[18] High allium vegetable consumption was associated with a reduced risk of gastric cancer in a meta-analysis of 19 case–control and two cohort studies (n = 543,220).[19] In a multicenter case–control study, a comparison of dietary data from 454 endometrial cancer cases and 908 controls found "a moderate protective role of allium vegetables on the risk of endometrial cancer."[20]

bioactive dose

Not known.

safety

Presumed safe when consumed in normal dietary quantities by non-allergic individuals.

Allspice (Pimenta dioica)

definition

Dried fruit of a Caribbean tree[21] that is ground into a reddish-brown powder and consumed as a spice. Allspice is used in Caribbean cooking as jerk seasoning; in Indian chutneys, biryani, and meat and poultry dishes; in Middle Eastern cooking; and is a standard ingredient in pumpkin pie. *P. dioica* contains numerous phytochemicals including phenolics, vanillin, eugenol, and terpenoids.[22] In traditional medicine, allspice has been used to treat hypertension, inflammation, pain, diarrhea, fever, cold, pneumonia, and bacterial infection.[22]

scientific findings

Laboratory studies have shown allspice to have antioxidant properties.[23,24] A review of allspice found its glycosides and polyphenols exerted antibacterial, hypotensive, antineuralgic, and analgesic properties in laboratory studies; in addition, *in vitro* and *in vivo* studies showed it to have anti-prostate-cancer and anti-breast-cancer properties, as well as to exhibit "selective antiproliferative and antitumor properties on human cancer cells and their animal models."[21]

bioactive dose

Not known.

safety

Presumed safe when consumed in normal dietary quantities by non-allergic individuals. There is insufficient reliable information available about the safety of allspice used in amounts greater than are normally found in food, especially during pregnancy and lactation.[5]

Almond (Prunus dulcis)

definition

Tree nut, also known as sweet almond, that is consumed raw, roasted, pureed as almond butter, in candy and baked products, and made into milk. In addition to protein and fiber, almonds are a source of α-tocopherol, manganese, magnesium, copper, phosphorus, riboflavin,[25] phytosterols, and polyphenolic compounds such as proanthocyanidins and lignans.[26] Almost 50% of almond weight is fat,[25] most of which is monounsaturated.[27]

scientific findings

When consumed as part of a low saturated fat diet, low cholesterol diet, 2.5–3.5 oz (70–100 g) of almonds reduced total cholesterol by 4%–11% and LDL cholesterol by 7%–12%, according to the results of five small human studies, two of which also found a 1.7%–3.5% increase in HDL cholesterol.[28] Perhaps due to their high content of bioavailable α-tocopherol, almond-supplemented diets may reduce LDL-cholesterol oxidation.[25] Despite nuts' general reputation for being high-calorie calorie, two randomized, controlled trials found that a low-calorie diet that included almonds did not increase body weight. In one of the studies (n = 123), overweight and obese individuals were randomly assigned to consume either an almond-supplemented low-calorie diet or a nut-free low-calorie diet. At 18 months, both groups experienced clinically significant and comparable weight loss.[29] In the second study (n = 65), subjects were randomized to a liquid formula-based weight-loss diet supplemented with almonds, or a liquid-formula-based-weight-loss diet supplemented with complex carbohydrates. At 24 weeks, greater reductions in weight were seen in the almond-supplemented group.[30] Both studies found improvements in blood lipids in almond-supplemented groups compared to control groups.[29,30] In a third, non–placebo-controlled study (n = 20), healthy women added almonds to their diet for 10 weeks, followed by a 3-week

A

washout period, followed by their usual diet without almonds for another 10 weeks. The study found that "10 weeks of daily almond consumption did not cause a change in body weight," which was attributed to "compensation for the energy contained in the almonds through reduced food intake from other sources."[31]

bioactive dose

Not known.

safety

Presumed safe when consumed in normal dietary quantities by non-allergic individuals.

Anise (Pimpinella anisum)

definition

Umbelliferous (umbrella-shaped) mint family plant whose volatile oils, including anethole, contribute to its licorice-like flavor and aroma.[5,32] Anise seeds are used as a spice and to flavor liquors. Anise has been used in folk medicine to treat nausea and ulcer.[33] Though anise seeds are commonly consumed after meals to freshen breath and to induce burping, no published reports were found to substantiate its mechanism of action to induce burping, which is thought to occur because a constituent in anise reduces the surface tension of the stomach contents, resulting in gas bubble coalescence and release.

scientific findings

An *in vitro* study demonstrated anti-*Helicobacter pylori* activity in an extract made from the seeds of *P. anisum*.[34] *P. anisum* has demonstrated antimicrobial, antifungal, antiviral, antioxidant, immunostimulant, muscle relaxant, analgesic, and anticonvulsant activity and reduced morphine dependence in laboratory studies.[35,36] Umbelliferous vegetables are considered to be among the foods and herbs having the highest anticancer activity.[37]

bioactive dose

Not known. An oral dose of one tablespoon of the tea taken several times a day has been used for antiflatulence.[5] The tea is prepared by steeping 1–2 teaspoons of the crushed seed for 10–15 min and then straining.[5]

safety

Presumed safe when consumed in normal dietary quantities by non-allergic individuals.

Anthocyanins

definition

Purple or red plant food pigments that serve as antioxidants, found in foods such as berries, black currant, blueberry, cherry, cranberry, eggplant, lingonberry, mulberry, lettuce, and strawberry.[38] Chemically classified as polyphenolic compounds, examples of anthocyanins include cyanidin, malvidin, and petunidin.[41] Used in folk medicine to treat liver dysfunction, hypertension, vision disorders, microbial infections, diarrhea, and other disorders.[39]

scientific findings

In laboratory research, anthocyanins demonstrated estrogenic activity that altered development of hormone-dependent disease symptoms; increased cytokine production, thus regulating immune response; reduced capillary permeability and fragility and strengthened membranes; exerted anti-inflammatory, antidiabetic, and antimicrobial properties; and demonstrated anticancer and antiproliferative capabilities.[39–43] A comprehensive review of eight prospective, controlled interventional and observational studies (n = 390,769 participants) found no evidence to suggest that high anthocyanin intake is inversely associated with colorectal adenomas.[44]

bioactive dose

Not known.

safety

Presumed safe when consumed in normal dietary quantities by non-allergic individuals.

Antioxidant

definition

Phytochemical that can prevent, inhibit, or repair damage caused by oxidative stress. Antioxidants may interfere with oxidation by inactivating a prooxidant compound, scavenging free radicals, acting as chelators to deactivate metal catalysts, repair oxidative damage, or stimulate the

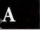

activity of antioxidant enzymes.[45,46] All plant foods are sources of anti-oxidants, which include carotenoids; vitamin C, vitamin E, and selenium; isothiocyanates; and phenolic compounds (flavonoids, stilbenes, phenolic acids, and lignans).[46]

scientific findings

Epidemiological data suggest that intake of foods rich in vitamin E, vitamin C, and β-carotene is associated with a decreased risk for coronary heart disease.[47] Studies support a beneficial effect of food-derived β-carotene, vitamin C, vitamin E, lutein, and xeaxanthin in delayed progression of advanced age-related macular degeneration; while other studies have reported inconclusive findings.[47] The U.S. Department of Agriculture has developed a rating scale to measure the antioxidant content of plant foods called the oxygen radical absorbance capacity.[48] A measure of anti-oxidant capacity of the diet called dietary total antioxidant capacity has been shown to be inversely associated with risks of developing common chronic diseases, and was found to be a good predictor of dietary and plasma antioxidant status in a sample of healthy, young adult men and women (n = 60 nonsmoking adults aged 16–25).[49]

bioactive dose

Not known and/or varies by antioxidant (see: Bioactive Dose for Selenium, Vitamin C, and Vitamin E—each has an RDA [recommended dietary allowance]. Note β-carotene has no RDA).

safety

Presumed safe when consumed in normal dietary quantities by non-allergic individuals. Varies by antioxidant (see: Safety for Selenium, Vitamin C, and Vitamin E—each has a UL [tolerable upper intake level]). β-carotene has no UL.

Apple (Domestica sylvestris)

definition

Popular fresh fruit of which there are thousands of varieties. Apples are also consumed dehydrated, dried, baked, as juice or cider, as applesauce, and in baked desserts. Apple pulp is high in the soluble fiber pectin.[50] Apple skins are a source of insoluble fiber and phytochemicals such as phloretin and the flavonoid quercetin.[51] Applesauce has been traditionally used to treat diarrhea as part of the BRAT (bananas–rice–applesauce–toast/tea) diet.[52]

A

scientific findings

Pectin may reduce diarrhea by stimulating epithelial growth in the colon.[53] Soluble fibers slow upper gastrointestinal transit time and alleviate diarrhea; on the other hand, the soluble fiber in apples increases fecal water content to promote water retention in stools, while insoluble fibers provide bulk, both actions of which promote laxation. Soluble fibers promote the excretion of cholesterol and bile acids, thereby helping to reduce serum cholesterol. Total and LDL cholesterol were reduced in a randomized, double-blind, placebo-controlled study (n = 71 healthy, moderately obese adults) in subjects ingesting 600 mg of apple polyphenols for 12 weeks, an effect not seen in the placebo group.[54] In a 1-year clinical trial (n = 160 postmenopausal women), consumption of 75 g dried apple (about two medium-sized apples) was found to significantly reduce atherogenic cholesterol levels in the third month.[55] A nonrandomized trial of healthy subjects (n = 23) found that apples, but not apple juice, significantly reduced total and LDL cholesterol.[56] Epidemiologic studies suggest an inverse relationship between apple consumption and colon cancer risk[57] and that regular consumption of one or more apples a day may reduce the risk for lung and colon cancer.[58] According to a review, "Exposure to apples and apple products has been associated with beneficial effects on risk, markers, and etiology of cancer, cardiovascular disease, asthma, and Alzheimer's disease" and preliminary data suggest an association of apples with improved cognitive outcomes related to normal aging, diabetes, weight management, bone health, pulmonary function, and gastrointestinal health.[59] A prospective, population-based cohort study (n = 20,069 men and women aged 20–65 years free of cardiovascular diseases at baseline) found that high intake of white-fleshed fruits may protect against stroke. Each 25-g/day increase in white fruit and vegetable consumption was associated with a 9% lower risk of stroke.[60] In a laboratory analysis, apple extracts showed strong antioxidant activity despite low total phenolic contents.[61]

bioactive dose

Not known.

safety

Presumed safe when consumed in normal dietary quantities by non-allergic individuals.

A

Apricot (Prunus armeniaca)

definition

Stone fruit member of the Rosaceae family that is consumed fresh, dried, canned, in jams and preserves, and as nectar. Apricots are good sources of β-carotene[62] and contain potassium, soluble and insoluble fiber,[63] and flavonoids.[64] In folk medicine, apricots have been used to treat hemorrhage, infertility, eye inflammation, and spasm.[65]

scientific findings

Apricots bound bile acids in an *in vitro* study.[66] Intestinal binding of bile acids by dietary soluble fiber reduces serum cholesterol levels in humans.

bioactive dose

Not known.

safety

Presumed safe when consumed in normal dietary quantities by non-allergic individuals.

Artichoke (Cynara scolymus)

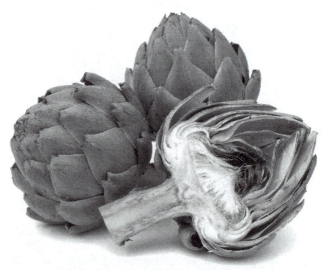

Artichoke. (Image from Binh Thanh Bui/Shutterstock.)

definition

Herb that is a good source of fiber (7 g per 1 medium artichoke) and a source of folate, calcium, and potassium,[67] in addition to caffeic acid and flavonoids.[68] Technically, the base of the flower petals (referred to as "leaves") are edible, and they are held in place by a core (artichoke "heart"), which is the main edible portion of the artichoke. Fresh artichokes can be steamed or braised, or, when purchased canned (either packed in salt water or with oil and other flavorings, such as vinegar), used as a salad vegetable.

scientific findings

A meta-analysis of three randomized, placebo-controlled clinical trials (n = 262 patients with hypercholesterolemia) concluded that artichoke leaf extract may have cholesterol-lowering potential.[69] In one trial, the total cholesterol level in participants receiving artichoke decreased from 7.16 to 6.86 mmol/L after 12 weeks and increased from 6.90 to 7.04 mmol/L in patients receiving placebo, the total difference being statistically significant.[69] A second trial found artichoke leaf extract reduced total cholesterol levels from 7.74 to 6.31 mmol/L, whereas the placebo reduced cholesterol from 7.69 to 7.03 mmol/L.[69] A third trial showed that artichoke leaf extract significantly reduced blood cholesterol compared with placebo in a subgroup of patients with baseline total cholesterol levels of more than 230 mg/dL.[69] In a 6-week, double-blind, randomized controlled trial (n = 247 patients with functional dyspepsia), a dose of 640 mg of artichoke leaf extract reduced dyspepsia compared to placebo.[70] In a randomized, crossover design study (n = 8 healthy subjects and n = 19 subjects with metabolic syndrome), glucose, insulin, and homocysteine levels were measured postprandially every 4 h after a meal containing boiled wild artichoke, white bread, refined olive oil, and lemon juice, and a control meal that did not contain the boiled artichoke. The boiled artichoke meal, compared with the control meal, reduced postprandial serum glucose and insulin response in normal subjects and had no effect in patients with metabolic syndrome or in homocysteine levels in either group.[71]

bioactive dose

Not known.

safety

Presumed safe when consumed in normal dietary quantities by non-allergic individuals.

A

Arugula (Eruca sativa)

definition

Also called rocket or roquette. Aromatic Brassicacea salad green. It may be finely chopped and combined with garlic, parmesan cheese, and other ingredients to make pesto. A good source of vitamin K[72] and glucosinolates.[73] *E. sativa* seed extract has been used to treat skin disorders in traditional Middle Eastern medicine.[74] Arugula seeds are used to grow microgreens used in salads and as a garnish.

scientific findings

Arugula (*E. sativa* cv. *Sky*) extract exhibited antioxidant properties *in vitro* in human colon cancer cells.[75]

bioactive dose

Not known.

safety

Presumed safe when consumed in normal dietary quantities by non-allergic individuals.

Asian pear (Pyrus pyrifolia)

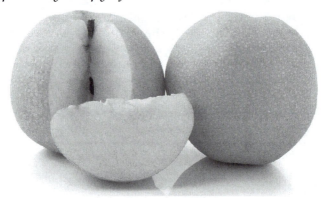

Asian pear. (Image from MRS.Siwaporn/Shutterstock.)

definition

Crisp-fleshed, juicy pear, sometimes called an Asian apple pear or Japanese pear. It resembles a yellow apple with rough, sandpaper-like skin, and it tastes like a watered-down apple.[76] A source of flavonoids, it contains 4 g of fiber per medium fruit.[77]

scientific findings

In laboratory research, *P. pyrifolia* cv. *Shingo* (Korean pear), a specific variety or cultivar of Asian pear, stimulated two key alcohol-metabolizing enzymes involved in alcohol detoxification.[78]

bioactive dose

Not known.

safety

Presumed safe when consumed in normal dietary quantities by non-allergic individuals.

Asparagus (Asparagus officinalis L.)

definition

Green shoot vegetable (the spears are "shoots") that is commonly eaten cooked by broiling or steaming. Asparagus is a good source of vitamin K and folate[79] and contains numerous phytochemicals including flavonoids[80] and saponins.[81] The mineral content (copper, iron, zinc, manganese, calcium, magnesium, sodium, potassium, and phosphorous) is higher in green asparagus than in other varieties, and nutrients are generally richest in the tips of the spears. Asparagus has been used in traditional medicine as a diuretic[82] and a contraceptive.[80]

scientific findings

In laboratory studies, asparagus has exhibited antifungal, antiviral, and antitumor properties attributed to steroidal saponins.[81] In an 8-week animal study, an asparagus extract reduced total and LDL cholesterol and raised HDL cholesterol in mice fed a high-fat diet to induce hyperlipidemia; in addition, antioxidative effects and normalization of animals' liver function tests were attributed to the asparagus extract.[83] The *Asparagus racemosus* species of asparagus, commonly used in the manufacture of dietary supplements of asparagus[84] exhibited diuretic properties in an experimental study of laboratory animals that compared asparagus to furosemide, a diuretic medication.[82]

bioactive dose

Not known. *A. racemosus* has been used medicinally as a tea prepared by steeping 40–60 g of the cut rhizome or root in 150 mL of boiling water for 5–10 min and then straining.[5]

safety

Presumed safe when consumed in normal dietary quantities by non-allergic individuals. Should not be consumed in quantities greater than are normally eaten in the diet during lactation due to a lack of safety information; or pregnancy due to its history of use as a contraceptive.[5] Eating asparagus caused urticaria, dysphagia, dyspnea, anaphylaxis, and skin lesions in sensitized individuals.[5]

Astaxanthin

definition

Naturally occurring antioxidant that imparts the characteristic pink pigment to shrimp, lobster, and salmon in the wild and added as a colorant to farm-raised crustaceans and salmon.[85] A 200-g portion of salmon contains approximately 1–7 mg of astaxanthin is rarely found in plant foods.[86]

scientific findings

In laboratory studies, astaxanthin reduced oxidative stress and inflammation, enhanced immune response, exhibited cardioprotective properties, and inhibited cancer cell growth.[86] An 8-week, randomized, double-blind, placebo-controlled study (n = 14 young healthy women), dietary astaxanthin supplementation decreased deoxyribonucleic acid (DNA) damage biomarkers and enhanced immune response.[85]

bioactive dose

Not known.

safety

Presumed safe when consumed in normal dietary quantities by non-allergic individuals.

Avocado (Persea americana)

definition

Fruit commonly consumed raw in salads and sushi and as the main ingredient in guacamole. Avocado is an excellent source of folate, is high in monounsaturated fat, and is a source of lutein, xeaxanthin, and an especially rich source of the β-sitosterol, supplying 114 mg per cup of commercial variety avocado and 175 mg per cup of California avocado.[88–91] Due to its high fat content, avocado is considered to be a high-calorie fruit.

scientific findings

The oils in avocado may theoretically promote absorption of fat-soluble vitamins that are consumed in the same meal. Consuming 200 g/day of avocado as part of a low-calorie diet did not compromise weight loss when subjects (n = 61, mean BMI [body mass index] of 32) substituted it for 30 g of mixed dietary fat.[92] In a controlled clinical trial (n = 15 normolipemic and 30 hypercholesterolemic subjects), all subjects received an avocado-enriched diet. The avocado-enriched diet reduced total cholesterol after 7 days in normolipemic subjects and significantly reduced total cholesterol in hyperlipemic subjects.[93]

bioactive dose

Not known.

safety

Presumed safe when consumed in normal dietary quantities by non-allergic individuals.

References

1. Seeram NP, Aviram M, Zhang Y, Henning SM, Feng L, Dreher M, Heber D. Comparison of antioxidant potency of commonly consumed polyphenol-rich beverages in the United States. *J Agric Food Chem.* 2008;56(4):1415–1422.
2. de Souza MO, Silva M, Silva ME, Oliveira P, Pedrosa ML. Diet supplementation with acai (*Euterpe oleracea* Mart.) pulp improves biomarkers of oxidative stress and the serum lipid profile in rats. *Nutrition.* 2010;26(7–8):804–810. doi: 10.1016/j.nut.2009.09.007. Epub 2009 Dec 22.
3. Mertens-Talcott SU, Rios J, Jilma-Stohlawetz P, Pacheco-Palencia LA, Meibohm B, Talcott ST, Derendorf H. Pharmacokinetics of anthocyanins and antioxidant effects after the consumption of anthocyanin-rich acai juice

A

and pulp (*Euterpe oleracea* Mart.) in human healthy volunteers. *Agric Food Chem*. 2008;56(17):7796–7802.

4. Udani JK, Singh BB, Singh VJ, Barrett ML. Effects of Açai (*Euterpe oleracea* Mart.) berry preparation on metabolic parameters in a healthy overweight population: A pilot study. *Nutr J*. 2011;10:45.

5. Jellin JM, Gregory PJ. *Natural Medicine Comprehensive Database*. Therapeutic Research Faculty. 2013. http://www.naturaldatabase.com. Accessed July 11, 2012.

6. US National Library of Medicine. National Institutes of Health. Medline Plus. Alfalfa. http://www.nlm.nih.gov/medlineplus/druginfo/natural/19. html. Accessed July 8, 2012.

7. Bora KS, Sharma A. Phytochemical and pharmacological potential of *Medicago sativa*: A review. *Pharm Biol*. 2011;49(2):211–220.

8. Mölgaard J, von Schenck H, Olsson AG. Alfalfa seeds lower low density lipoprotein cholesterol and apolipoprotein B concentrations in patients with type II hyperlipoproteinemia. *Atherosclerosis*. 1987;65(1–2):173–179.

9. Malinow MR, Connor WE, McLaughlin P, Stafford C, Lin DS, Livingston AL, Kohler GO, McNulty WP. Cholesterol and bile acid balance in Macaca fascicularis. Effects of alfalfa saponins. *J Clin Invest*. 1981;67(1): 156–162.

10. Story JA, LePage SL, Petro MS, West LG, Cassidy MM, Lightfoot FG, Vahouny GV. Interactions of alfalfa plant and sprout saponins with cholesterol in vitro and in cholesterol-fed rats. *Am J Clin Nutr*. 1984;39:917–929.

11. DerMardersian A, Beutler J, eds. *The Review of Natural Products*, 5th edn. St. Louis MO: Wolters Kluwer Health; 2008.

12. US Department of Agriculture. Agricultural Research Service. Phytochemical Database. *Allium cepa*/onion. http://www.pl.barc.usda.gov/usda_plant/plant_detail.cfm?code=7124465071244650&plant_id=396&ThisName=ps721. Accessed January 1, 2013.

13. Formica JV, Regelson W. Review of the biology of quercetin and related bioflavonoids. *Food Chem Toxicol*. 1995;33(12):1061–1080.

14. Bianchini F, Vainio H. Allium vegetables and organosulfur compounds: Do they help prevent cancer? *Environ Health Perspect*. 2001;109(9):893–902.

15. Powolny AA, Singh SV. Multitargeted prevention and therapy of cancer by diallyl trisulfide and related Allium vegetable-derived organosulfur compounds. *Cancer Lett*. 2008;269(2):305–314.

16. US Department of Agriculture. Agricultural Research Service. National Nutrient Database for Standard Reference Release. Onions, raw. http://ndb.nal.usda.gov/ndb/foods/show/3065?man=&lfacet=&count=&max=35&qlookup=onion&offset=&sort=&format=Abridged&reportfmt=other&rptfrm=&ndbno=&nutrient1=&nutrient2=&nutrient3=&-subset=&totCount=&measureby=&_action_show=Apply+Changes&Qv=1&Q5824=0.062&Q5825=1&Q5826=1&Q5827=1&Q5828=1&Q5829=1&Q5830=1&Q5831=1&Q5832=1&Q5833=10.0. Accessed February 19, 2015.

17. Hsing AW, Chokkalingam AP, Gao YT, Madigan MP, Deng J, Gridley G, Fraumeni JF Jr. Allium vegetables and risk of prostate cancer: A population-based study. *J Natl Cancer Inst*. 2002;94(21):1648–1651.

18. Grant WB. A multicountry ecologic study of risk and risk reduction factors for prostate cancer mortality. *Eur Urol*. 2004;45(3):271–279.

19. Zhou Y, Zhuang W, Hu W, Liu GJ, Wu TX, Wu XT. Consumption of large amounts of Allium vegetables reduces risk for gastric cancer in a meta-analysis. *Gastroenterology.* 2011;141(1):80–89.

20. Galeone C, Pelucchi C, Dal Maso L, Negri E, Montella M, Zucchetto A, Talamini R, La Vecchia C. Allium vegetables intake and endometrial cancer risk. *Public Health Nutr.* 2009;12(9):1576–1579.

21. Zhang L, Lokeshwar BL. Medicinal properties of the Jamaican pepper plant *Pimenta dioica* and allspice. *Curr Drug Targets.* 2012;13(14):1900–1906. Epub 2012 November 6.

22. US Department of Agriculture. Agricultural Research Service. Beltsville Agricultural Research Center. Medicinal Plants Database. *Pimenta dioica*/allspice. http://www.pl.barc.usda.gov/usda_plant/plant_home.cfm. Accessed October 28, 2011.

23. Padmakumari KP, Sasidharan I, Sreekumar MM. Composition and antioxidant activity of essential oil of pimento (*Pimenta dioica* (L) Merr.) from Jamaica. *Nat Prod Res.* 2011;25:152–160. doi: 10.1080/14786419.2010.526606.

24. Kikuzaki H, Sato A, Mayahara Y, Nobuji Nakatani N. Galloylglucosides from berries of *Pimenta dioica. J Nat Prod.* 2000;63(6):749–752.

25. Chen CY, Lapsley K, Blumberg J. A nutrition and health perspective on almonds. *J Sci Food Agric.* 2006;86:2245–2250.

26. Bolling BW, Chen CY, McKay DL, Blumberg JB. Tree nut phytochemicals: Composition, antioxidant capacity, bioactivity, impact factors. A systematic review of almonds, Brazils, cashews, hazelnuts, macadamias, pecans, pine nuts, pistachios and walnuts. *Nutr Res Rev.* 2011;24(2):244–275.

27. US Department of Agriculture. Agricultural Research Service. Nutrient Data Laboratory. Nuts, almonds, dry roasted, without salt added. http://ndb.nal.usda.gov/ndb/foods/show/3617?fg=&man=&lfacet=&format=&count=&max=25&offset=&sort=&qlookup=almond. Accessed June 27, 2013.

28. Academy of Nutrition and Dietetics Evidence Analysis Library. What is the relationship between consuming almonds and cholesterol levels in patients with hyperlipidemia? Academy of Nutrition and Dietetics. http://andevidencelibrary.com/conclusion.cfm?conclusion_statement_id=250983&highlight=almonds&home=1. Accessed May 6, 2013.

29. Foster GD, Leh Shantz K, Vander Veur SS, Oliver T, Lent MR, Virus A, Szapary PO, Rader DJ, Zemel BS, Gilden-Tsai A. A randomized trial of the effects of an almond-enriched, hypocaloric diet in the treatment of obesity. *Am J Clin Nutr* 2012;96:249–254.

30. Wien MA, Sabaté JM, Iklé DN, Cole SE, Kandeel Fr. Almonds vs complex carbohydrates in a weight reduction program. *Int J Obes Relat Metab Disord.* 2007;98(3):651–656. Epub 2007 April 20.

31. Hollis J, Mattes R. Effect of chronic consumption of almonds on body weight in healthy humans. *Br J Nutr.* 2007;98(3):651–656. Epub 2007 April 20.

32. US Department of Agriculture. Agricultural Research Service. Phytochemical Database. *Pimpinella anisum.* http://www.pl.barc.usda.gov/usda_plant/plant_home.cfm. Accessed November 21, 2011.

33. Ashraffodin Ghoshegir S, Mazaheri M, Adibi P. *Pimpinella anisum* in the treatment of functional dyspepsia: A double-blind, randomized clinical trial. *J Res Med Sci: The Official Journal of Isfahan University of Medical Sciences.* 2015;20:13–21.

34. Mahady GB, Pendland SL, Stoia A, Hamill FA, Fabricant D, Dietz BM, Chadwick LRE. In vitro susceptibility of *Helicobacter pylori* to botanical extracts used traditionally for the treatment of gastrointestinal disorders. *Phytother Res.* 2005;19(11):988–991.

35. Shojaii A, Abdollahi Fard M. Review of pharmacological properties and chemical constituents of *Pimpinella anisum*. *ISRN Pharm.* 2012;2012:510795. doi: 10.5402/2012/510795. Epub 2012 July 16.

36. Lee JB, Yamagishi C, Hayashi K, Hayashi T. Antiviral and immunostimulating effects of lignin–carbohydrate–protein complexes from *Pimpinella anisum*. *Biosci Biotechnol Biochem.* 2011;75(3):459–465. Epub 2011 March 7.

37. Craig WJ. Phytochemicals: Guardians of our health. *J Am Diet Assoc.* 1997;97(10 Suppl 2):S199–204.

38. Balk E, Chung M, Raman G, Tatsioni A, Chew P, Ip S, DeVine D, Lau J. B Vitamins and berries and age-related neurodegenerative disorders. *Evidence Report/Technology Assessment No.* 134. (Prepared by Tufts-New England Medical Center Evidence-based Practice Center under Contract No. 290-02-0022.) AHRQ Publication No. 06-E008. Rockville, MD: Agency for Healthcare Research and Quality; 2006.

39. Lila MA. Anthocyanins and human health: An in vitro investigative approach. *J Biomed Biotechnol.* 2004;5:306–313. http://jbb.hindawi.com.

40. Borissova P, Valcheva S, Belcheva A. Antiinflammatory effect of flavonoids in the natural juice from *Aronia melanocarpa*, rutin and rutin–magnesium complex on an experimental model of inflammation induced by histamine and serotonin. *Acta Physiol Pharmacol Bulg.* 1994;20(1):25–30.

41. Boniface R. Effect of anthocyanins on human connective tissue metabolism in the human. *Klin Montsbl Augenheilkd.* 1996;209(6):368–377.

42. Cisowska A, Wojnicz D, Hendrich AB. Anthocyanins as antimicrobial agents of natural plant origin. *Nat Prod Commun.* 2011;6(1):149–156.

43. Pei-Ni Chena P-N, Chub S-C, Chiouc H-L, Kuoa W-H, Chiang C-L, Hsieha Y-S. Mulberry anthocyanins, cyanidin 3-rutinoside and cyanidin 3-glucoside, exhibited an inhibitory effect on the migration and invasion of a human lung cancer cell line. *Cancer Lett.* 2006;235(2):248–259.

44. Jin H, Leng Q, Li C. Dietary flavonoid for preventing colorectal neoplasms. *Cochrane Database Syst Rev.* 2012;8:CD009350. doi: 10.1002/14651858. CD009350.pub2.

45. Shahidi F. Natural antioxidants: An overview. In: Shahidi F, ed. *Natural Antioxidants. Chemistry, Health Effects and Applications.* Champaign, IL: AOCS Press; 1996:1–11.

46. Parletta N, Milteb CM, Meyer BJ. Nutritional modulation of cognitive function and mental health. *J Nutr Biochem.* 2013;24:725–743.

47. Academy of Nutrition and Dietetics Evidence Analysis Library. What is the relationship between eating foods rich in antioxidants and cardiovascular disease? Academy of Nutrition and Dietetics. http://andevidencelibrary. com/conclusion.cfm?conclusion_statement_id=123&highlight=vitamin%20 E&home=1&auth=1. Accessed May 6, 2013.

48. Miwa S, Nakamura M, Okuno M, Miyazaki H, Watanabe J, Ishikawa-Takano Y, Miura M, Takase N, Hayakawa S, Kobayashi S. Production of starch with antioxidative activity by baking starch with organic acids. *Biosci Biotechnol Biochem.* 2011;75(9):1649–1653. Epub 2011 September 7.

49. Wang Y, Yang M, Lee SG, Davis CG, Koo SI, Chun OK. Dietary total anti-oxidant capacity is associated with diet and plasma antioxidant status in healthy young adults. *J Acad Nutr Diet*. 2012;112(10):1626–1635. doi: 10.1016/j.jand.2012.06.007.

50. American Heart Association. Healthy Diet Goals. http://www.heart.org/HEARTORG/GettingHealthy/NutritionCenter/HealthyDietGoals/Healthy-Diet-Goals_UCM_310436_SubHomePage.jsp. Accessed March 30, 2013.

51. Le Marchand L, Murphy SP, Hankin JH, Wilkens LR, Kolonel LN. Intake of flavonoids and lung cancer. *J Natl Cancer Inst*. 2000;92(2):154–160.

52. Salfi SF, Holt K. The role of probiotics in diarrheal management. *Holist Nurs Pract*. 2012;26(3):142–149. doi: 10.1097/HNP.0b013e31824ef5a3.

53. Schultz AA, Ashby-Hughes B, Taylor R, Gillis DE, Wilkins M. Effects of pectin on diarrhea in critically ill tube-fed patients receiving antibiotics. *Am J Crit Care*. 2000;9(6):403–411.

54. Nagasako-Akazome Y, Kanda T, Ohtake Y, Shimasaki H, Kobayashi T. Apple polyphenols influence cholesterol metabolism in healthy subjects with relatively high body mass index. *J Oleo Sci*. 2007;56(8):417–428.

55. Chai SC, Hooshmand S, Saadat RL, Payton ME, Brummel-Smith K, Arjmandi BH. Daily apple versus dried plum: Impact on cardiovascular disease risk factors in postmenopausal women. *J Acad Nutr Diet*. 2012;112(8):1158–1168. doi: 10.1016/j.jand.2012.05.005.

56. Ravn-Haren G, Dragsted LO, Buch-Andersen T, Jensen EN, Jensen RI, Nemeth-Balogh M, Paulovicsova B et al. Intake of whole apples or clear apple juice has contrasting effects on plasma lipids in healthy volunteers. *Eur J Nutr*. 2013;52(8):1875–1889. Epub 2012 December 28.

57. Koch TC, Briviba K, Watzl B, Fähndrich C, Bub A, Rechkemmer G, Barth SW. Prevention of colon carcinogenesis by apple juice in vivo: impact of juice constituents and obesity. *Mol Nutr Food Res*. 2009;53(10):1289–1302.

58. Gerhauser C. Cancer chemopreventive potential of apples, apple juice, and apple components. *Planta Med*. 2008;74(13):1608–1624. doi: 10.1055/s-0028-1088300. Epub 2008 October 14.

59. Hyson DA. A comprehensive review of apples and apple components and their relationship to human health. *Adv Nutr*. 2011;2(5):408–420. doi: 10.3945/an.111.000513. Epub 2011 September 6.

60. Oude Griep LM, Verschuren WM, Kromhout D, Ocké MC, Geleijnse JM. Stroke. Colors of fruit and vegetables and 10-year incidence of stroke. *Stroke*. 2011;42(11):3190–3195. Epub 2011 September 15.

61. Kähkönen MP, Hopia AI, Vuorela HJ, Rauha J-P, Pihlaja K, Kujala TS, Heinonen M. Antioxidant activity of plant extracts containing phenolic compounds. *J Agric Food Chem*. 1999;47(10):3954–3962.

62. US Department of Agriculture. Agricultural Research Center. Nutrient Data Laboratory. Apricot. http://www.nal.usda.gov/fnic/foodcomp/search/index.html. Accessed October 3, 2011.

63. Whitney ER, DeBruyne LK, Pinna K, Rolfes SR. *Nutrition for Health & Healthcare*, 4th edn. Belmont, CA: Cengage; 2011: Appendix A.

64. US Department of Agriculture. Agricultural Research Service. Beltsville Agricultural Research Center. *Prunus armeniaca*/apricot. http://www.pl.barc.usda.gov/usda_plant/plant_home.cfm. Accessed October 10, 2011.

65. Yi D, Yi N, Mavi A. Antioxidant and antimicrobial activities of bitter and sweet apricot (*Prunus armeniaca* L.) kernels. *Braz J Med Biol.* 2009;42(4):346–352.
66. Kahlon TS, Smith GE. In vitro binding of bile acids by bananas, peaches, pineapple, grapes, pears, apricots and nectarines. *Food Chem.* 2007;101(3):1046–1051.
67. US Department of Agriculture. Agricultural Research Service. Nutrient Data Laboratory. Artichokes (Globe or French), raw. Globe or French. http://ndb. nal.usda.gov/ndb/foods/show/2807?fg=&man=&lfacet=&format=&count= &max=25&offset=&sort=&qlookup=artichoke. Accessed December 23, 2012.
68. US Department of Agriculture. Agricultural Research Service. Medicinal Plants Database. *Cynara scolymus.* http://www.pl.barc.usda.gov/usda_plant/plant_home.cfm. Accessed November 14, 2011.
69. Wider B, Pittler MH, Thompson-Coon J, Ernst E. Artichoke leaf extract for treating hypercholesterolaemia. *Cochrane Database Syst Rev.* 2009;7(4):CD003335.
70. Holtmann G, Adam B, Haag S, Collet W, Grünewald E, Windeck T. Efficacy of artichoke leaf extract in the treatment of patients with functional dyspepsia: A six-week placebo-controlled, double-blind, multicentre trial. *Aliment Pharmacol Ther.* 2003;18(11–12):1099–1105.
71. Nomikos T, Detopoulou P, Fragopoulou E, Pliakis E, Antonopoulou S. Boiled wild artichoke reduces postprandial glycemic and insulinemic responses in normal subjects but has no effect on metabolic syndrome patients. *Nutr Res.* 2007;27(12):741–749.
72. US Department of Agriculture. Agricultural Research Service. Nutrient Data Laboratory. Arugula, raw. http://ndb.nal.usda.gov/ndb/foods/show /3551?qlookup=arugula&fg=&format=&man=&lfacet=&max=25&new=1. Accessed December 31, 2012.
73. US Department of Agriculture. Agricultural Research Service. Phytochemical Database. *Eruca sativa*/arugula, rocket salad. http://www. pl.barc.usda.gov/usda_plant/plant_home.cfm. Accessed October 28, 2011.
74. Yehuda H, Khatib S, Susan I, Musa R, Vaya J, Tamir S. Potential skin antiinflammatory effects of 4-methylthiobutylisothiocyanate (MTBI) isolated from rocket (*Eruca sativa*) seeds. *Biofactors.* 2009;35(3):295–305. doi: 10.1002/biof.32.
75. Jin J, Koroleva OA, Gibson T, Swanson J, Magan J, Zhang Y, Rowland IR, Wagstaff C. Analysis of phytochemical composition and chemoprotective capacity of rocket (*Eruca sativa* and *Diplotaxis tenuifolia*) leafy salad following cultivation in different environments. *J Agric Food Chem.* 2009;57(12):5227–5234. doi: 10.1021/jf9002973.
76. Produce for Better Health Foundation. Fruit and Veggies Matter. Asian pear. http://www.fruitsandveggiesmatter.gov/month/asian_pear.html. Accessed June 5, 2011.
77. US Department of Agriculture. Agricultural Research Service. Nutrient Data Laboratory. Asian pear. http://ndb.nal.usda.gov/. Accessed January 21, 2012.
78. Lee HS, Isse T, Kawamoto T, Woo HS, Kim AK, Park JY, Yang M. Effects and action mechanisms of korean pear (*Pyrus pyrifolia* cv. *Shingo*) on alcohol detoxification. *Phytother Res.* 2012;26(11):1753–1758. doi: 10.1002/ptr.4630. Epub 2012 March 26.
79. US Department of Agriculture. Agricultural Research Center. Nutrient Data Laboratory. Asparagus, cooked, boiled, drained. http://www.nal.usda.gov/ fnic/foodcomp/cgi-bin/measure.pl. Accessed October 3, 2011.

80. US Department of Agriculture. Agricultural Research Service. Phytochemical Database. *Asparagus oficinalis*/asparagus. http://www.pl.barc.usda.gov/usda_plant/plant_detail.cfm?code=84204419842044198420441984204419842 04419842044198420441984204419842044198420441984204419842044198420441984204 419842044198420441984204419842044198420441984204419842044198420441984204 419842044198420441984204419842044198420441984204419842044198420441984204 4198420441984204419&plant_id=470&y1s27=&ThisName=ps721. Accessed May 15, 2013.

81. Wang L, Wang X, Yuan X, Zhao B. Simultaneous analysis of diosgenin and sarsapogenin in *Asparagus officinalis* byproduct by thin-layer chromatography. *Phytochem Anal*. 2011;22(1):14–17.

82. Kumar MC, Udupa AL, Sammodavardhana K, Rthnakar UP, Shvetha U, Kodancha GP. Acute toxicity and diuretic studies of the roots of *Asparagus racemosus* Willd in rats. *West Indian Med J*. 2010;59(1):3–6.

83. Zhu X, Zhang W, Pang X, Wang J, Zhao J, Qu W. Hypolipidemic effect of n-butanol extract from *Asparagus officinalis* L. in mice fed a high-fat diet. *Phytother Res*. 2011;25(8):1119–1124.

84. Patil D, Gautam M, Gairola S, Jadhav S. Patwardhan B. HPLC/tandem mass spectrometric studies on steroidal saponins: An example of quantitative determination of Shatavarin IV from dietary supplements containing *Asparagus racemosus*. *J AOAC Int*. 2014;97(6):1497–1502.

85. Higuera-Ciapara I, Félix-Valenzuela L, Goycoolea FM. Astaxanthin: A review of its chemistry and applications. *Crit Rev Food Sci Nutr*. 2006;46(2):185–196.

86. Park JS, Chyun JH, Kim YK, Line LL, Chew BP. Astaxanthin decreased oxidative stress and inflammation and enhanced immune response in humans. *Nutr Metab (London)*. 2010;7:18. doi: 10.1186/1743-7075-7-18.

87. Huang J-C, Zhong Y-J, Liu J, Sandmann G, Chen F. Metabolic engineering of tomato for high-yield production of astaxanthin. *Metab Engineer* 2013;17:59–67.

88. US Department of Agriculture. Agricultural Research Service. Nutrient Data Laboratory. Avocados, raw, all commercial varieties. http://ndb.nal.usda.gov/ndb/foods/show/2175?fg=&man=&lfacet=&format=&count=&max=25&offset=&sort=&qlookup=avocado. Accessed December 31, 2012.

89. Dreher ML, Davenport AJ. Hass avocado composition and potential health effects. *Crit Rev Food Sci Nutr*. 2013;53(7):738–750. doi: 10.1080/10408398.2011.556759.

90. US Department of Agriculture. Agricultural Research Service. National Nutrient Database. Avocado http://ndb.nal.usda.gov/ndb/nutrients/report/nutrientsfrm?max=25&offset=0&totCount=0&nutrient1=641&nutrient2=&nutrient3=&subset=0&fg=9&sort=f&measureby=m. Accessed March 23, 2015.

91. US Department of Agriculture Agricultural Research Service. USDA Database for the Isoflavone Content of Selected Foods Release 2.0. http://www.ars.usda.gov/SP2UserFiles/Place/80400525/Data/isoflav/Isoflav_R2.pdf. Accessed March 1, 2015.

92. Pieterse Z, Jerling JC, Oosthuizen W, Kruger HS, Hanekom SM, Smuts CM, Schotte AE. Substitution of high monounsaturated fatty acid avocado for mixed dietary fats during an energy-restricted diet: Effects on weight loss, serum lipids, fibrinogen, and vascular function. *Nutr*. 2005;21(1):67–75.

93. López Ledesma R, Frati Munari AC, Hernández Dominguez BC, Cervantes Montalvo S, Hernández Luna MH, Juárez C, Morán Lira S. Monounsaturated fatty acid (avocado) rich diet for mild hypercholesterolemia. *Arch Med Res*. 1996;27(4):519–523.

B

Banana (Musa paradisiaca)

definition

Among the most commonly eaten fresh fruits, banana is a good source of pectin, potassium, vitamin C, and vitamin B6, and contains serotonin and 2-pentanone.[1-4] Bananas are routinely recommended to patients to maintain or restore blood potassium levels because one large (8–9" long) banana supplies approximately 500 mg of potassium.[2] Bananas have a low glycemic index.[5] They have been traditionally recommended for diarrhea management as part of the pediatric BRAT (bananas–rice–applesauce–toast) diet.[6]

scientific findings

Green bananas and pectin significantly reduced diarrhea in a small, double-blind clinical trial (n = 62 boys aged 5–12 months with persistent diarrhea [≥ 14 days]) randomly assigned to receive, for seven days, either a rice-based diet (n = 21); a rice-based diet with 250 g/L of cooked green banana (n = 22); or a rice-based diet with 4 g/kg of pectin (n = 19). Diarrhea significantly improved in the banana- and pectin-supplemented group compared to the rice-only group.[7] Possible mechanisms for bananas to maintain normal stool consistency include that pectin may stimulate epithelial growth in the colon to reduce diarrhea[8] and/or that soluble fiber slows gastrointestinal (GI) transit time, increasing the likelihood of nutrient absorption. Banana pulp had a cholesterol-lowering effect in rats, which was attributed to both its soluble and insoluble fibers.[9] An experimental study found that 2-pentanone inhibited biomarkers of colon cancer in human colon cancer cells.[4]

bioactive dose

Not known.

B

safety

Presumed safe when consumed in normal dietary quantities by non-allergic individuals. A case of acute pancreatitis possibly resulting from banana allergy has been reported.[10] Excessive eating of bananas (up to 20 bananas/day), with no other foods for 2 years by a case subject with anorexia nervosa, resulted in hyperdopaminemia, defined as whole blood dopamine exceeding the normal range of 0.5–6.2 ng/mL.[11]

Basil, sweet (Ocimum basilicum)

definition

Mint family herb that contains phenolics and terpenoids, such as stigmasterol and β-sitosterol.[12] When consumed in a significant quantity rather than in small quantities as a culinary herb, for example in a 1/4-cup portion as pesto (a paste made with sweet basil, garlic, parmesan cheese, and walnuts used to coat cooked pasta), sweet basil provides a significant amount of vitamin K.[13] Sweet basil is used fresh or dried in flavoring many foods. Thai basil is a different variety of sweet basil, which has pointed (not rounded) leaves and is dark green in color with purple pigments, especially on its stems, whereas, sweet basil is uniformly grass-green in color. Although sweet basil is grown domestically, Thai basil is native to Southeast Asian cooking and is commonly sold in Asian markets.

scientific findings

In laboratory studies, sweet basil cultivars exhibited antioxidant and free radical scavenging activity attributed to its phenolic components.[14–16]

bioactive dose

Not known.

safety

Presumed safe when consumed by nonallergic individuals in normal dietary quantities.

Beer

definition

Alcoholic beverage made from fermenting a grain, such as barley, and adding hops, also a grain, to impart the characteristic bitter flavor.

Twelve ounces of regular (5% alcohol) beer provides approximately 350 cal, 13–14 g of alcohol (ethanol), 10 g of carbohydrate, negligible amounts of vitamins, such as niacin (1% DV [daily value]), potassium (3% DV), manganese (2% DV), and selenium (3% DV),[17–19] and polyphenols, which beer has less of than wine.[20] Beer consumption dates to at least 5000–7000 BC when wet grains combined with yeast in the air causing fermentation.

scientific findings

Polyphenols, such as xanthohumol, and phytochemical metabolites in beer have exhibited anti-inflammatory, antithrombotic, antiatherogenic, antioxidant, anticarcinogenic, estrogenic, and antiviral properties in experimental research (*in vitro*, cell culture, enzyme assay).[20] A meta-analysis of 26 studies examining beer and vascular risk found evidence of an inverse association between light-to-moderate beer consumption and vascular risk.[21] A systematic review of more than 35 observational studies examining the effect of beer on body weight found insufficient scientific evidence to assess whether beer intake at moderate levels (<500 mL/day or less than two 12-oz beers) is associated with general or abdominal obesity, but concluded that "higher intake, may be positively associated with abdominal obesity."[22] Beer's probiotic effects are due, in part, to the yeast used to make beer, *Saccharomyces cerevisiae*. *S. cerevisiae* reduced abdominal pain in irritable bowel syndrome (IBS) in a small, randomized, controlled, clinical trial 9 (n = 179 adults with irritable bowel syndrome).[23]

bioactive dose

"Moderate consumption" has been defined as no more than one drink (12 oz of regular beer) per day for women and no more than two drinks (24 oz of regular beer) per day for men.[18]

safety

Presumed safe when consumed in normal dietary quantities by non-allergic individuals. Heavy beer drinking (≥2 drinks/day) was associated with increased risk of colorectal cancer in a meta-analysis that included 12 case control and nine cohort studies, while light or moderate beer drinking was not.[24] The findings of a meta-analysis of 17 case–control and six cohort studies suggest that high consumption of beer (and other alcoholic beverages) was associated with an increased lung cancer risk.[25]

Beet (Beta vulgaris)

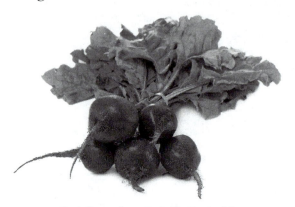

Beet. (Image from yamix/Shutterstock.)

definition

Also known as red beet or sugar beet. Root vegetable that is a good source of folate and potassium, a fair, but not good source of iron, and a source of anthocyanin, betaine, phenolics, flavonoids, and terpenoids.[26] Its above-ground portion, the beet greens, are rich in fiber, magnesium, and vitamin K. Fresh beets are roasted, baked, or boiled; canned beets are a common salad bar vegetable and may be pickled and served cold; and when very thinly sliced may be consumed raw as a salad ingredient. Beet greens are typically sautéed.

scientific findings

B. vulgaris exhibited antioxidant properties in a laboratory analysis.[27] Pre-exercise beet juice in athletes postponed fatigue and increased endurance and enhanced low- and high-intensity aerobic performance but did not reduce muscular fatigue during 30 s of intense anaerobic exercise.[28]

bioactive dose

Not known.

safety

Presumed safe when consumed in normal dietary quantities by non-allergic individuals. Approximately 10% or more of people may experience beeturia, pink or red urine, following the ingestion of beets, which may be associated with iron deficiency.[29,30]

β-carotene

definition

Vitamin A precursor present in rich amounts in yellow- and orange-fleshed fruits and vegetables, certain red fruits and vegetables, and dark green vegetables. Good sources include carrots, pumpkin, and spinach. Cooking a fruit or vegetable may enhance its β-carotene bioavailability.[31]

scientific findings

Laboratory studies suggest β-carotene functions as an antioxidant.[32] Observational epidemiological studies suggest an association between higher dietary levels of fruits and vegetables containing β-carotene and a lower risk of lung cancer.[33]

safety

Presumed safe when consumed in normal dietary quantities by non-allergic individuals. No UL has been established for β-carotene and "no adverse effects except for carotenodermia have been reported from consumption of food β-carotene."[32] Carotenodermia, the yellow discoloration of the skin, is thought to be harmless when it occurs due to the intake of food carotenoids.[32]

β-glucan

definition

Bioactive polysaccharide found naturally in foods that contain yeast, fungi, including mushrooms, certain bacteria, seaweeds,[34] and grains such as oats. β-glucans in cereals are soluble fibers.

scientific findings

Regular consumption of β-glucans contributes to maintenance of normal blood cholesterol concentrations.[35] Yeast-derived β-glucans dosed at 7.5 g twice daily, significantly reduced total cholesterol concentrations by 6%–8% in patients with hypercholesterolemia after 7–8 weeks of treatment.[36] In a meta-analysis, ingesting β-glucans derived from barley in doses of 3–10 g/day significantly reduced total and LDL cholesterol over 4–6 weeks of treatment without significantly affecting HDL cholesterol.[36] Adding β-glucans, as during food enrichment, may adversely affect β-glucan structure or solubility, decreasing its ability to reduce cholesterol levels[36]: A barley product highly enriched with β-glucans (75% by weight) exhibited altered ability to significantly reduce total cholesterol.[36]

There is insufficient reliable information available about the effectiveness of β-glucans for uses other than cholesterol lowering.[36]

bioactive dose

Consumption of >3 g of β-glucans daily from oats or barley may be associated with the maintenance of normal blood cholesterol levels in adults who have normal or mild elevations of their total cholesterol levels.[35]

safety

Presumed safe when consumed in normal dietary quantities by non-allergic individuals. There is some evidence that 15 g/day of yeast-derived β-glucans can be used safely for up to 8 weeks.[36]

Bitter orange (Citrus aurantium)

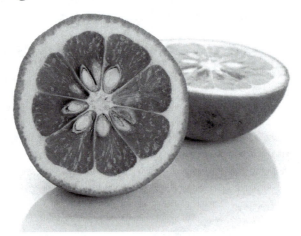

Bitter orange. (Image from Laitr Keiows/Shutterstock.)

definition

Also known as Seville orange or sour orange. Orange that resembles a navel orange, but is too sour to be popular for eating in the United States.[37] Used to make marmalade, relishes, candy, and condiments.[38] Bitter orange has been used in traditional medicine for nausea, indigestion, and constipation; current folk or traditional uses of bitter orange are for heartburn, loss of appetite, nasal congestion, and weight loss, and is also applied to the skin to treat fungal infections such as ringworm and athlete's foot.[39]

scientific findings

There is little evidence to support the use of bitter orange for any physiological effect or health condition.[39] Bitter orange peel extract is used in place of ephedra in many herbal weight-loss products.[39] Though studies have evaluated bitter orange extract in supplemental form in combination with other weight-targeted ingredients (and results have been inconclusive),[36] the use of bitter orange as a food in weight reduction has not been evaluated.[38]

bioactive dose

Not known.

safety

Presumed safe when consumed in normal dietary quantities by nonallergic individuals. According to a review, *C. aurantium* contains 6′,7′-dihydroxybergamottin and bergapten, both of which inhibit cytochrome P450-3A, and would be expected to increase serum levels of many drugs.[38] Bitter orange contains the chemical synephrine (oxedrine),[38] which is similar to the main chemical in ephedra, an FDA (Food and Drug Administration)-banned substance that causes high blood pressure and is linked to heart attack and stroke.[40]

Blackcurrant (Ribes nigrum)

definition

Also spelled black currant. High-vitamin C berry that is a significant source of anthocyanins. Used to make liqueurs.

scientific findings

The effect of blackcurrant anthocyanins on progression of glaucoma was evaluated in a placebo-controlled, double-blind trial (n = 38 glaucoma subjects) in which subjects taking eye drops were randomized to receive either oral blackcurrant anthocyanins (n = 19) or a placebo (n = 19) for 2 years. In the blackcurrant anthocyanins group, an insignificant improvement in ocular blood flow, but not intraocular pressure, was observed, whereas no effect occurred in the placebo group.[40]

bioactive dose

Not known.

safety

Presumed safe when consumed in normal dietary quantities by non-allergic individuals.

Black pepper (Piper nigrum)

definition

Ground, dried fruit of the *P. nigrum* vine that is among the most-used culinary seasonings. Usually consumed in such minute quantities that its nutrient contribution is nominal; however, one teaspoon of black ground pepper supplies 1% DV for calcium and 5% DV for vitamin K.[41] Contains the phytochemical piperine.[42]

scientific findings

In laboratory studies, black pepper exhibited antioxidant and free-radical-scavenging properties.[42,43] Piperine displayed beneficial, protective effects against inflammation and alveolar bone loss, supported bone microstructures, and prevented collagen fiber degradation in an experimental periodontitis study.[44]

bioactive dose

Not known.

safety

Presumed safe when consumed in normal dietary quantities by non-allergic individuals.

Blueberry (Vaccinium corymbosum, Vaccinium angustifolium)

definition

Common sweet berry that is eaten fresh, frozen, dried, as a preserve, and as a constituent of mixed juice beverages. Blueberries contain vitamin A, vitamin C, potassium, thiamin, riboflavin, vitamin B6, and folate, and are a rich source of fiber,[45] in addition to tannin and flavonoids, such as anthocyanins and proacyanidins.[46]

scientific findings

There is inadequate scientific research to evaluate the effectiveness of blueberry in any physiologic affect or health condition.[45] Blueberries have higher total antioxidant capacity relative to other fruits due to their antho-cyanin and procyanidin constituents; however, berry anthocyanins have been found to have a low bioavailability.[47] An *in vitro* study found that despite their low bioavailability, blueberries were a potent *in vivo* anti-oxidant at very low concentrations.[48] One portion of blueberries (300 g) improved cell antioxidant defense against DNA damage in a small, ran-domized crossover design study (n = 10 young healthy men).[48] According to a review, anthocyanins from blueberry extract were able to cross the blood–brain barrier in a rat study that found brain anthocyanins to be positively associated with learning performance, though factors other than anthocyanins could also have contributed to the neurocognitive effects seen in the study.[45] While many fruits may increase bladder irrita-tion in interstitial cystitis, blueberries are among a handful of fruits that reportedly do not.[49]

bioactive dose

Not known.

safety

Presumed safe when consumed in normal dietary quantities by non-allergic individuals.

Bok choi (Brassica campestris)

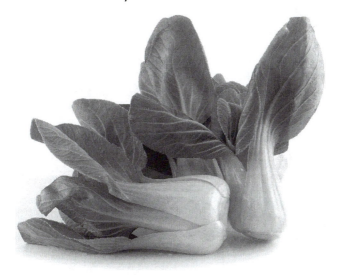

Bok choi. (Image from SOMMAI/Shutterstock.)

definition

Also called pak choi. Hardy, green and white leaf vegetable usually prepared by stir-frying or sauteing. Bok choi is a source of calcium, vitamin K, potassium, and vitamin C,[50] in addition to isothiocyanates and indoles.[51]

scientific findings

See *Brassica vegetables.*

bioactive dose

Not known.

safety

Presumed safe when consumed in normal dietary quantities by non-allergic individuals.

Boron

definition

Trace mineral found in avocado, peanut butter, peanuts, prune and grape juice, chocolate products, wine, pecans, and raisin bran cereal.[52]

scientific findings

Little data are available on the biologic functions of boron[52] beyond that it plays a role in metabolic processes related to bone.[53] Diets high in boron provide approximately 3.25 mg boron per 2000 kcal/day; diets low in boron provides 0.25 mg boron per 2000 kcal/day.[36]

bioactive dose

No RDA has been established for boron.

safety

A tolerable upper limit of 20 mg has been established.[52]

Brassica vegetables (Brassica oleracea)

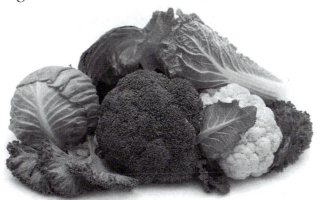

Brassica vegetables. (Image from Serg64/Shutterstock.)

definition

Also called cruciferous or mustard family vegetables. Genus consisting of many common species, such as broccoli, cauliflower, Brussels sprouts, cabbage, kale, and others, that contain compounds known to have antioxidant effects, such as glucosinolates, flavonoids, and vitamin C[54,55] and have been widely studied for anticancer effects.

scientific findings

High consumption of brassica vegetables may be associated with decreased risk of cancers of the lung, stomach, colon, and rectum, according to a review of six cohort studies and 74 case–control studies evaluating brassica consumption and cancer risk; importantly, though, this research did not separate out whether vegetables generally could be responsible for the effect versus specifically brassica vegetables.[56] Epidemiological research suggests that eating about 1.75 cups of cruciferous vegetables decreases the risk of developing bladder cancer by about 30% in men and women.[36] Some epidemiological research suggests that consumption of brassica vegetables is associated with a reduced risk of prostate cancer; however, other epidemiological research has found no association.[36] Sulforaphane and indole-3-carbinol, types of glucosinolates, have been shown in laboratory research to regulate genes that prevent cancer cell proliferation and viability.[57]

bioactive dose

Not known.

safety

Presumed safe when consumed in normal dietary quantities by non-allergic individuals. A case–control study (n = 293 cases of thyroid cancer and 354 population controls) in Melanesian women found that consumption of an average of one serving (50–80 g) of cruciferous vegetables daily was associated with thyroid cancer among women with low iodine intake (<96 µg/day).[58] Raw brassica (cruciferous) vegetables contain goitrogens that interfere with iodine utilization, thereby affecting the functionality of the thyroid, which depends on iodine to make thyroid hormones, however, cooking destroys goitrogens.[59]

Brazil nut (Bertholletia excelsa)

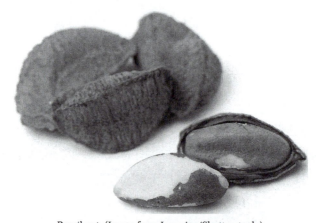

Brazil nut. (Image from Jessmine/Shutterstock.)

definition

Crescent-shaped oily white nut that is large in comparison to other nuts, weighing approximately 5 g, and is sourced from a tree native to the Amazon rainforest.[60] Typically eaten raw, straight out of the shell, Brazil nuts are a particularly rich source of the mineral selenium, supplying 290 µg of selenium per 1 nut[61]—more than 3 × the selenium daily reference value of 70 µg. Though they are high in fat (most of which is polyunsaturated and monounsaturated), providing 3 g of fat per nut and 30 cal, Brazil nuts also supply magnesium, copper, manganese, vitamin E, and thiamin.[62,63]

scientific findings

Brazil nuts have been used to correct selenium deficiency.[64] In a small, nonrandomized human trial (n = 37 obese, selenium-deficient women with hypercholesterolemia), one Brazil nut daily for 8 weeks corrected selenium deficiency and significantly improved HDL cholesterol levels.[61]

bioactive dose

Not known.

safety

Presumed safe when consumed in normal dietary quantities by non-allergic individuals.

Broccoli (Brassica oleracea L. var. italica)

definition

Hardy green vegetable whose thick, edible stalks and flowering heads (florets) are eaten raw or cooked. A good source of fiber, magnesium, potassium, vitamin C, folate, and carotenoids, it is also a good source of calcium: a broccoli stalk with floret (150 g) supplies 70 mg (7% DV) of calcium.[65] Phytochemical components include glucosinolates, phenolic acids, and flavonoids.[66]

scientific findings

More than 50% of the calcium in broccoli is absorbed compared to approximately 30% absorption of the calcium in dairy products.[67] Glucosinolate in broccoli was shown to be antimicrobial against *Staphylococcus aureus* in a laboratory study.[68] Epidemiological research suggests that consumption of broccoli is associated with a modestly reduced risk of breast cancer in premenopausal women but not in postmenopausal women.[36] Epidemiological research suggests consumption of broccoli might be associated with a reduced risk of colorectal and stomach cancer.[69] A laboratory study found that broccoli soluble fiber prevented *Escherichia coli* translocation in Crohn's disease cells, which may have implications in preventing Crohn's disease by limiting access of harmful bacteria to vulnerable intestinal cells.[69]

bioactive dose

Not known.

safety

Presumed safe when consumed in normal dietary quantities by nonallergic individuals. Recent laboratory studies indicate that broccoli extracts and/or glucosinolate-derived degradation products might have undesirable genotoxic effects, the relevance of which to human health is not yet known.[70]

Brussels sprouts (*Brassica oleracea* var. *gemmifera* DC.)

definition

Brassicaceae vegetable that resembles a greenish-yellow miniature cabbage. It can be cooked by steaming, sautéing, roasting, or broiling after being coated with olive oil, and is a source of vitamin K, lutein, xeaxanthin and the antioxidant glutathione.[71,72]

scientific findings

Rats induced to develop mammary cancer that were fed a 20% brussels sprout diet had a 13% incidence of tumor, whereas, those fed a casein–cornstarch diet had a 77% incidence of tumor. Tumors regressed in rats switched from the casein-cornstarch diet to the brussels sprouts diet after 6 weeks; but in the 10th week of the study, 100% of rats developed tumors. Rats fed the 20% brussels sprout diet during tumor initiation exhibited a 67% incidence of fibroadenomas, whereas rats fed the casein-cornstarch diet during initiation, but switched later to the brussels sprouts diet, showed over a 90% incidence of adenocarcinomas.[73]

bioactive dose

Not known.

safety

Presumed safe when consumed in normal dietary quantities by non-allergic individuals.

References

1. Yapo BM. Pineapple and banana pectins comprise fewer homogalacturonan building blocks with a smaller degree of polymerization as compared with yellow passion fruit and lemon pectins: Implication for gelling properties. *Biomacromolecules.* 2009;10(4):717–721. doi: 10.1021/bm801490e.

2. US Department of Agriculture. Agricultural Research Service. Nutrient Data Laboratory. Bananas, raw. http://ndb.nal.usda.gov/ndb/foods/show/2178. Accessed March 30, 2013.

3. Feldman JM, Lee EM. Serotonin content of foods: Effect on urinary excretion of 5-hydroxyindoleacetic acid. *Am J Clin Nutr*. 1985;41:639–643.

4. Pettersson J, Karlsson PC, Göransson U, Rafter JJ, Bohlin L. The flavouring phytochemical 2-pentanone reduces prostaglandin production and COX-2 expression in colon cancer cells. *Biol Pharm Bull*. 2008;31(3):534–547.

5. Whitney E, DeBruyne LK, Pinna K, Rolfes SR. *Nutrition for Health and Health Care*, 5th edn. Belmont CA: Cengage Learning; 2011.

6. Salfi SF, Holt K. The role of probiotics in diarrheal management. *Holistic Nurs Pract*. 2012;26(3):142–149. doi: 10.1097/HNP.0b013e31824ef5a3.

7. Rabbani GH, Teka T, Saha SK, Zaman B, Majid N, Khatun M, Wahed MA, Fuchs GJ. Green banana and pectin improve small intestinal permeability and reduce fluid loss in Bangladeshi children with persistent diarrhea. *Dig Dis Sci*. 2004;49(3):475–484.

8. Schultz AA, Ashby-Hughes B, Taylor R, Gillis DE, Wilkins M. Effects of pectin on diarrhea in critically ill tube-fed patients receiving antibiotics. *Am J Crit Care*. 2000;9(6):403–411.

9. Horigome T, Sakaguchi E, Kishimoto C. Hypocholesterolaemic effect of banana (*Musa sapientum* L. var. cavendishii) pulp in the rat fed on a cholesterol-containing diet. *Br J Nutr*. 1992;68(1):231–244.

10. Inamura H, Kashiwase Y, Morioka J, Kurosawa M. Acute pancreatitis possibly caused by allergy to bananas. *Investig Allergol Clin Immunol*. 2005;15(3):222–224.

11. Tazoe M, Narita M, Sakuta R, Nagai T, Narita N. Hyperkalemia and hyperdopaminemia induced by an obsessive eating of banana in an anorexia nervosa adolescent. *Brain Dev*. 2007;29(6):369–372. Epub 2006 December 27.

12. USDA Agricultural Research Service Herbs and Spices Database. http://www.pl.barc.usda.gov/usda_index.cfm. Accessed October 25, 2011.

13. USDA National Nutrient Database. Basil. http://www.nal.usda.gov/fnic/foodcomp/cgi-bin/list_nut_edit.pl. Accessed November 25, 2011.

14. Henning SM, Zhang Y, Seeram NP, Lee RP, Wang P, Bowerman S, Heber D. Antioxidant capacity and phytochemical content of herbs and spices in dry, fresh and blended herb paste form. *Int J Food Sci Nutr*. 2011;62(3):219–225. Epub 2010 December 1.

15. Kaurinovic B, Popovic M, Vlaisavljevic S, Trivic S. Antioxidant capacity of *Ocimum basilicum* L. and *Origanum vulgare* L. extracts. *Molecules*. 2011;16(9):7401–7414.

16. Nguyen PM, Kwee EM, Niemeyer ED. Potassium rate alters the antioxidant capacity and phenolic concentration of basil (*Ocimum basilicum* L.) leaves. *Food Chem*. 2010;123(14):1235–1241.

17. Pennington JAT (ed.). Alcohol (ethanol) content of alcoholic beverages. *Bowe's & Church's Food Values of Portions Commonly Used*, 17th edn. Philadelphia, PA: Lippincott Williams & Wilkins; 1998: 315.

18. US Department of Health and Human Services. US Food and Drug Administration. *Guidance for Industry: A Food Labeling Guide* (14. Appendix F: Calculate the Percent Daily Value for the Appropriate Nutrients). http://www.fda.gov/Food/GuidanceRegulation/GuidanceDocuments

RegulatoryInformation/LabelingNutrition/ucm064928.htm. Accessed January 30, 2015.

19. US Department of Agriculture. Agricultural Research Service. National Nutrient Database. Beer, regular per 12 ozs. http://ndb.nal.usda.gov/ndb/nutrients/report/nutrientsfrm?max=25&offset = 0&totCount = 0&nutrient1 = 317&nutrient2 = &nutrient3=&subset=0&fg=&sort=f&measureby=m. Accessed January 25, 2015.

20. Arranz S, Chiva-Blanch G, Valderas-Martínez P, Medina-Remón A, Lamuela-Raventós RM, Estruch R. Wine, beer, alcohol and polyphenols on cardiovascular disease and cancer. *Nutrients*. 2012;4(7):759–781.

21. Costanzo S, Di Castelnuovo A, Donati MB, Iacoviello L, de Gaetano G. Wine, beer or spirit drinking in relation to fatal and non-fatal cardiovascular events: A meta-analysis. *Eur J Epidemiol*. 2011;26(11):833–850. doi: 10.1007/s10654-011-9631-0. Epub 2011 November 11.

22. Bendsen NT, Christensen R, Bartels EM, Kok FJ, Sierksma A, Raben A, Astrup A. Is beer consumption related to measures of abdominal and general obesity? A systematic review and meta-analysis. *Nutr Rev*. 2013;71(2):67–87. doi: 10.1111/j.1753-4887.2012.00548.x. Epub 2012 December 13.

23. De Chambruna GP, Neut C, Chaub A, Cazaubielf M, Perering F, Justeng P, Desreumaux P. A randomized clinical trial of *Saccharomyces cerevisiae* versus placebo in the irritable bowel syndrome. *Dig Liver Dis*. 2015;47:119–124.

24. Zhang C, Zhong M. Consumption of beer and colorectal cancer incidence: A meta-analysis of observational studies. *Cancer Causes Control*. 2015;26(4):549–560. Epub 2015 February 13.

25. Chao C. Associations between beer, wine, and liquor consumption and lung cancer risk: A meta-analysis. *Cancer Epidemiol Biomarkers Prev*. 2007;16(11): 2436–2447.

26. US Department of Agriculture. National Nutrient Database. Beets, cooked. http://ndb.nal.usda.gov/ndb/foods/show/2901?manu=&fgcd=. Accessed April 3, 2015.

27. Jiratanan T, Liu RH. Antioxidant activity of processed table beets (*Beta vulgaris* var, conditiva) and green beans (*Phaseolus vulgaris* L.). *J Agric Food Chem*. 2004;52(9):2659–2670.

28. Clark N. Eating in the Athlete's Kitchen Part 4. US Olympic Committee. http://www.teamusa.org/USA-Taekwondo/Features/2015/February/11/Eating-in-the-Athletes-Kitchen-Pt-4. Accessed March 24, 2015.

29. Mitchell SC. Food idiosyncrasies: Beetroot and asparagus. *Drug Metab Dispos*. 2001;29(4):539–543.

30. Sotos JG. Beeturia and iron absorption. *Lancet*. 1999;354:1032.

31. Mayne ST. Beta-carotene, carotenoids, and disease prevention in humans. *FASEB J*. 1996;10:690–701.

32. Institute of Medicine. *Dietary Reference Intakes for Vitamin C, Vitamin E, Selenium and Carotenoids*. Washington DC: National Academy Press; 2000.

33. Cortés-Jofré M, Rueda JR, Corsini-Muñoz G, Fonseca-Cortés C, Caralloso M, Bonfill Cosp X. Drugs for preventing lung cancer in healthy people. *Cochrane Database Syst Rev*. 2012;10:CD002141. doi: 10.1002/14651858.

34. Du B, Bian Z, Xu B. Skin health promotion effects of natural beta-glucan derived from cereals and microorganisms: A review. *Phytother Res*. 2014; 28(2):159–166. doi: 10.1002/ptr.4963. Epub 2013 March 11.

35. EFSA Panel on Dietetic Products, Nutrition and Allergies (NDA). Scientific opinion on the substantiation of health claims related to beta glucans and maintenance of normal blood cholesterol concentrations (ID 754, 755, 757, 801, 1465, 2934) and maintenance or achievement of a normal body weight (ID 820, 823) pursuant to Article 13(1) of Regulation (EC) No 1924/2006. *EFSA J.* 2009;7(9):1254 [18pp.]. doi: 10.2903/j.efsa.2009.1254. Available online: www.efsa.europa.eu/efsajournal.

36. Jellin JM, Gregory PJ. *Natural Medicine Comprehensive Database.* Therapeutic Research Faculty; 2013. http://www.naturaldatabase.com. Accessed July 11, 2012.

37. Fugh Berman A, Myers A. *Citrus aurantium,* an ingredient of dietary supplements marketed for weight loss: Current status of clinical and basic research. *Exp Biol Med.* 2004;229(8):698–704.

38. Der Marderosian A, Beutler JA. *The Review of Natural Products,* 5th edn. St. Louis, MO: Wolters Kluwer Health; 2008.

39. National Institutes of Health. National Center for Complementary and Alternative Medicine. Herbs at a Glance. Bitter orange. http://nccam.nih.gov/health/bitterorange/D390_Herbs.pdf. Accessed June 4, 2011.

40. Ohguro H, Ohguro I, Katai M, Tanaka S. Two-year randomized, placebo-controlled study of black currant anthocyanins on visual field in glaucoma. *Ophthalmologica.* 2012;228(1):26–35. doi: 10.1159/000335961. Epub 2012 February 22.

41. US Department of Agriculture. Agricultural Research Service. National Nutrient Database. Spices, pepper, black. http://ndb.nal.usda.gov/ndb/foods/show/261?fgcd=&manu=&lfacet=&format=&count=&max=35&offset=&sort=&qlookup=+black+pepper. Accessed August 25, 2015.

42. Vijayakumar RS, Surya D, Nalini N. Antioxidant efficacy of black pepper (*Piper nigrum* L.) and piperine in rats with high fat diet induced oxidative stress. *Redox Rep.* 2000;9(2):105–110.

43. Gülçin I. The antioxidant and radical scavenging activities of black pepper (*Piper nigrum*) seeds. *Int J Food Sci Nutr.* 2005;56(7):491–499.

44. Dong Y, Huihui Z, Li C. Piperine inhibit inflammation, alveolar bone loss and collagen fibers breakdown in a rat periodontitis model. *J Periodontal Res.* 2015; March 2 [Epub ahead of print]. doi: 10.1111/jre.12262.

45. US National Library of Medicine. National Institutes of Health. Medline Plus. Blueberry. http://www.nlm.nih.gov/medlineplus/druginfo/natural/1013.html. Accessed April 4, 2013.

46. Balk E, Chung M, Raman G, Tatsioni A, Chew P, Ip S, DeVine D, Lau J. B vitamins and berries and age-related neurodegenerative disorders. Evidence Report/Technology Assessment No. 134. (Prepared by Tufts-New England Medical Center Evidence-based Practice Center under Contract No. 290-02-0022). *AHRQ* Publication No. 06-E008. Rockville, MD: Agency for Healthcare Research and Quality; April 2006.

47. Bornsek SM, Ziberna L, Polak T, Vanzo A, Ulrih NP, Abram V, Tramer F, Passamonti S. Bilberry and blueberry anthocyanins act as powerful intracellular antioxidants in mammalian cells. *Food Chem.* 2012;134(4):1878–1884. doi: 10.1016/j.foodchem.2012.03.092. Epub 2012 March 30.

48. Del Bo C, Riso P, Campolo J, Møller P, Loft S, Klimis-Zacas D, Brambilla A, Rizzolo A, Porrini M. A single portion of blueberry (*Vaccinium*

corymbosum L) improves protection against DNA damage but not vascular function in healthy male volunteers. *Butr Res.* 2013;33(3):220–227. doi: 10.1016/j.nutres.2012.12.009. Epub 2013 February 1.

49. Cranston C. Interstitial cystitis—chronic, common, and sometimes complicated to treat. *Am Nurse Today.* 2010;5(1):19–24.
50. USDA Agricultural Research Service. National Nutrient Database. Cabbage, Chinese (pak choi), raw. http://ndb.nal.usda.gov/ndb/foods/show/2943?fg=&man=&lfacet=&format=&count=&max=25&offset=&sort=&qlookup=bok+choi. Accessed May 1, 2013.
51. Fowke JH, Morrow JD, Motley S, Bostick RM, Ness RM. Brassica vegetable consumption reduces urinary F2-isoprostane levels independent of micronutrient intake. *Carcinogenesis.* 2006;27(10):2096–2102.
52. Institute of Medicine. *Dietary Reference Intakes for Vitamin A, Vitamin K, Arsenic, Boron, Chromium, Copper, Iodine, Iron, Manganese, Molybdenum, Nickel, Silicon, Vanadium and Zinc.* Washington DC: Institute of Medicine; 2001.
53. Palacios C. The role of nutrients in bone health, from A to Z. *Crit Rev Food Sci Nutr.* 2006;46(8):621–628.
54. Zhang Y. Allyl isothiocyanate as a cancer chemopreventive phytochemical. *Mol Nutr Food Res.* 2010;54(1):127–135.
55. Bhandari SR, Kwak JH. Chemical composition and antioxidant activity in different tissues of brassica vegetables. *Molecules.* 2015;20(1):1228–1243. doi: 10.3390/molecules20011228.
56. Van Poppel G, Verhoeven DT, Verhagen H, Goldbohm RA. Brassica vegetables and cancer prevention. Epidemiology and mechanisms. *Adv Exp Med Biol.* 1999;472:159–168.
57. Royston KJ, Tollefsbol TO. The epigenetic impact of cruciferous vegetables on cancer prevention. *Curr Pharmacol Rep.* 2015;1(1):46–51.
58. Truong T, Baron-Dubourdieu D, Rougier Y, Guénel P. Role of dietary iodine and cruciferous vegetables in thyroid cancer: A countrywide case–control study in New Caledonia. *Cancer Causes Control.* 2010;21(8):1183–1192. Epub 2010 April 2.
59. Greer, MA. Goitrogens in foods. *Am J Clin Nutr.* 1957;5(4):440–444.
60. Taniwaki MH, Pitt JI, Iamanaka BT, Sartori D, Copetti MV, Balajee A, Fungaro MH, Frisvad JC. *Aspergillus bertholletius* sp. nov. from Brazil nuts. *PLoS One.* 2012;7(8):e42480. doi: 10.1371/journal.pone.0042480. Epub 2012 August 27.
61. Cominetti C, de Bortoli MC, Garrido AB Jr, Cozzolino SM. Brazilian nut consumption improves selenium status and glutathione peroxidase activity and reduces atherogenic risk in obese women. *Nutr Res.* 2012;32(6):403–407. doi: 10.1016/j.nutres.2012.05.005. Epub 2012 June 12.
62. Produce for Better Health Foundation. Fruit & Veggies More Matters. Brazil Nuts: Nutrition. Selection. Storage. http://www.fruitsandveggiesmorematters.org/brazil-nuts. Accessed May 19, 2013.
63. US Department of Agriculture. Agricultural Research Service. Nutrient Data Laboratory. Brazil nuts, dried, unblanched. http://ndb.nal.usda.gov/ndb/foods/show/3621. Accessed May 21, 2013.
64. Stockler-Pinto MB, Lobo J et al. Effect of Brazil nut supplementation on plasma levels of selenium in hemodialysis patients: 12 months of follow-up. *J Renal Nutr.* 2012;22(4):434–439. doi: 10.1053/j.jrn.2011.08.011. Epub 2012 January 3.

65. US Department of Agriculture. Agricultural Research Service. Nutrient Data Laboratory. Broccoli, raw. http://ndb.nal.usda.gov/ndb/foods/show/2857. Accessed May 21, 2013.
66. Domínguez-Perles R, Martínez-Ballesta MC, Carvajal M, García-Viguera C, Moreno DA. Broccoli-derived by-products—A promising source of bioactive ingredients. *J Food Sci*. 2010;75(4):C383–C392.
67. Whitney E, Rolfes SR. Water and the major minerals. *Understanding Nutrition*, 12th edn. Belmont CA: Wadsworth Cengage Learning; 2011: 404.
68. Survay NS, Kumar B, Jang M, Yoon DY, Jung YS, Yang DC, Park SW. Two novel bioactive glucosinolates from broccoli (*Brassica oleracea* L. var. italica) florets. *Bioorg Med Chem Lett*. 2012;22(17):5555–5558. doi: 10.1016/j.bmcl.2012.07.016. Epub 2012 July 14.
69. Roberts CL, Keita AV, Duncan SH, O'Kennedy N, Söderholm JD, Rhodes JM, Campbell BJ. Translocation of Crohn's disease *Escherichia coli* across M-cells: Contrasting effects of soluble plant fibres and emulsifiers. *Gut*. 2010;59(10):1331–1339. doi: 10.1136/gut.2009.195370. Epub 2010 September 2.
70. Latté KP, Appel KE, Lampen A. Health benefits and possible risks of broccoli—An overview. *Food Chem Toxicol*. 2011;49(12):3287–3309. Epub 2011 August 28.
71. US Department of Agriculture. Agricultural Research Service. National Nutrient Database. Brussels sprouts. http://www.nal.usda.gov/fnic/food-comp/cgi-bin/list_nut_edit.pl. Accessed November 24, 2011.
72. Zacharis CK, Tzanavaras PD, Zotou A. Ethyl propiolate as a post-column derivatization reagent for thiols: Development of a green liquid chromatographic method for the determination of glutathione in vegetables. *Anal Chim Acta*. 2011;690(1):122–128. Epub 2011 February 24.
73. Munson L, Anderson JL, Stoewsand GS. Protective effect of dietary Brussels sprouts against mammary carcinogenesis in Sprague-Dawley rats. *Cancer Lett*. 1988;39(2):199–207.

C

Cabbage (Brassica oleracea var. capitata)

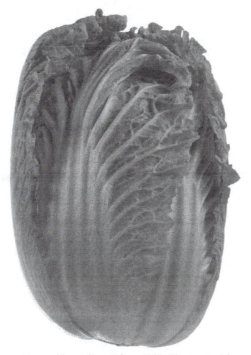

Napa cabbage. (Image from Kellis/Shutterstock.)

definition

Firm-leafed *Brassica* vegetable that may be consumed raw, cooked, or pickled and fermented to make sauerkraut (white or red cabbage) or kimchee (napa cabbage). Both white cabbage (pale green in color) and red cabbage (magenta and white in color) are good sources of vitamin C and vitamin K, and all members of the *Brassica* genus contain glucosinolates and antioxidants; additionally, red cabbage is a good source of vitamin A.[1,2] In traditional medicine, cabbage juice has been used to treat peptic ulcer.[3,4]

scientific findings

An experimental study found that cabbage juice extract significantly inhibited gastric ulcer formation in different animal models due to its ability to stimulate the synthesis of mucus, increase pH, and decrease hydrogen ions in the stomach.[4] Brassinin in cabbage exerted chemopreventive properties during the initiation and promotion phases of carcinogenesis in a laboratory study.[5] In a case–control study (n = 697 newly diagnosed bladder cancer cases compared to n = 708 healthy controls matched to cases by age, gender, and ethnicity), median isothiocyanate (ITC) intake from cabbage family vegetables containing ITCs was lower in bladder cancer cases compared to healthy controls. Median ITC intake was statistically significantly lower in bladder cancer cases (1.41½-cup servings of cabbage family vegetables) than in healthy controls (who consumed 1.76½-cup servings of cabbage family vegetables). Controls' intake was significant for including cole slaw (from green and red cabbage) and sauerkraut.[6]

bioactive dose

Not known. For gastric pain and hyperacidity, a dose of 1 teaspoon of cabbage juice 3 times daily before meals has been used.[7]

safety

Presumed safe when consumed in normal dietary quantities by non-allergic individuals. Goitrogens in raw cabbage can interfere with iodine utilization and thyroid function[8]; cooking cabbage destroys goitrogens.[9]

Caffeine

definition

One of the most commonly ingested alkaloids worldwide,[10] tastes bitter and is a nervous system stimulant and diuretic. Over 60 different plants contain natural caffeine, including coffee beans, tea, kola nuts (used to flavor cola), and cacao pods (used to make chocolate products). Caffeine is also produced synthetically for use in foods and drugs.[11] The average adult ingests 200 mg/day.[11] Caffeine content in 8 ounces of common beverages include coffee, 95–200 mg (with darker roasts containing less caffeine than lighter roasts because caffeine is lost during roasting in a process called sublimation[7]); black tea, 40–120 mg; and green tea, 15–60 mg.[7]

scientific findings

Caffeine ingestion improves mental alertness and prevents fatigue.[7] Taking caffeine orally in combination with analgesics is effective for treating simple headache and migraine headache.[7] Caffeine is an ergogenic aid.

bioactive dose

A dose of 250 mg has been used for headache; 150–600 mg has been used for fatigue; 2–10 mg/kg or more has been used for athletic performance.[7]

safety

Presumed safe when consumed in normal dietary quantities by non-allergic individuals. Caffeine can blunt appetite and cause headache, dizziness, nervousness, irritability, trouble sleeping, and dependence. Tolerance varies by individual, but amounts greater than 250–300 mg/day have been associated with tachyarrhythmias, sleep disturbances, and other side effects.[7] Amounts less than 200 mg/day have not been associated with clinically important adverse fetal effects and are generally recognized to be safe during pregnancy, but pregnant women should address caffeine use with their physician.[11] Consumption of caffeine in amounts over 200 mg/day is associated with increased risk of miscarriage.[7] Breast milk concentrations of caffeine are thought to be approximately 50% of maternal serum concentrations, and caffeine consumption in large amounts is possibly unsafe during lactation as caffeine can cause sleep disturbances, irritability, and increased bowel activity in breast-fed infants exposed to caffeine.[7] Large amounts of caffeine may cause or worsen fibrocystic breast disease.[12]

Calcium

definition

Major mineral element of skeleton and teeth, present in the body in quantities of 1100–1200 g, that is also necessary for nerve transmission, muscle contraction, blood clotting, blood pressure maintenance, and other functions.[13] Good sources of calcium include dairy products; certain dark green leafy vegetables, such as bok choi, broccoli, kale, and watercress; tofu made with calcium sulfate; canned fish containing edible bones, such as sardines; almonds and pistachios; and calcium-fortified beverages such as orange juice, almond milk, rice milk, and soy milk. Efficiency of calcium absorption decreases as people age.[13]

scientific findings

Adequate calcium intake is associated with optimal bone development and bone mineral density. Some studies have found that consuming the recommended amount of calcium can reduce the risk of developing hypertension.[14] "Many clinical trials and observational studies show that intake of dietary calcium modestly reduces blood pressure in patients with or without hypertension, usually around 1–2 mmHg," and further, "calcium may be more effective at lowering blood pressure in certain people, such as those who are salt-sensitive and those with low baseline dietary calcium intake"[7]; however, the evidence does not support a strong relationship between increased calcium intake and blood pressure reduction in healthy and hypertensive adults.[15] "Obesity often coexists with low calcium intake and [low] vitamin D [intake] insufficiency," but current evidence from randomized clinical trials do not support that calcium and vitamin D accelerates weight or fat loss in obesity.[16]

bioactive dose

The RDA for calcium is 1000 mg for 19–50 year-old adults.

safety

The UL for calcium is 2500 mg, an amount that would require dietary intake of more than eight 8-oz. servings of milk. High calcium intake may interfere with the absorption of minerals and is associated with hypercalcemia and milk-alkali syndrome. Doses >1000–1300 mg/day for adults have also been associated with an increased risk of myocardial infarction.[7] High calcium intake suppresses vitamin D activity.[17] High intake of calcium from supplements, but not foods, is associated with the development of kidney stones.[14] To prospectively examine whether calcium intake influenced risk of prostate cancer, the Health Professionals Follow Up Study (n = 47,781 men) followed subjects free of cancer at baseline in 1986 through 1994. Consumption of calcium was related to higher risk of total, advanced, and metastatic prostate cancer, especially at intakes exceeding 2000 mg/day.[17]

Cantaloupe (Cucumis melo)

definition

Orange-fleshed melon consumed fresh; a good source of fiber and vitamins A, C, and E[18]; cantaloupe also supplies nonprovitamin A carotenoids, phenolics, and terpenoids.[19]

scientific findings

Cantaloupe extract reduced diabetes-induced renal oxidative stress, a precursor of diabetic nephropathy, in mice.[20] A case–control study (n = 438 Chinese women age matched to n = 438 controls) that examined dietary intake and breast cancer risk found that consumption of the "watermelon/papaya/cantaloupe" fruit group was significantly inversely associated with breast cancer risk; further, other constituents of cantaloupe, including vitamins C and E and fiber were inversely associated with breast cancer risk.[21]

bioactive dose

Not known.

safety

Presumed safe when consumed in normal dietary quantities by non-allergic individuals.

Canthaxanthin

definition

Type of xanthophyll carotenoid closely related chemically to β-carotene[22] and presumed to be a human antioxidant. Found naturally in plant and animal foods such as mushrooms[23] and trout[24] and added to foods such as farmed salmon as a colorant.[25] In addition, canthaxanthin has come to be used widely as a drug, food, and cosmetic colorant.[26]

scientific findings

Canthaxanthin scavenged free radicals in a laboratory study.[27] A cross-sectional study (n = 235 women) investigating the comparative plasma levels of dietary antioxidants, including canthaxanthin, in a target group of women (n = 95 women with cervical intraepithelial neoplasia or cervical cancer) versus in a control group (n = 40) found that plasma canthaxanthin was found to be lower in women with cervical cancer and cervical intraepithelial neoplasia versus the control group.[28]

bioactive dose

Not known.

safety

Presumed safe when consumed in normal dietary quantities by nonallergic individuals. An experimental study found that canthaxanthin may be associated with the formation of undesirable crystals in the macula lutea membranes of the retina,[26] a condition termed canthaxanthin retinopathy, while other carotenoids have not been reported to cause this phenomenon.[22] An acceptable daily intake of 0.00–0.03 mg/kg body weight has been established for canthaxanthin.[29] Canthaxanthin is likely safe when used orally in amounts commonly found naturally in foods, but likely unsafe when used in amounts higher than those commonly found naturally in foods.[7]

Caper (Capparis spinosa)

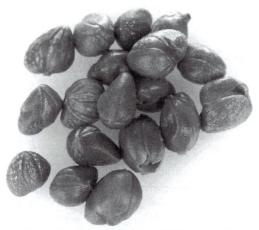

Caper. (Image from Africa Studio/Shutterstock.)

definition

Unopened flower bud of the *Capparis spinosa* shrub that is pickled and used as a pungent, salty condiment eaten in small quantities due to its strong flavor. Capers contain numerous phytochemicals, including phenolics, tocopherols, sterols, alkaloids, glucosinolates, and fatty acids.[30] Traditionally used as a diuretic, astringent, and antidiabetic, antihyperlipidemic, and antirheumatic agent.[30]

scientific findings

There is inadequate scientific evidence to support traditional uses of capers. Laboratory studies have demonstrated its antioxidant and anti-inflammatory effects.[31,32] In an experimental study, caper extract demonstrated potent lipid-lowering properties in diabetic rats.[33]

bioactive dose

Not known.

safety

Presumed safe when consumed in normal dietary quantities by non-allergic individuals.

Capsaicin

definition

Vanilloid compound[34] that is the active ingredient in *Capsicum frutescens* (see Pepper, chili). Contact causes irritation and burning sensation. Known for its thermogenic properties,[35] capsaicin causes sweating, followed by a cooling of body temperature through the evaporation of sweat. Its name may derive from the Greek *kapto*, meaning "to bite," or the Latin *capsa*, meaning box, referring to the fact that the pepper pod is hollow.[36]

scientific findings

In a small, placebo-controlled study (n = 11 heartburn sufferers) designed to evaluate capsaicin's effects on gastrointestinal parameters related to heartburn, subjects were given a meal followed by a placebo, and, on another occasion, a meal followed by a 5-mg capsaicin capsule. Capsaicin significantly decreased time to peak heartburn onset (120 min vs. 247 min).[37] In an experimental study, capsaicin improved endothelial cell function *in vitro*, which the authors hypothesized may have implications for cardiovascular health.[38] Epidemiological data revealed that the consumption of foods containing capsaicin was associated with a lower prevalence of obesity,[39] and capsaicin is being investigated for its role in weight management due to its mildly thermogenic properties.[39,40] While capsaicin is used topically in medicines, no studies were found to justify its topical use when sourced from food, and therefore, topical use of capsaicin is not addressed.

bioactive dose

Not known.

C

safety

Presumed safe when consumed in normal dietary quantities by non-allergic individuals. Capsaicin is known to cause an extreme burning sensation.

Carambola (Averrhoa carambola)

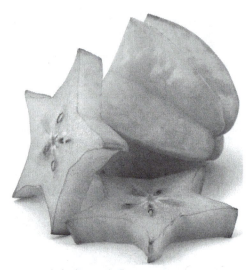

Carambola. (Image from EM Arts/Shutterstock.)

definition

Also called star fruit. Yellow, star-shaped fruit of the Oxalidaceae family that is popular in Asian cultures, and contains 3 g of fiber, 40 mg of vitamin C, and approximately 140 mg of potassium per cup,[41] in addition to polyphenolic antioxidants.[42]

scientific findings

Insoluble fibers in star fruit experimentally adsorbed glucose, retarded glucose diffusion, postponed the release of glucose from starch, and inhibited the activity of α-amylase *in vitro*, mechanisms that may be hypoglycemic in human beings.[43]

bioactive dose

Not known.

safety

Presumed safe when consumed in normal dietary quantities by non-allergic individuals. Carambola is associated with considerable adverse effects, including neurotoxicity and nephrotoxicity, and should not be used by uremic patients.[44]

Caraway (Carum carvi)

definition

Aromatic herb whose crescent-shaped seed is commonly used to make rye bread and distilled to produce an essential oil used to flavor cheese, sausage, and other products. Source of the phytochemicals quercetin and limonene.[45] Herbal products formulated for abdominal discomfort and pain frequently contain caraway oil. Caraway contains the monoterpene carvone; foods containing carvone have a history of use as carminatives.[45]

scientific findings

Caraway essential oils inhibited colon carcinogenesis in rats.[46] Carvone exhibited antinociceptive (analgesic) and anti-inflammatory activities in a laboratory study.[47]

bioactive dose

Not known.

safety

Presumed safe when consumed in normal dietary quantities by non-allergic individuals. Pregnant women should avoid medicinal use of caraway oil because it may stimulate menstruation.[7]

Carnitine

definition

Also called L-carnitine (the form found in food that is the active form in the body found in skeletal and cardiac muscle). Dietary sources of carnitine include meats, especially red meats; dairy products; breads; and vegetables.[48] The average adult consumes 60–180 mg of carnitine per day, while those eating a vegan diet take in 10–12 mg a day.[48] Healthy

C

people do not need to consume carnitine from food because it is made *in vivo* from lysine and methionine via the liver and kidney in quantities that are probably sufficient to meet daily requirements[49] (such nutrients are considered to be "nonessential" dietary compounds). Body levels of carnitine can be low in certain disease states; for example, some preterm infants, who cannot synthesize sufficient carnitine, require carnitine supplementation.[48]

scientific findings

Carnitine transports long-chain fatty acids into the mitochondria for oxidation and energy production and transports waste compounds out of the mitochondria.[48] There is scientific agreement on carnitine supplementation for carnitine deficiency.[48] Primary carnitine deficiency is a genetic condition that prevents the body from using certain fats for energy, signs and symptoms of which typically appear during infancy or early childhood and can include encephalopathy, cardiomyopathy, confusion, vomiting, muscle weakness, and hypoglycemia.[48]

bioactive dose

Not known.

safety

Presumed safe when consumed in normal dietary quantities by non-allergic individuals.

Carnosol

definition

Phytochemical found in common herbs, such as rosemary, sage, parsley, and oregano.[50]

scientific findings

Carnosol exhibited antioxidant,[51] anti-inflammatory, and chemoprotective properties in laboratory studies.[52]

bioactive dose

Not known.

safety

Presumed safe when consumed in normal dietary quantities by non-allergic individuals.

Carotenoids

definition

Subclass of terpenoids that includes two distinct types of molecules, the carotenes and the xanthophylls. More than 600 types of naturally occurring carotenoids have been identified, of which approximately 50 have provitamin A activity.[53] Carotenoid sources include fruits, vegetables, and oils.[54]

scientific findings

Numerous observational studies have found that people who ingest more carotenoids in their diets have a reduced risk of several chronic diseases, including cancer, cardiovascular disease, age-related macular degeneration, and cataract.[53] Major public health benefits could be achieved by increasing consumption of carotenoid-rich foods, the primary source of which is fruits and vegetables.[55]

safety

No UL has been established for carotenoids and no adverse effects except for carotenodermia, the yellow discoloration of the skin, is thought to occur from ingesting excessive amounts of dietary β-carotene. Carotenodermia is harmless when it occurs due to the intake of food sources of carotenoids.[56]

bioactive dose

Not known.

safety

Presumed safe when consumed in normal dietary quantities by non-allergic individuals.

Carrot (Daucus carota L.)

definition

Typically orange root vegetable widely recognized for its role in vision
because its provitamin A carotenoids maintain the cornea and make
rhodopsin. It is a good source of insoluble fiber,[57] and different cultivars
contain different phytochemicals, for example, purple carrots are rich in
anthocyanins.[55] Commonly eaten fresh and as part of processed foods,
carrots are among the 10 most economically important vegetable crops
grown worldwide.[58]

scientific findings

Daucus carota exhibited anticancer and antioxidant activities in laboratory
research.[58] In an experimental study, its oil suppressed proliferation and
induced apoptosis of human colon adenocarcinoma cells.[58] Consumption
of carrot juice led to a marked increase in β-carotene and α-carotene in
fecal markers, which in turn showed high dose-dependent cytotoxic and
antiproliferative effects on colon adenocarcinoma cells in a small randomized, cross-over design study (n = 22 healthy young men).[59]

bioactive dose

Not known.

safety

Presumed safe when consumed in normal dietary quantities by non-
allergic individuals.

Catechin

definition

Polyphenol flavonoids that have strong antioxidant properties and can
protect against oxidative damage.[60] Found in tea (black, oolong, and
green), apples, pears, chocolate, and broad beans.[61] Types of catechins
include epicatechin, epicatechin gallate, and epigallocatechin gallate.

scientific findings

A number of human observational studies found that tea catechins were
associated with a reduced risk of stroke.[62] A beneficial effect of a high intake
of catechins against chronic obstructive pulmonary disease was seen in a

large observational trial (n = 13,651 adults) in which dietary intake of catechins and pulmonary function were estimated in three Dutch cities from 1994 to 1997. In this study, total catechin intake was positively associated with pulmonary function and inversely associated with chronic cough.[63] The Netherlands Cohort Study (n = 4280 men and women aged 55–69 years at baseline) assessed the association between body mass index and catechins over a 14-year period. Women with the highest intake of total catechins experienced a significantly lower increase in body mass index while no significant differences in body mass index change were observed in men.[61] To evaluate the effect of a high catechin intake and the incidence of and mortality from ischemic heart disease and stroke, data from the Zutphen Elderly Study, a prospective cohort study of 806 men aged 65–84 years at baseline in 1985, were evaluated. Catechin intake was inversely associated with ischemic heart disease mortality but was not associated with the incidence of myocardial infarction or stroke incidence.[64] Catechins exhibited the following properties in laboratory studies: antioxidant; antiproliferative; vascular protective (antihypertensive, anti-inflammatory, antithrombogenic, lipid lowering); and monoamine oxidase inhibitory.[65,66]

bioactive dose

Not known.

safety

Presumed safe when consumed in normal dietary quantities by nonallergic individuals. Experimental data in animal models suggest that catechins are not teratogenic.[7]

Cauliflower (Brassica oleracea)

definition

Brassica vegetable consumed raw or cooked that is an excellent source of vitamins C and K[67] and a source of glucosinolates.

scientific findings

In a laboratory study, an antioxidant in cauliflower neutralized free radical activity and inhibited the peroxidation of linolenic acid.[68]

bioactive dose

Not known.

C

safety

Presumed safe when consumed in normal dietary quantities by non-allergic individuals.

Celery (Apium graveolens)

definition

Salad herb and umbelliferous vegetable that is commonly sautéed or added cooked or uncooked for its characteristic flavor and crisp texture. Source of fiber and numerous phytochemicals, including flavonoids such as quercetin, flavonols, and flavones.[69,70] Celery and celery seed have been traditionally used as carminatives.

scientific findings

Umbelliferous vegetables are considered to be among the foods and herbs having the highest anticancer activity.[71]

bioactive dose

Not known. The carminative dose of celery seed is 1–4 g[72]; however, neither dose nor efficacy has been proven.

safety

Presumed safe when consumed in normal dietary quantities by non-allergic individuals. When celery oil or seeds are used orally in amounts larger than are normally consumed in the diet, celery may have uterine stimulant or abortifacient effects[7] and should be avoided during pregnancy. Celery consumption has been associated with allergic reactions.[73,74]

Chamomile (Matricaria recutita [German chamomile], Chamomilla recutita [Roman chamomile])

definition

Herb consumed as tea. One of the most popular single ingredient herbal teas,[75] chamomile is caffeine-free, supplies negligible nutrients, and is a source of the phytochemical apigenin.[76,77] German chamomile is the most commonly consumed type of chamomile tea in the United States.[75]

Chamomile is in use today as a traditional remedy for sleeplessness, anxiety, and gastrointestinal conditions such as upset stomach, gas, and diarrhea, although studies examining chamomile alone are lacking for many of these uses.[75]

scientific findings

A randomized, double-blind, placebo-controlled study (n = 57 subjects with anxiety) found significant reductions in total Hamilton Depression Rating scores for chamomile for 8 weeks for all participants versus placebo.[78] In a laboratory analysis, apigenin demonstrated anti-inflammatory, antioxidant, and anticarcinogenic properties.[76]

bioactive dose

Not known.

safety

Presumed safe when consumed in normal dietary quantities by non-allergic individuals. Allergic reactions and anaphylaxis have been reported in people who have eaten or come into contact with chamomile products.[75,7]

Cheese

definition

High-protein, low-carbohydrate dairy group food that, depending on type, is generally high or moderately high in fat calories, a good source of calcium, providing approximately 200 mg of calcium per 1–1.5-ounce serving.[79] Unlike milk, cheese is not routinely fortified with vitamin D but is a source of potassium, phosphorus, riboflavin, niacin, and vitamin B12.[80]

scientific findings

Eating cheese can be an effective strategy for preventing cavities when consumed in combination with cariogenic foods,[81] possibly because chewing stimulates saliva flow, which washes away sugars and/or cariogenic bacteria, or because nutrients in cheese, including protein, calcium, and phosphorus, neutralize plaque acids.[81,82] Even in the presence of sucrose, cheeses such as aged cheddar, Swiss, blue, Monterey Jack, mozzarella, brie, gouda, and American processed cheese may prevent plaque pH from dropping to a level conducive to cavity formation.[82] Constituents in cheese, including calcium, may help to meet the RDA for calcium and perform functions such as maintaining normal blood pressure (calcium relaxes blood vessels), in which calcium is thought to play a role due to its ability to relax blood vessels.[83,84] Fermented cheeses such as Camembert contain prebiotic and probiotic bacteria.[85]

bioactive dose

Not known.

safety

Presumed safe when consumed in normal dietary quantities by non-allergic individuals.

Cherimoya (Annona cherimola)

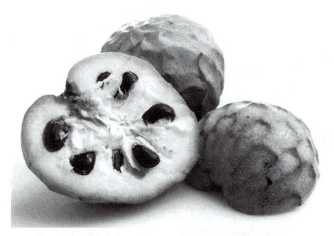

Cherimoya. (Image from EsHanPhot/Shutterstock.)

definition

Green-skinned fruit with yellowish, creamy flesh and large black inedible seeds. It is thought to be native to South America but is grown in California.[86] Cherimoya's flavor has been described as succulent and custard-like and like a blend of banana, pineapple, papaya, peach, and strawberry.[87] It can be made into juice or used to make fruit salad. Cherimoya has been used in traditional Mexican medicine for its anti-anxiety, anticonvulsant, and tranquilizing properties.[88]

scientific findings

In an animal study, *Annona cherimola* extract administered intraperitoneally significantly decreased plasma total cholesterol, triglycerides, and LDL-cholesterol, and increased HDL-cholesterol levels.[88] Cherimoya is a source of fiber, magnesium, potassium, cyptoxanthin, lutein, and xeaxanthin.[89]

bioactive dose

Not known.

safety

Presumed safe when consumed in normal dietary quantities by non-allergic individuals.

Cherry (Prunus avium)

definition

Also called sweet cherry. Common small Rosaceae family fruit, to which apples also belong, known for sweetness. Eaten fresh, dried, and canned. One cup of raw sweet cherries is a good source of vitamin C.[90] Cherries are a source of the phytochemicals phenolics and anthocyanins.[91]

scientific findings

In an animal model of arthritis, cherry anthocyanins exhibited anti-inflammatory and antioxidative effects.[92]

bioactive dose

Not known.

safety

Presumed safe when consumed in normal dietary quantities by non-allergic individuals.

Chicory (Cichorium intybus)

definition

Perennial with a periwinkle blue flower that grows in the wild. The leaves are used raw in salads, the roots are boiled and eaten, and roasted, ground roots may be used to enhance the richness of coffee.[93] Fructans (natural, low-calorie sweeteners) are sourced from the chicory plant (see also *fructans*).

scientific findings

In a laboratory study, *Cichorium intybus* exhibited antioxidant properties.[94]

bioactive dose

Not known.

safety

Presumed safe when consumed in normal dietary quantities by non-allergic individuals. Chicory is possibly unsafe when used orally in excessive amounts because it may induce menstruation or miscarriage.[7]

Chive (Allium schoenoprasum)

definition

Long green leaves of a bulbous allium vegetable, hollow and similar to those of an onion, but smaller in diameter.[95] Used as a culinary herb fresh or dried.

scientific findings

In a population study (n = 238 men with confirmed cases of prostate cancer compared to n = 471 male control subjects), intake of allium vegetables, including chives, was inversely associated with the risk of prostate cancer: men in the highest of three intake categories of total allium vegetables (>10.0 g/day) had a statistically significantly lower risk of prostate cancer than those in the lowest category (<2.2 g/day).[96]

bioactive dose

Not known.

safety

Presumed safe when consumed in normal dietary quantities by non-allergic individuals.

Chocolate (Theobroma cacao)

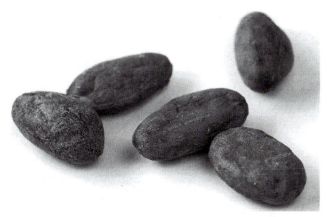

Cacao bean. (Image from eversummerphoto/Shutterstock.)

definition

Confection made from the cacao bean that could be made with or without milk, the latter of which is flavonoid rich. High in fat, a 160-g (6-ounce) bar of dark chocolate is an excellent source of iron, potassium, and magnesium, and a good source of zinc.[97] Chocolate products and cocoa are "among the most concentrated sources of the procyanidin flavonoids catechin and epicatechin."[98]

scientific findings

Intake of flavonoid-rich foods and risk for cardiovascular disease are inversely related, possibly due to flavonoid-induced changes in oxidant defense, vascular reactivity, and platelet reactivity.[98] A meta-analysis of 13 randomized, controlled trials published between 1955 and 2001 in which treated groups consumed an average daily flavanol intake ranging from 30 mg to 1000 mg[99] showed that dark chocolate reduced systolic hypertension or diastolic prehypertension (note: there are approximately 50 mg of flavanols in a 100-g portion of dark chocolate and approximately 13 mg of flavanols in a 100-g portion of milk chocolate).[100] In another study, active treatment with cocoa products for 2–18 weeks reduced mean systolic and diastolic blood pressure across all trials in a meta-analysis of 10 randomized controlled trials (n = 297) of healthy normotensive adults or patients with prehypertension/stage 1 hypertension.[101] A review concluded that the evidence about cocoa or chocolate and blood pressure is unclear and the results of six studies published through 2007 are conflicting.[102]

bioactive dose

For cardiovascular disease prevention, 19–54 g of cocoa per day or 46–100 g of dark chocolate per day has been used.[7]

safety

Presumed safe when consumed in normal dietary quantities by non-allergic individuals.

Choline

definition

Vitamin, which serves as a precursor for the neurotransmitter acetylcholine, is necessary for *de novo* synthesis of phospholipids and participates as a methyl donor in the conversion of homocysteine to methionine.[103,104] Betaine is its metabolite. The average adult consumes 730–1040 mg of choline a day in food sources such as milk, liver, eggs, peanuts, and orange juice.[103,104]

scientific findings

Preconception dietary intakes of choline between 350.56 and 544.36 mg or more were associated with reduced risk of neural tube defects in an epidemiological study (n = 424 mothers of children with neural tube defects and n = 440 mothers of nonneural tube defect-affected children).[104] Neural tube defect risk estimates were lowest for women whose diet 3 months prior to conception were rich in choline, possibly due to the impact of choline deficiency on folate metabolism.[104] Dietary supplements of choline are not addressed in this guide.

bioactive dose

The AI for adults aged 19–50 years is 425–550 mg, and for pregnant women is 450 mg/day.

safety

An UL of 3.5 g of choline has been established for adults.

Chromium

definition

Trace mineral necessary for insulin action[105] is referred to as the glucose tolerance factor.[95] Broccoli contains 11 mcg per 1/2 cup; grape juice supplies

8 mcg per 1 cup; dried basil supplies 2 mcg per tablespoon; and green beans supply 1 mcg per 1/2 cup.[105] Eating a variety of whole grains, fruits, vegetables, meats, milk, and milk products provides adequate amounts of chromium.[105]

scientific findings

Chromium may improve insulin sensitivity, which can modify the risk of diabetes and cardiovascular disease,[106] but a deficiency can have the opposite effect. Symptomatic chromium deficiency is considered to be rare but can occur due to malnutrition.[95,105] Symptoms include severe glucose intolerance and weight loss.[95] Chromium deficiency impairs the body's ability to use glucose to meet its energy needs and raises the body's insulin requirements.[105] Chromium status is difficult to measure. The assessment of toenail chromium has been used to determine chromium status in the research setting.[106] Diabetic men with CVD had lower toenail chromium than healthy control subjects in a cross-sectional analysis comparing men with diabetes only (n = 688), diabetes with prevalent CVD (n = 198), and healthy control subjects (n = 361).[106]

bioactive dose

The AI for chromium is 25–35 µg.

safety

No UL has been established for chromium.

Cilantro (Coriandrum sativum)

definition

Coriander leaves and soft stems are chopped and used in Latin cooking, for example, in salsa or to garnish bean-and-rice dishes. Cilantro is grown from coriander seed. It is a source of vitamin A and vitamin K, and contains numerous phytochemicals, including caffeic acid, chlorogenic acid, quercetin, and limonene.[107,108]

scientific findings

Laboratory studies have shown coriander essential oils to have antioxidant and hepatoprotective properties.[109] Coriander extract exerted anti-anxiety activity in a laboratory study.[110]

bioactive dose

Not known.

safety

Presumed safe when consumed in normal dietary quantities by non-allergic individuals.

Cinnamon (Cinnamomum cassia)

definition

Spice sourced from the bark of a tropical tree native to Asia that is used as a flavorful stick or in ground form to flavor fruity or savory dishes. Contains the phytochemical cinnamaldehyde.[111]

scientific findings

In animal models, cinnamon exhibited hypoglycemic, antimicrobial, antifungal, antiviral, antioxidant, antitumor, blood pressure-lowering, cholesterol-lowering, lipid-lowering, gastroprotective, and anticholinesterase properties.[112,113] A few clinical trials have shown conflicting results regarding the effects of cinnamon in the treatment of diabetes, and additional randomized controlled clinical trials are needed before therapeutic recommendations can be made for the use of cinnamon as an effective treatment in humans.[7]

bioactive dose

Not known.

safety

Presumed safe when consumed in normal dietary quantities by non-allergic individuals.

Citrus fruit

definition

Juicy, segmented fruits of the genus *Citrus* that are good sources of vitamin C and folate and are among the best sources of flavonoids (e.g., naringenin, hesperidin, nobiletin, and tangeretin). The skin, peel, or rinds of citrus fruits are rich in essential oils and contain more phytochemical compounds on a per gram basis than the edible interior flesh.[114] Otherwise, inedible fruit peels are consumed, for example, when lemon peel is scraped and added to recipes as lemon "zest"; a small piece of lime is twisted to expel its juice and the peel is added to a beverage (lime "twist"); or sour orange rind is included in marmalade. Citrus rinds contain a variety of phytochemicals, including carotenoids, flavanone glycosides, and flavonoids.[115]

scientific findings

Consumption of citrus fruit and citrus juice was inversely related to the risk of pancreatic cancer, according to an observational study (n = 384 cases and 983 controls).[116] A prospective analysis (n = 185,885 older adults participating in the Multiethnic Cohort Study) showed consuming citrus fruits was inversely associated with the risk of invasive bladder cancer in women, but not in men (in addition, women with the highest intakes of nutrients rich in citrus fruits, including C and folate had a lower risk of bladder cancer).[117] Epidemiological research suggests citrus flavonoid-containing foods attenuate cardiovascular diseases; experimental and a limited number of clinical studies have shown properties in citrus fruit to be lipid-lowering, insulin-sensitizing, antihypertensive, and anti-inflammatory; citrus flavonoids blunt the inflammatory response in metabolically important tissues, including liver, adipose tissue, kidney, and the aorta; and in animal models, citrus flavonoids show marked suppression of atherogenesis through improved metabolic parameters and also through direct impact on the vessel wall.[118] Results from epidemiologic and experimental studies suggest that citrus may have a role in promoting vascular health, although clinical trial data are lacking.[119] Citrus bioflavonoid and a related metabolite, hesperidin, exerted antiviral effects on human cell lines.[120] Nobiliten, a bioflavonoid found in citrus flesh and peel, has exhibited anti-inflammatory effects in laboratory studies.[121–123] Tangeretin, a flavone found in citrus peel,[124] has been shown to have anti-atherogenic and anti-inflammatory properties[125] and chemoprotective properties in leukemia cells[126] and colon cancer cells.[124] Carvone exhibited antinociceptive and anti-inflammatory activities in a laboratory study.[48] Flavonoids exert cardioprotective and anticarcinogenic properties *in vitro* and *in vivo*.[127]

safety

Presumed safe when consumed in normal dietary quantities by non-allergic individuals. Consuming citrus or coming into physical contact with citrus peel has resulted in allergic reaction. Citrus flavonoids have low or no cytotoxicity to healthy, normal cells.[128]

Clove (Eugenia caryophyllata)

definition

Spice sourced from an evergreen tree commonly used in fruit-based dishes, such as pumpkin pie and mulled wine (wine to which mulling spices, such as cinnamon and cloves, have been added). Clove oil, which contains eugenol, is most popularly known as being a toothache remedy topically; however, according to FDA, efficacy is lacking for this use. In addition to eugenol, other phytochemical components in clove include phenolics.[129]

scientific findings

Clove was shown to have anti-inflammatory effects in a laboratory study.[130] Clove is not effective for common uses: vomiting, upset stomach, nausea, gas, or diarrhea.[131] Clove also has mild topical anesthetic properties, but has not been clinically proven to be effective for toothache.[131]

bioactive dose

Not established.

safety

Presumed safe when consumed in normal dietary quantities by non-allergic individuals. Ingesting clove oil has been linked to reports of coagulopathy, liver damage, and other serious side effects in infants and children.[131]

Coconut (Cocos nucifera)

definition

Large Arecaceae family nut. The flesh of coconuts, a source of potassium and saturated fat,[132] in addition to flavonoid and saponin, is used in shredded form in baked products. Coconut water, which contains 400 mg of potassium per cup, making it a good source of potassium, and coconut oil have become popular products. Coconut milk is an emulsion of grated coconut meat.[7] Coconut has been used in traditional medicine for the treatment of metabolic disorders and particularly as an anti-inflammatory, antimicrobial, and analgesic.[133,134]

scientific findings

The saturated medium-chain triglycerides in coconut oil increase total serum cholesterol, but affect HDL-cholesterol levels favorably.[135] Diets rich in coconut oils have been shown to reduce coronary artery disease risk factors, such as tissue plasminogen activator antigen and lipoprotein(a)[135]; however, current recommendations are to limit saturated fats, including coconut oil to no more than 7% of calories.[136] Lauric acid, the most abundant fatty acid in coconut oil, is effective in preventing tooth decay and plaque buildup.[135] Saponin and polyphenols in coconut were attributed with anti-inflammatory and antinociceptive properties in an animal study.[137] The predominate fat in coconut, medium-chain triglyceride, is easier to digest and absorb than long-chain triglycerides and therefore may be useful in fat malabsorption.

bioactive dose

Not known.

safety

Presumed safe when consumed in normal dietary quantities by nonallergic individuals.

Coenzyme Q10

definition

Also called Co Q10. Fat-soluble antioxidant[138] synthesized in the body that occurs in virtually all cells—it is ubiquitous—hence it is also known as "ubiquinone." A participant in ATP generation in aerobic metabolism that is essential for electron and proton transport in the mitochondrial respiratory chain.[139] It is present in highest quantities in the heart, liver, kidney, and pancreas.[7] The richest sources include meat, fish, nuts, and some oils, while dairy products, vegetables, fruits, and cereals provide smaller amounts.[140] The average dietary intake of Co Q10 is 3–6 mg.[138]

scientific findings

Primary deficiency is caused by genetic mutations that affect Co Q10 biosynthesis. Secondary deficiency may be linked to the use of statins to treat hyperlipidemia.[141] Coenzyme Q10 deficiency is thought to be a rare condition, the symptoms of which include weakness, fatigue, and seizures.[142] Low blood levels of ubiquinone have been found in cancer patients with myeloma, lymphoma, and cancers of the breast, lung, prostate, pancreas, colon, kidney, and head and neck.[143] Not enough evidence exists to demonstrate the benefits or harm of supplemental coenzyme Q10 and its use in cardiovascular disease.[144]

bioactive dose

Not known.

C

safety

Presumed safe when consumed in normal dietary amounts by non-allergic individuals.

Coffee (Coffea arabica)

definition

Popular beverage made from brewing the roasted seeds of the coffee plant that is drunk to improve mental alertness and prevent fatigue. The average adult ingests 200 mg of caffeine per day.[11] Caffeine content in 8 ounces of common beverages includes coffee, 95–200 mg (with darker roasts containing less caffeine due to sublimation during roasting).[7] Coffee provides numerous phytochemicals, including chlorogenic acids and other polyphenols.[145]

scientific findings

Epidemiology suggests that polyphenols exert cardioprotective effects and laboratory studies suggest that polyphenols exert antioxidant, vasodilatory, anti-inflammatory, antifibrotic, antiapoptotic, and metabolic effects.[146] Coffee consumption was inversely associated with the prevalence of type 2 diabetes mellitus in several observational studies.[147,148] Coffee consumption may also be protective against the development of gallstones.[149] Epidemiological evidence suggests that drinking more than 3 cups of coffee daily may significantly reduce the risk of rectal cancer.[7] Chlorogenic acid protected cells from oxidative damage in a laboratory study,[150] induced growth of beneficial microorganisms in colon cancer cells in an *in vitro* study,[151] and, along with other polyphenols, has been postulated to exert preventive effects against cardiovascular disease and type 2 diabetes.[151]

bioactive dose

The typical dose of caffeine for headache or restoring mental alertness is up to 250 mg/day, about 2 cups of coffee.[7]

safety

Presumed safe when consumed in normal dietary quantities by nonallergic individuals. Four to seven 5-ounce cups of caffeinated coffee per day provide approximately 600 mg of caffeine, which is considered to be excessive for most people.[11] Even 250–300 mg/day has been associated with significant adverse effects, such as tachyarrhythmias and sleep disturbances.[7] Coffee consumption has been associated with hyperhomocysteinemia in some observational studies.[152]

Copper

definition

Trace mineral found in shellfish, nuts, beans, organ meats, and whole grains[54] that functions as a component of a number of metalloenzymes and that is involved in red blood cell formation, immunity, and in the maintenance of blood vessels, nerves, and bones.[54] The average dietary intake of copper by U.S. women is 1.0–1.1 mg/day (1000–1100 µg), and men consume 1.2–1.6 mg/day (1200–1600 µg).[7]

scientific findings

Copper deficiency, although rare, causes normocytic, hypochromic anemia, leukopenia, and neutropenia.[54] Copper toxicity is also rare in the U.S. population.[153] Measurement of copper status is difficult.[153]

bioactive dose

The RDA for adults aged 19–50 years is 1000 µg.

safety

An UL of 10,000 µg has been established.

Corn (Zea mays)

definition

Poaceae family fruit that is sometimes eaten as a starchy vegetable (e.g., corn on the cob) and other times as a grain (e.g., popcorn).[154] Corn is a source of potassium, phosphorus, fiber, xeaxanthin, and ferulic acid.[155] It is deficient in the amino acids lysine and tryptophan. Eaten cooked, canned, frozen, and used to make oil, flour, starch, and other food products, such as high-fructose corn syrup. Traditional medicinal applications of *Zea mays* include use as a diuretic and for treating dropsy, hypertension, hemorrhage, warts, and diabetes.[155]

scientific findings

Zea mays exhibited antioxidant properties and slowed glucose absorption in a laboratory study.[156]

bioactive dose

Not known.

C

safety

Presumed safe when consumed in normal dietary quantities by non-allergic individuals.

Coumaric acid (p-coumarate)

definition

Polyphenolic compound called a cinnaminate found in many foods, including beer, carrots, cereal brans, garlic, mung bean, peanuts, strawberry, raspberry, spinach, wine, and vinegar.[157–159]

scientific findings

In laboratory animals, coumaric acid reduced LDL cholesterol levels.[160] Phenolic compounds have exhibited antioxidant properties *in vitro*.[161]

bioactive dose

Not known.

safety

Presumed safe when consumed in normal dietary quantities by non-allergic individuals.

Coumarin

definition

Chemical compound found in milk, vodka, cinnamon (*Cassia cinnamon*) and products flavored with cinnamon such as liqueurs.[162]

scientific findings

An experimental study found coumarins in lemon peel inhibited free radical generation.[163]

bioactive dose

Not established.

safety

Presumed safe when consumed in normal dietary quantities by nonallergic individuals. Coumarin may be toxic when used at high doses for long periods of time. It has hepatotoxic and carcinogenic properties[164]; therefore, a European Tolerable Daily Intake has been set at 0.1 mg/kg of body weight.[164] According to a European survey, intake of coumarin may approach the tolerable daily intake when foods flavored with cinnamon are heavily used.[164]

Cranberry (Vaccinium macrocarpon)

definition

Bitter fruit of an evergreen shrub that is consumed as a fruit or juice cocktail, dried, and fresh or canned as cranberry sauce. Cranberry is a source of vitamin C, choline, vitamin A, and vitamin K,[165] and proanthocyanidin. Some practice guidelines currently recommend consumption of pure cranberry–lingonberry juice as an option for preventing recurrent urinary tract infection (UTI).[166]

scientific findings

Daily doses of 120–4000 mL/day of cranberry juice or 400 mg of cranberry extract were used to help prevent UTIs[72] based on the results of small studies that theorized cranberry prevents bacteria from sticking to the cells that line the bladder.[167] A review including 24 studies (n = 4473 subjects) concluded that cranberry juice cannot currently be recommended for the prevention of UTIs, and that although some small studies demonstrated a small benefit for women with recurrent UTIs, there were no statistically significant differences when the results of a much larger study were included.[168]

bioactive dose

Not known.

safety

Presumed safe when consumed in normal dietary quantities by non-allergic individuals.

Cryptoxanthin, β-cryptoxanthin

definition

Xanthophyll carotenoids are found in foods such as oranges, tangerines, yellow pepper, papaya, pumpkin, zucchini, and corn.[169–171]

scientific findings

β-cryptoxanthin is one of the five carotenoids that predominate in human plasma[172] and serves as an antioxidant and a source of vitamin A.[55] In a laboratory study, it exhibited antitumor effects.[170]

bioactive dose

Not known.

safety

Presumed safe when consumed in normal dietary quantities by non-allergic individuals.

Cumin (Cuminum cyminum)

definition

Seed that is used whole or ground into a spice in Indian and Middle Eastern cooking. Though it would be consumed in miniscule amounts, cumin is a source of calcium, magnesium, potassium, iron, zinc, phosphorus, and selenium and numerous antioxidants.[173] Traditionally used for the treatment and management of sleep disorders, indigestion, and hypertension.[174]

scientific findings

Cumin has demonstrated antihyperglycemic and antihypertensive properties in animal studies.[174,175]

bioactive dose

Not known.

safety

Presumed safe when consumed in normal dietary quantities by non-allergic individuals. Safrole, a natural mutagenic compound, which is degraded by cooking, is a constituent of cumin.[173]

References

1. US Department of Agriculture. Agricultural Research Service. Nutrient Data Lab. Cabbage, raw. http://ndb.nal.usda.gov/ndb/foods/show/2874. Accessed May 25, 2013.

2. Velasco P, Francisco M, Moreno DA, Ferreres F, García-Viguera C, Cartea ME. Phytochemical fingerprinting of vegetable *Brassica oleracea* and *Brassica napus* by simultaneous identification of glucosinolates and phenolics. *Phytochem Anal.* 2011;22(2):144–152.

3. Cheney G. Rapid healing of peptic ulcers in patients receiving fresh cabbage juice. *Calif Med.* 1949;70:1:1–6.

4. Júnior LC, Niero R, Andrade SF. Gastroprotective activity of hydroalcoholic extract obtained from the leaves of *Brassica oleracea* var. *acephala* DC in different animal models. *J Ethnopharmacol.* 2011;138(2):503–507. doi: 10.1016/j. jep.2011.09.046. Epub 2011 October 1.

5. Mehtz RG, Liu J, Constantinoul A, Thomas CF, Hawthorne M, You M, Gerhäuser C, Pezzuto JM, Moon RC, Moriarty RM. Cancer chemopreventive activity of brassinin, a phytoalexin from cabbage. *Carcinogenesis.* 1995;16(2):399–404.

6. Zhao H1, Lin J, Grossman HB, Hernandez LM, Dinney CP, Wu X. Dietary isothiocyanates, GSTM1, GSTT1, NAT2 polymorphisms and bladder cancer risk. *Int J Cancer.* 2007 May 15;120(10):2208–2213.

7. Jellin JM, Gregory PJ. Natural Medicine Comprehensive Database. Therapeutic Research Faculty. 2013. http://www.naturaldatabase.com. Accessed July 11, 2012.

8. Grosvenor MB, Smolin LA. *Visualizing Nutrition.* Hoboken, NJ: John Wiley & Sons; 2010.

9. Greer MA. Goitrogens in foods. *Am J Clin Nutr.* 1957;5(4):440–444.

10. Dworzański W, Opielak G, Burdan F. Side effects of caffeine. *Pol Merkur Lekarski.* 2009;27(161):357–361.

11. US Food and Drug Administration. Medicines in my Home: Caffeine and your body. http://www.fda.gov/downloads/Drugs/ResourcesForYou/Consumers/BuyingUsingMedicineSafely/UnderstandingOver-the-CounterMedicines/UCM205286.pdf. Accessed November 28, 2011.

12. National Institutes of Health. Medline Plus. Caffeine in the diet. http://www.nlm.nih.gov/medlineplus/ency/article/002445.htm. Accessed March 12, 2011.

13. Whitney E, DeBruyne LK, Pinna K, Rolfes SR. *Nutrition for Health and Health Care,* 4th edn. Belmont, CA: Cengage Learning; 2011.

14. National Institutes of Health. Office of Dietary Supplements. Calcium Fact Sheet. http://ods.od.nih.gov/factsheets/Calcium-QuickFacts. Accessed November 29, 2011.

15. Academy of Nutrition and Dietetics. HTN: Minerals (2007). http://www.andeal.org/topic.cfm?menu=5285&cat=2777. Accessed 25 February, 2015.

16. Soares MJ, Ping-Delfos CS, Ghanbari MH. Calcium and vitamin D for obesity: A review of randomized controlled trials. *Eur J Clin Nutr.* 2011;65(9):994–1004.

17. Giovannucci E, Rimm EB, Wolk A, Ascherio A, Stampfer MJ, Colditz GA, Willett WC. Calcium and fructose intake in relation to risk of prostate cancer. *Cancer Res.* 1998;58:442.

18. US Department of Agriculture. Agricultural Research Service. National Nutrient Database. Cantaloupe, raw. http://ndb.nal.usda.gov/ndb/foods/show/2290. Accessed December 6, 2011.

19. US Department of Agriculture. Agricultural Research Service. Phytochemical Database. *Cucumis melo.* http://www.pl.barc.usda.gov/usda_plant/plant_detail.cfm?code=69685564&plant_id=446&y1s27=Honeydew&ThisName=ps721. Accessed December 6, 2011.

20. Naito Y, Akagiri S, Uchiyama K, Kokura S, Yoshida N, Hasegawa G, Nakamura N et al. Reduction of diabetes-induced renal oxidative stress by a cantaloupe melon extract/gliadin biopolymers, oxykine, in mice. *Biofactors.* 2005;23(2):85–95.

21. Zhang CX, Ho SC, Chen YM, Fu JH, Cheng SZ, Lin FY. Greater vegetable and fruit intake is associated with a lower risk of breast cancer among Chinese women. *Int J Cancer.* 2009;125(1):181–188.

22. deWolff FA. Nutritional toxicology: The significance of natural toxins. *Human Toxicol.* 1988;(7):443–447.

23. US Department of Agriculture. Agricultural Research Service. Phytochemical Database. Canthaxanthin. Accessed July 5, 2013.

24. Torrissen OJ. Pigmentation of salmonids: Interactions of astaxanthin and canthaxanthin on pigment deposition in rainbow trout. *Aquaculture.* 1989;79(1–4):363–374.

25. Baker, RMT. Canthaxanthin in aquafeed applications: Is there any risk? *Trends Food Sci Tech.* 2001;12(7): 240–243.

26. Sujak A. Interactions between canthaxanthin and lipid membranes— Possible mechanisms of canthaxanthin toxicity. *Cell Mol Biol Lett.* 2009;14(3):395–410. Epub 2009 February 12.

27. Yiki V. Biological functions and activities of animal carotenoids. *Pure Appl Chem.* 1991;63(1):141–146.

28. Palan PR, Mikhail MS Goldberg GL, Basu J, Runowicz CD, Romney SL. Plasma levels of beta-carotene, lycopene, canthaxanthin, retinol, and alpha- and tau-tocopherol in cervical intraepithelial neoplasia and cancer. *Clin Cancer Res.* 1996;2(1):181–185.

29. International Programme on Chemical Safety. World Health Organization. Safety Evaluation of Certain Food Additives and Contaminants WHO Food Additives Series: 44. Prepared by the Fifty-Third Meeting of the Joint FAO/WHO Expert Committee on Food Additives (JECFA) World Health Organization, Geneva, 2000. IPCS—International Programme on Chemical Safety Evaluation of National Assessments of Intake of Canthaxanthin. http://www.inchem.org/documents/jecfa/jecmono/v44jec22.htm. Accessed November 1, 2011.

30. US Department of Agriculture. Agricultural Research Service. Phytochemical Database. http://ndb.nal.usda.gov/ndb/foods/show/273?qlookup=caper&fg=&format=&man=&lfacet=&max=25&new=1. Accessed July 05, 2013.

31. Yang T, Wang C, Chou G, Cheng X, Wang Z. A new antioxidant compound from *Capparis spiniosa* [sic]. *Pharm Biol.* 2010;48(5):589–594. Accessed June 25, 2011.

32. Zhou H, Jinn R, Kang J, Huang X, Li Y, Zhuang C, Yang F et al. Antiinflammatory effects of caper (*Capparis spinosa* L.) fruit aqueous extract and the isolation of main phytochemicals. *J Agric Food Chem.* 2010;22:58(24):12717–12721.

33. Eddouks M, Lemhadria A, Michel J-B. Hypolipidemic activity of aqueous extract of *Capparis spinosa* L. in normal and diabetic rats. *J Ethnopharmacol.* 2005;98(3):345–350.

34. Szallasi A. Vanilloid (capsaicin) receptors in health and disease. *Am J Clin Pathol.* 2002;118:110–121.

35. Galgani JE, Ravussin E. Effect of dihydrocapsiate on resting metabolic rate in humans. *J Clin Nutr.* 2010;92(5):1089–1093. Epub 2010 September 8.

36. Szallasi A, Blumber PM. Vanilloid (capsaicin) receptors and mechanisms. *Pharmacol Rev*. 1999;51(2):159–212.

37. Rodriguez-Stanley S, Collings KL, Robinson M, Owen W, Miner PB Jr. The effects of capsaicin on reflux, gastric emptying and dyspepsia. *Aliment Pharmacol Ther*. 2000;14(1):129–134.

38. Chularojmontri L, Suwatronnakorn M, Wattanapitayakul SK. Influence of capsicum extract and capsaicin on endothelial health. *J Med Assoc Thai*. 2010;93:S92–101.

39. Lopez HL, Ziegenfuss TN, Hofheins JE, Habowski SM, Arent SM, Weir JP, Ferrando AA. Eight weeks of supplementation with a multi-ingredient weight loss product enhances body composition, reduces hip and waist girth, and increases energy levels in overweight men and women. *J Int Soc Sports Nutr*. 2013;10(1):22. doi: 10.1186/1550-2783-10-22.

40. Lee J, Li Y, Li C, Li D. Natural products and body weight control. *North Am J Med Sci*. 2011;3:13–19.

41. US Department of Agriculture. Agricultural Research Service. National Nutrient Database. Star fruit, fresh, 1 cup, raw. http://ndb.nal.usda.gov/ ndb/foods/show/2223?fgcd=&manu=&lfacet=&format=&count=&max=35 &offset=&sort=&qlookup=carambola. Accessed February 25, 2015.

42. Shui G, Leong LP. Analysis of polyphenolic antioxidants in star fruit using liquid chromatography and mass spectrometry. *J Chromatogr*. 2004;1022(1–2):67–75.

43. Chau CF, Chen C-H, Lin C-Y. Insoluble fiber-rich fractions derived from *Averrhoa carambola*: Hypoglycemic effects determined by *in vitro* methods. *Food Sci Technol LEB*. 2004;37(3):331–335.

44. Tse KC, Yip PS, Lam MF, Choy BY, Li FK, Lui SL, Lo WK, Chan TM, Lai KN. Star fruit intoxication in uraemic patients: Case series and review of the literature. *Intern Med J*. 2003;33(7):314–316.

45. US Department of Agriculture. Agricultural Research Service. Phytochemical Database. Carum carvi/caraway. http://ndb.nal.usda.gov/ndb/ foods/show/225?fg=&man=&lfacet=&format=&count=&max=25&offset= &sort=&qlookup=caraway. Accessed July 5, 2013.

46. Dadkhah A, Allameh A, Khalafi H, Ashrafihelan J. Inhibitory effects of dietary caraway essential oils on 1,2-dimethylhydrazine-induced colon carcinogenesis is mediated by liver xenobiotic metabolizing enzymes. *Nutr Cancer*. 2011;63(1):46–54.

47. de Sousa DP, Camargo EA, Oliveira FS, de Almeida RN. Anti-inflammatory activity of hydroxydihydrocarvone. *Z Naturforsch C*. 2010;65(9–10):543–550.

48. National Institutes of Health. Office of Dietary Supplement Fact Sheets. Carnitine. http://ods.od.nih.gov/factsheets/carnitine. Accessed April 7, 2011.

49. Institute of Medicine Food and Nutrition Board. *Recommended Dietary Allowances*, 10th edn. Washington, DC: National Academy Press; 1989.

50. US Department of Agriculture. Agricultural Research Service. Phytonutrient Database. http://www.pl.barc.usda.gov/usda_plant/plant_home.cfm. Accessed December 3, 2012.

51. Frankel EN, Wen Huang S-W, Aeschbah R, Prior E. Antioxidant activity of a rosemary extract and its constituents, carnosic acid, carnosol, and rosmarinic acid, in bulk oil and oil-in-water emulsion. *J Agric Food Chem*. 1996;44(1):131–135.

52. Johnson JJ. Carnosol: A promising anti-cancer and anti-inflammatory agent. *Cancer Lett.* 2011;305(1):1–7.

53. Mayne ST. Beta-carotene, carotenoids, and disease prevention in humans. *FASEB J.* 1996;10:690–701.

54. Institute of Medicine. *Dietary References Intakes for Vitamin A, Vitamin K, Aresenic, Boron, Chromium, Copper, Iodine, Iron, Manganese, Molybdenum, Nickel, Silicon, Vanadium, and Zinc.* Washington DC: Institute of Medicine; 2001.

55. Xu ZS, Huang Y, Wang F, Song X, Wang GL, Xiong AS. Transcript profiling of structural genes involved in cyanidin-based anthocyanin biosynthesis between purple and non-purple carrot (*Daucus carota* L.) cultivars reveals distinct patterns. *BMC Plant Biol.* 2014;14:262. doi: 10.1186/s12870-014-0262-y.

56. DeBruyne LK, Pinna K. *Nutrition for Health and Healthcare*, 5th edn. Belmont, CA: Wadsworth Cengage Learning; 2014.

57. Klosterbuer A, Roughead ZF, Slavin J. Benefits of dietary fiber in clinical nutrition. *Nutr Clin Pract.* 2011;26(5):625–635.

58. Shebaby WN, Bodman-Smith KB, Mansour A, Mroueh M, Taleb RI, El-Sibai M, Daher CF. *Daucus carota* pentane-based fractions suppress proliferation and induce apoptosis in human colon adenocarcinoma HT-29 cells by inhibiting the MAPK and PI3K pathways. *J Med Food.* 2015;18(7):745–752. Epub 2015 January 19.

59. Schnabele K, Briviba K, Bub A, Roser S, Pool-Zobel BL, Rechkemmer G. Effects of carrot and tomato juice consumption on faecal markers relevant to colon carcinogenesis in humans. *Br J Nutr.* 2008;99(3):606–613. doi: 10.1017/S0007114507819143.

60. Tseng HC, Wang MH, Soung HS, Chang Y, Kuo-Chi C. (-)Epigallocatechin-3-gallate prevents the reserpine-induces impairment of short-term social memory in rats. *Behav Pharmacol* 2015 Jul 20 [Epub ahead of print].

61. Hughes LAE, Arts ICW, Ambergen T, Brants HAM, Dagnelie PC, Goldbohm RA, van den Brandt PA, Wijenber MP. Higher dietary flavone, flavonol, and catechin intakes are associated with less of an increase in BMI over time in women: A longitudinal analysis from the Netherlands Cohort Study. *Am J Clin Nutr.* 2008(88)5:1341–1352.

62. Arab L, Liebeskind DS. Tea, flavonoids and stroke in man and mouse. *Arch Biochem Biophys.* 2010;501(1):31–36.

63. Tabak C, Arts IC, Smit HA, Heederik D, Kromhout D. Chronic obstructive pulmonary disease and intake of catechins, flavonols, and flavones: The MORGEN Study. *Am J Respir Crit Care Med.* 2001;164(1):61–64.

64. Arts IC, Hollman PC, Feskens EJ, Bueno de Mesquita HB, Kromhout D. Catechin intake might explain the inverse relation between tea consumption and ischemic heart disease: The Zutphen Elderly Study. *Am J Clin Nutr.* 2001;74(2):227–232.

65. Babu PV, Liu D. Green tea catechins and cardiovascular health: An update. *Curr Med Chem.* 2008;15(18):1840–1850.

66. Reimann HJ, Lorenz W, Fischer M, Frölich R, Meyer HJ, Schmal A. Histamine and acute haemorrhagic lesions in rat gastric mucosa: Prevention of stress ulcer formation by (+)-catechin, an inhibitor of specific histidine decarboxylase *in vitro*. *Agents Actions.* 1977;7(1):69–73.

67. US Department of Agriculture. Agricultural Research Service. Nutrient Data Lab. Cauliflower, raw. http://ndb.nal.usda.gov/ndb/foods/show/2893? fg=&man=&lfacet=&format=&count=&max=25&offset=&sort=&qlookup= cauliflower. Accessed May 3, 2013.

68. Koksal E, Gulcin I. Antioxidant activity of cauliflower (*Brassica oleracea* L.). *Turk J Agric For.* 2008;32:65–78.

69. Crozier AK, Lean MEJ, McDonald MS, Black C. Quantitative analysis of the flavonoid content of commercial tomatoes, onions, lettuce, and celery. *J Agric Food Chem.* 1997;45(3);590–595.

70. Zhang Y, Li Y, Cao C, Cao J, Zhang Y, Wang C, Wang J, Zhang X, Zhao X. Dietary flavonol and flavone intakes and their major food sources in Chinese adults. *Nutr Cancer.* 2010;62(8):1120–1127.

71. Craig WJ. Phytochemicals: Guardians of our health. *J Am Diet Assoc.* 1997;97(10 Suppl 2):S199–204.

72. Der Marderosian A, Beutler JA. *The Review of Natural Products.* 5th edn. St. Louis, MO: Wolters Kluwer Health; 2008;383–386.

73. Pałgan K, Götz-Żbikowska M, Tykwińska M, Napiórkowska K, Bartuzi Z. Celery—Cause of severe anaphylactic shock. *Postepy Hig Med Dosw* (Online). 2012;66:132–134. doi: 10.5604/17322693.986123.

74. Chen JY, Quirt J, Lee KJ. Proposed new mechanism for food and exercise induced anaphylaxis based on case studies. *Allergy Asthma Clin Immunol.* 2013;9(1):11. doi: 10.1186/1710-1492-9-11.

75. National Institutes of Health National Center for Complementary and Alternative Medicine. Chamomile. https://nccih.nih.gov/health/ chamomile. Accessed March 4, 2011.

76. McKay DL, Blumberg JB. A review of the bioactivity and potential health benefits of chamomile tea (*Matricaria recutita* L.). *Phytother Res.* 2001; 20(7):519–530.

77. Patel D1, Shukla S, Gupta S. Apigenin and cancer chemoprevention: Progress, potential and promise (review). *Int J Oncol.* 2007;30(1):233–245.

78. Amsterdam JD, Shults J, Soeller I, Mao JJ, Rockwell K, Newberg AB. Chamomile (*Matricaria recutita*) may provide antidepressant activity in anxious, depressed humans: An exploratory study. *Altern Ther Health Med.* 2012;18(5):44–49.

79. National Dairy Council. Dairy's Unique Nutrient Combination. http://www.nationaldairycouncil.org/HealthandWellness/Pages/ DairysUniqueNutrientCombination.aspx. Accessed June 25, 2011.

80. Dairy Nutrients and Health Benefits. http://www.choosemyplate.gov/ foodgroups/dairy-why.html. Accessed January 6, 2015.

81. Herod EL. The effect of cheese on dental caries: A review of the literature. *Aust Dent J.* 1991;36(2):120–125.

82. American Dental Hygienists Association Continuing Education Course 7. Diet and Nutrition Implications for Oral Health. Anticariogenic Foods. http://www.adha.org/ce-course-7#foods. Accessed December 3, 2011.

83. Huang WY, Davidge ST, Wu J. Bioactive natural constituents from food sources—Potential use in hypertension prevention and treatment. *Crit Rev Food Sci Nutr.* 2013;53(6):615–630. doi: 10.1080/10408398.2010.550071.

84. Cichosz G, Czeczot H. Calcium—Essential for everybody. *Pol Merkur Lekarski.* 2014;36(216):407–411.

85. Schlienger JL, Paillard F, Lecerf JM, Romon M, Bonhomme C, Schmitt B, Donazzolo Y et al. Effect on blood lipids of two daily servings of Camembert cheese. An intervention trial in mildly hypercholesterolemic subjects. *Int J Food Sci Nutr*. 2014;65(8):1013–1018.

86. California Rare Fruit Growers. Cherimoya. http://www.crfg.org/pubs/ff/cherimoya.html. Accessed March 12, 2015.

87. Produce for Better Health. Cherimoya. http://www.fruitsandveggiesmorematters.org/get-to-know-the-succulent-cherimoya. Accessed August 23, 2015.

88. Martínez-Vázquez M, Estrada-Reyes R, Araujo Escalona AG, Ledesma Velázquez I, Martínez-Mota L, Moreno J, Heinze G. Antidepressant-like effects of an alkaloid extract of the aerial parts of *Annona cherimolia* in mice. *J Ethnopharmacol*. 2012;139(1):164–170. doi: 10.1016/j.jep.2011.10.033. Epub 2011 November 9.

89. US Department of Agriculture. Agricultural Research Service. Nutrient Database. Cherimoya, raw. Accessed http://ndb.nal.usda.gov/ndb/foods/show/2225?fg=&man=&lfacet=&count=&max=35&sort=&qlookup=cherimoya&offset=&format=Full&new=&measureby=. Accessed March 1, 2015.

90. US Department of Agriculture. Agricultural Research Service. Nutrient Data Lab. Cherries, raw, sweet. http://ndb.nal.usda.gov/ndb/foods/show/2201?fg=&man=&lfacet=&format=&count=&max=25&offset=&sort=&qlookup=cherries. Accessed May 1, 2013.

91. Hanbali LB, Ghadieh RM, Hasan HA, K Nakhal Y, Haddad JJ. Measurement of antioxidant activity and antioxidant compounds under versatile extraction conditions: I. The immuno-biochemical antioxidant properties of sweet cherry (*Prunus avium*) extracts. *Antiinflamm Antiallergy Agents Med Chem*. 2013;12(2):173–187.

92. He YH, Zhou J, Wang YS, Xiao C, Tong Y, Tang JC, Chan AS, Lu AP. Anti-inflammatory and anti-oxidative effects of cherries on Freund's adjuvant-induced arthritis in rats. *Scand J Rheumatol*. 2006;35(5):356–358.

93. Pollen Library.com. Chicory Endive (Chicorium). http://www.orleanscoffee.com/explore_coffee/what_is_chicory.html. Accessed July 27, 2013.

94. Sultana S, Perwaiz S, Iqbal M, Athar M. Crude extracts of hepatoprotective plants, *Solanum nigrum* and *Cichorium intybus* inhibit free radical-mediated DNA damage. *J Ethnopharmacol*. 1995;45(3):189–192.

95. North Carolina State University Cooperative Extension. Chive. http://content.ces.ncsu.edu/chives/ Accessed August 23, 2015.

96. Hsing AW, Chokkalingam AP, Gao YT, Madigan MP, Deng J, Gridley G, Fraumeni JF Jr. Allium vegetables and risk of prostate cancer: A population-based study. *J Natl Cancer Inst*. 2002;94(21):1648–1651.

97. US Department of Agriculture. Agricultural Research Service. Nutrient Data Laboratory. Chocolate, dark, 45%–59% cacao solids. http://ndb.nal.usda.gov/ndb/foods/show/6227?fg=&man=&lfacet=&format=&count=&max=25&offset=&sort=&qlookup=dark+chocolate+candy. Accessed May 1, 2013.

98. Keen CL. Chocolate: Food as medicine/medicine as food. *J Am Coll Nutr*. 2001;20(5 Suppl):436S–439S; discussion 440S–442S.

99. Ried K, Sullivan T, Fakler P, Frank OR, Stocks NP. Does chocolate reduce blood pressure? A meta-analysis. *BMC Med*. 2010;28(8):39.

100. US Department of Agriculture. Agricultural Research Service. USDA Database for the Flavonoid Content of Selected Foods. Beltsville, MD. March 2003:23.

101. Desch S, Schmidt J, Kobler D, Sonnabend M, Eitel I, Sareban M, Rahimi K, Schuler G, Thiele H. Effect of cocoa products on blood pressure: Systematic review and meta-analysis. *Am J Hypertens.* 2010;23(1):97–103. Epub 2009 November 12.

102. Academy of Nutrition and Dietetics Evidence Analysis Library: "HTN: Cocoa and Chocolate (2007)". www.andealorg/topic.cfm?menu-5285&cat = 2791. Accessed February 25, 2015.

103. *Dietary Reference Intakes for Thiamin, Riboflavin, Niacin, Vitamin B6, Folate, Vitamin B12, Pantothenic Acid, Biotin and Choline.* Washington DC: Institute of Medicine; 1998.

104. Shaw GM, Carmichael SL, Yang W, Selvin S, Schaffer DM. Periconceptional dietary intake of choline and betaine and neural tube defects in offspring. *Am J Epidemiol.* 2004;160(2):102–109.

105. National Institutes of Health Office of Dietary Supplements. Dietary Supplement Fact Sheet: Chromium. http://ods.od.nih.gov/factsheets/Chromium-HealthProfessional/. Accessed February 8, 2011.

106. Rajpathak S, Rimm EB, Li T, Morris JS, Stampfer MJ, Willett WC, Hu FB. Lower toenail chromium in men with diabetes and cardiovascular disease compared with healthy men. *Diabetes Care.* 2004;27(9):2211–2116.

107. US Department of Agriculture. Agricultural Research Service. Nutrient Data Lab. Coriander (leaves), raw. http://ndb.nal.usda.gov/ndb/foods/sho w/2917?fg=&man=&lfacet=&format=&count=&max=25&offset=&sort=& qlookup=cilantro. Accessed May 1, 2013.

108. US Department of Agriculture. Agricultural Research Service. Phytochemical Database. http://www.pl.barc.usda.gov/usda_plant/plant_ detail.cfm?code=69685564&plant_id=403&y1s27=Cilantro&ThisName= ps721. Accessed December 6, 2011.

109. Samojlik I, Lakić N, Mimica-Dukić N, Daković-Svajcer K, Bozin B. Antioxidant and hepatoprotective potential of essential oils of coriander (*Coriandrum sativum* L.) and caraway (*Carum carvi* L.) (Apiaceae). *J Agric Food Chem.* 2010;58(15):8848–8853.

110. Mahendra P, Bisht S. Anti-anxiety activity of *Coriandrum sativum* assessed using different experimental anxiety models. *Indian J Pharmacol.* 2011;43(5):574–577.

111. US Department of Agriculture. Agricultural Research Service. Phytochemical Database. Cinnamon. http://www.pl.barc.usda.gov/usda_plant/ plant_detail.cfm?code=69685564&plant_id=55&ThisName=ps721. Accessed May 1, 2013.

112. Bandara T, Uluwaduge I, Jansz ER. Bioactivity of cinnamon with special emphasis on diabetes mellitus: A review. *Int J Food Sci Nutr.* 2012;63(3): 380–386. Epub 2011 October 19.

113. Boğa M, Hacıbekiroğlu I, Kolak U. Antioxidant and anticholinesterase activities of eleven edible plants. *Pharm Biol.* 2011;49(3):290–295. Epub 2011 February 2.

114. Andreotti C, Ravaglia D, Ragaini A, Costa G. Phenolic compounds in peach (*Prunus persica*) cultivars at harvest and during fruit maturation. *Ann Appl Biol.* 2008;153(1):11–23.

115. Bermejo A, Llosá MJ, Cano A. Analysis of bioactive compounds in seven citrus cultivars. *Food Sci Technol Int.* 2011;17(1):55–62. Epub 2011 February 7.

116. Jansen RJ, Robinson DP, Stolzenberg-Solomon RZ, Bamlet WR, de Andrade M, Oberg AL, Hammer TJ et al. Fruit and vegetable consumption is inversely associated with having pancreatic cancer. *Cancer Cause Control.* 2011;22(12):1613–1625. Epub 2011 September 14.

117. Park SY, Ollberding NJ, Woolcott CG, Wilkens LR, Henderson BE, Kolonel LN. Fruit and vegetable intakes are associated with lower risk of bladder cancer among women in the multiethnic cohort study. *J Nutr.* 2013;143(8):1283–1292. Epub 2013 June 5.

118. Assini JM, Mulvihill EE, Huff MW. Citrus flavonoids and lipid metabolism. *Curr Opin Lipidol.* 2013;24(1):34–40. doi: 10.1097/MOL.0b013e32835c07fd.

119. Dow CA, Wertheim BC, Patil BS, Thomson CA. Daily consumption of grapefruit for 6 weeks reduces urine F2-isoprostanes in overweight adults with high baseline values but has no effect on plasma high-sensitivity C-reactive protein or soluble vascular cellular adhesion molecule 1. *J Nutr.* 2013;143(10):1586–1592. doi: 10.3945/jn.113.175166. Epub 2013 July 31.

120. Kaul TN, Middleton E Jr, Ogra PL. Antiviral effect of flavonoids on human viruses. *J Med Virol.* 1985;15(1):71–79.

121. Lin N, Sato T, Takayama Y, Mimaki Y, Sashida Y, Yano M, Ito A. Novel anti-inflammatory actions of nobiletin, a citrus polymethoxy flavonoid, on human synovial fibroblasts and mouse macrophages. *Biochem Pharmacol.* 2003;65(12):2065–2071.

122. Murakami A, Nakamura Y, Ohto Y, Yano M, Koshiba T, Koshimizu K, Tokuda H, Nishino H, Ohigashi H. Suppressive effects of citrus fruits on free radical generation and nobiletin, an anti-inflammatory polymethoxy-flavonoid. *Biofactors.* 2000;12(1–4):187–192.

123. Cui Y, Wu J, Jung SC, Park DB, Maeng YH, Hong JY, Kim SJ et al. Anti-neuroinflammatory activity of nobiletin on suppression of microglial activation. *Biol Pharm Bull.* 2010;33(11):1814–1821.

124. Pan M-H, Wei-Jen Chen W-J, Lin-Shiau S-Y, Ho C-T, Lin J-K. Tangeretin induces cell-cycle G1 arrest through inhibiting cyclin-dependent kinases 2 and 4 activities as well as elevating Cdk inhibitors p21 and p27 in human colorectal carcinoma cells. *Carcinogenesis.* 2002;23(10):1677–1684.

125. Chong SY, Wu MY, Lo YC. Tangeretin sensitizes SGS1-deficient cells by inducing DNA damage. *J Agric Food Chem.* 2013;61(26):6376–6382. doi: 10.1021/jf401831e. Epub 2013 June 25.

126. Hirano T, Abe K, Gotoh M, Oka K. Citrus flavone tangeretin inhibits leukaemic HL-60 cell growth partially through induction of apoptosis with less cytotoxicity on normal lymphocytes. *Br J Cancer.* 1995;72:1380–1388.

127. Zamora-Ros R, Knaze V, Luján-Barroso L, Slimani N, Romieu I, Fedirko V, Santucci de Magistris M et al. Estimated dietary intakes of flavonols, flavanones and flavones in the European prospective investigation into cancer and nutrition (EPIC) 24 hour dietary recall cohort. *Br J Nutr.* 2011;106(12):1915–1925.

128. Hwang SL, Shih PH, Yen GC. Neuroprotective effects of citrus flavonoids. *J Agric Food Chem.* 2012;60(4):877–885. Epub 2012 January 6.

129. US Department of Agriculture. Agricultural Research Service. Phytochemical Database. *Syzygium aromaticum.* http://www.pl.barc.usda.gov/usda_plant/plant_detail.cfm?code=6968556469685564&plant_id=475&ThisName=ps721. Accessed December 30, 2012.

130. Öztürk A, Özbek H. The anti-inflammatory activity of *Eugenia caryophylatta* essential oil: An animal model of anti-inflammatory activity. *Eur J Gen Med.* 2005;2(4):159–163.

131. National Institutes of Health National Center for Complementary and Alternative Medicine. Clove. http://www.nlm.nih.gov/medlineplus/druginfo/natural/251.html. Accessed February 8, 2011.

132. US Department of Agriculture. Agricultural Research Service. National Nutrient Database. Coconut, raw per 1/4 cup. http://ndb.nal.usda.gov/ndb/foods/show/3688?man=&lfacet=&count=&max=35&qlookup=coconut&offset=&sort=&format=Abridged&reportfmt=other&rptfrm=&ndbno=&nutrient1=&nutrient2=&nutrient3=&subset=&totCount=&measureby=&_action_show=Apply+Changes&Qv=1&Q6931=0.25&Q6932=1&Q6933=1. Accessed February 26, 2015.

133. Deb-Mandal M, Mandal S. Coconut (*Cocos nucifera* L.: Arecaceae): In health promotion and disease prevention. *Asian Pac J Trop Med.* 2011 Mar;4(3):241–7. doi: 10.1016/S1995-7645(11)60078-3. Epub 2011 April 12.

134. Lima EB, Sousa CN, Meneses LN, Ximenes NC, Santos Júnior MA, Vasconcelos GS, Lima NB, Patrocínio MC, Macedo D, Vasconcelos SM. *Cocos nucifera* (L.) (Arecaceae): A phytochemical and pharmacological review. *Braz J Med Biol Res.* 2015 August 18. pii: S0100-879X2015005054773. [Epub ahead of print]

135. Lawrence GD. Dietary fats and health: Dietary recommendations in the context of scientific evidence. *Adv Nutr.* 2013;4:294–302.

136. The American Heart Association. Tropical Oils. http://www.heart.org/HEARTORG/GettingHealthy/NutritionCenter/HealthyEating/Tropical-Oils_UCM_306031_Article.jsp. Accessed February 28, 2015.

137. Naskar S, Mazumder UK, Pramanik G, Saha P, Haldar PK, Gupta M. Evaluation of antinociceptive and anti-inflammatory activity of hydromethanol extract of *Cocos nucifera* L. *Inflammopharmacology.* 2013;21(1):31–35. doi: 10.1007/s10787-012-0135-7. Epub 2012 April 17.

138. Kizhakekuttu TJ, Widlansky ME. Natural antioxidants and hypertension: Promise and challenges. *Cardiovasc Ther.* 2010;28(4):e20–32. doi: 10.1111/j.1755-5922.2010.00137.x. Epub 2010 March 29.

139. Xie LX, Williams KJ, He CH, Weng E, Khong S, Rose TE, Kwon O, Bensinger SJ, Marbois BN, Clarke CF. Resveratrol and para-coumarate serve as ring precursors for coenzyme Q biosynthesis. *J Lipid Res.* 2015;56(4):909–919. Epub 2015 February 14.

140. Pravst I, Zmitek K, Zmitek J. Coenzyme Q10 contents in foods and fortification strategies. *Crit Rev Food Sci Nutr.* 2010;50(4):269–280. doi: 10.1080/10408390902773037.

141. Potgieter M, Pretorius E, Pepper MS. Primary and secondary coenzyme Q10 deficiency: The role of therapeutic supplementation. *Nutr Rev.* 2013;71(3): 180–188. doi: 10.1111/nure.12011. Epub 2013 January 30.

142. US National Library of Medicine. National Institutes of Health. Medline Plus. Coenzyme Q10. http://www.nlm.nih.gov/medlineplus/druginfo/natural/938.html. Accessed January 28, 2012.

143. Shekelle P, Hardy ML, Coulter I, Udani J, Spar M, Oda K, Jungvig LK et al. Effect of the supplemental use of antioxidants vitamin C, vitamin E, and coenzyme Q10 for the prevention and treatment of cancer. Evidence Report/Technology

Assessment Number 75. (Prepared by Southern California Evidence-based Practice Center under Contract No. 290-97-0001.) AHRQ Publication No. 04-E003. Rockville, MD: Agency for Healthcare Research and Quality. August 2003.

144. Academy of Nutrition and Dietetics Evidence Analysis Library. What is the relationship between supplemental coenzyme Q10 and cardiovascular disease? http://andevidencelibrary.com/default.cfm?library = EBG&home = 1. Accessed July 16, 2013.

145. US Department of Agriculture. Agricultural Research Service. Phytonutrient Database. Coffee. http://www.pl.barc.usda.gov/usda_plant/plant_detail .cfm?code=69685564&plant_id=387&ThisName=ps721. Accessed May 1, 2013.

146. Lecour S, Lamont KT. Natural polyphenols and cardioprotection. *Mini Rev Med Chem.* 2011;11(14):1191–1199. Epub 2011 October 28.

147. Lin WY, Pi-Sunyer FX, Chen CC, Davidson LE, Liu CS, Li TC, Wu MF, Li CI, Chen W, Lin CC. Coffee consumption is inversely associated with type 2 diabetes in Chinese. *Eur J Clin Invest.* 2011;41(6):659–666. doi: 10.1111/j.1365-2362.2010.02455.x. Epub 2011 January 12.

148. Machado LM, da Costa TH, da Silva EF, Dórea JG. Association of moderate coffee intake with self-reported diabetes among urban Brazilians. *Int J Environ Res Public Health.* 2011;8(8):3216–3231. Epub 2011 August 3.

149. Shaffer EA. Gallstone disease: Epidemiology of gallbladder stone disease. *Best Pract Res Clin Gastroenterol.* 2006;20(6):981–996.

150. Hoelzl C, Knasmüller S, Wagner KH, Elbling L, Huber W, Kager N, Ferk F et al. Instant coffee with high chlorogenic acid levels protects humans against oxidative damage of macromolecules. *Mol Nutr Food Res.* 2010;54(12):1722–1733.

151. Mills CE, Tzounis X, Oruna-Concha MJ, Mottram DS, Gibson GR, Spencer JP. *In vitro* colonic metabolism of coffee and chlorogenic acid results in selective changes in human faecal microbiota growth. *Br J Nutr.* 2015;113(8): 1220–1227. Epub 2015 March 26.

152. Kim HJ, Kim MK, Kim JU, Ha HY, Choi BY. Major determinants of serum homocysteine concentrations in a Korean population. *J Korean Med Sci.* 2010;25(4):509–516. Epub 2010 March 19.

153. National Institutes of Health. Determinants of Copper Needs Across the Life Span. https://ods.od.nih.gov/News/Copper.aspx. Accessed August 23, 2015.

154. Walker, A-M. Corn, Is it a fruit, vegetable or grain? http://ucanr.edu/sites/ MarinMG/files/141899.pdf. Accessed March 19, 2015.

155. US Department of Agriculture. Agricultural Research Service. Phytochemical database. Xeaxanthin. http://www.pl.barc.usda.gov/usda_chem/ achem_detail.cfm?code=28969643&chemical_id=1258&ThisName=sd1. Accessed January 29, 2011.

156. Lee CH, Garcia HS, Parkin KL. Bioactivities of kernel extracts of 18 strains of maize (*Zea mays*). *J Food Sci.* 2010;75(8):C667–672. doi: 10.1111/j.1750-3841.2010.01784.x. Epub 2010 September 20.

157. Clifford MN. Chlorogenic acids and other cinnamates—Nature, occurrence and dietary burden. *J Sci Food Agric.* 1999;79(3):362–372.

158. Pai TV, Sawant SY, Ghatak AA, Chaturvedi PA, Gupte AM, Desai NS. Characterization of Indian beers: Chemical composition and antioxidant potential. *J Food Sci Technol.* 2015;52(3):1414–1423.

159. Dejan Stojković D, Petrović J, Soković M, Glamočlija J, Kukić-Marković J, Petrović S. *In situ* antioxidant and antimicrobial activities of naturally occurring caffeic acid, *p*-coumaric acid and rutin, using food systems. *J Sci Food Agric.* 2013;93(13):3205–3208.

160. Zang LY, Cosma G, Gardner H, Shi X, Castranova V, Vallyathan V. Effect of antioxidant protection by *p*-coumaric acid on low-density lipoprotein cholesterol oxidation. *Am J Physiol Cell Physiol.* 2000;279(4):C954–960.

161. Shaheen UY. *p*-Coumaric acid ester with potential antioxidant activity from the genus *Salvia. Free Radicals Antioxid.* 2011;1(1):23–27.

162. US Department of Agriculture. Agricultural Research Service. Phytochemical Database. Coumarin. http://www.pl.barc.usda.gov/usda_chem/achem_query_result.cfm?code=69685564&ThisName=chem. Accessed December 6, 2011.

163. Miyake Y, Murakami A, Sugiyama Y, Isobe M, Koshimizu K, Ohigashi H. Identification of coumarins from lemon fruit (*Citrus limon*) as inhibitors of *in vitro* tumor promotion and superoxide and nitric oxide generation. *J Agric Food Chem.* 1999;47(8):3151–3317.

164. Abraham K, Wöhrlin F, Lindtner O, Heinemeyer G, Lampen A. Toxicology and risk assessment of coumarin: Focus on human data. *Mol Nutr Food Res.* 2010;54(2):228–239. doi: 10.1002/mnfr.200900281.

165. US Department of Agriculture. Agricultural Research Service. Nutrient Data Lab. Cranberry sauce. http://www.nal.usda.gov/fnic/foodcomp/cgi-bin/list_nut_edit.pl. Accessed November 24, 2011.

166. Society of Obstetricians and Gynaecologists of Canada. SOGC clinical practice guidelines. The detection and management of vaginal atrophy. Number 145, May 2004. *Int J Gynaecol Obstet.* 2005;88(2):222–228.

167. National Institutes of Health. National Center for Complementary and Alternative Medicine. Herbs at a Glance Cranberry. http://nccam.nih.gov/health/cranberry/ataglance.htm. Accessed June 1, 2011.

168. Jepson RG, Williams G, Craig JC. Cranberries for preventing urinary tract infections. *Cochrane Database Syst Rev.* 2012;10:CD001321. doi: 10.1002/14651858.CD001321.pub5.

169. US Department of Agriculture. Agricultural Research Service. Phytonutrient database. Betacryptoxanthin. http://www.pl.barc.usda.gov/usda_chem/achem_detail.cfm?code=69685564&chemical_id=1257&ThisName=sd1Cryptoxanthin. Accessed June 25, 2011.

170. Kohnoa H, Taimaa M, Sumidaa T, Azumac Y, Ogawad H, Tanakaa T. Inhibitory effect of mandarin juice rich in β-cryptoxanthin and hesperidin on 4-(methylnitrosamino)-1-(3-pyridyl)-1-butanone-induced pulmonary tumorigenesis in mice. *Cancer Lett.* 2001;174(2):141–150. doi:10.1016/S0304-3835(01)00713-3.

171. Wingerath T, Stahl W, Sies H. β-Cryptoxanthin selectively increases in human chylomicrons upon ingestion of tangerine concentrate rich in β-cryptoxanthin esters. *Arch Biochem Biophys.* 1995;342(2):385–390. doi:10.1006/abbi.1995.0052.

172. Haegele AD, Gillette C, O'Neill C, Wolfe P, Heimendinger J, Sedlacek S, Thompson HJ. Plasma xanthophyll carotenoids correlate inversely with indices of oxidative DNA damage and lipid peroxidation. *Cancer Epidemiol Biomarkers Prev.* 2000;9:421–425.

173. Katti K, Chanda N, Shukla R, Zambre A, Subramanian T, Kulkarni RR, Kannan R, Katti KV. Green nanotechnology from cumin phytochemicals: Generation of biocompatible gold nanoparticles. *Int J Green Nanotechnol Biomed.* 2009;1(1):B39–B52.

174. Kalaivani P, Saranya RB, Ramakrishnan G, Ranju V, Sathiya S, Gayathri V, Thiyagarajan LK, Venkhatesh JR, Babu CS, Thanikachalam S. *Cuminum cyminum,* a dietary spice, attenuates hypertension via endothelial nitric oxide synthase and NO pathway in renovascular hypertensive rats. *Clin Exp Hypertens.* 2013;35(7):534–542. Epub 2013 February 12.

175. Roman-Ramos R, Flores-Saenz JL, Alarcon-Aguilar FJ. Anti-hyperglycemic effect of some edible plants. *J Ethnopharmacol.* 1995;48(1):25–32.

D

Dairy foods group

definition

Foods produced from milk are good sources of protein, riboflavin, vitamin B12, calcium, magnesium, potassium, and when fortified, vitamins A and D.[1] One serving of dairy food supplies approximately 300 mg of calcium and includes 1 cup of vitamin-D-fortified milk/rice milk/almond milk/soy milk; 1.5 oz of hard, natural cheese such as cheddar, or 2 oz of processed cheese such as American Cheese; 8 oz of yogurt or frozen yogurt; or 2 cups of cottage cheese. Only vitamin-D-fortified milk and other dairy products expressly labeled "fortified with vitamin D" are sources of vitamin D.

scientific findings

Meeting the recommended servings of dairy products is necessary to maintain adequate bone mineral density and is especially important for bone mineralization during childhood and adolescence. Adequate intake of reduced- and non-fat dairy products is associated with a reduced risk of cardiovascular disease and type 2 diabetes.[2]

bioactive dose

Three servings of dairy foods are recommended daily for people aged 19–50. This amount meets the calcium RDA, but not the vitamin D RDA.

safety

Presumed safe when consumed in normal dietary quantities by non-allergic individuals.

Dandelion (Taraxacum officinale)

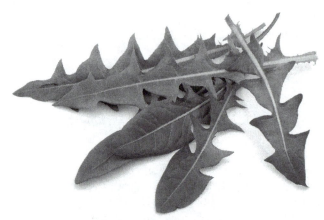

Dandelion. (Image from Volosina/Shutterstock.)

definition

Bitter dark green leaf named for its toothed leaf margins (*dent de leon* means "lion's tooth"). A good source of calcium and an excellent source of vitamins C and K.[3] It also supplies numerous phytochemicals including taraxasterol.[4] The root is a source of triterpenes, steroids, and inulin.[5] Regarded by some to be a garden weed, it is more commonly eaten as a salad green in Europe than in the United States. In traditional medicine, dandelion has been used as a diuretic and, in Chinese, Arabian, and Native American traditional medicine, to treat cancer.[6,7]

scientific findings

In a small, non–placebo-controlled, nonrandomized pilot study (n = 17), urinary volume and fluid intake were recorded to establish baseline values for urinary frequency and urinary excretion ratio (urination volume:fluid intake) at intervals. Subjects were dosed with 8 mL of dandelion extract three times a day for 1 day. The study found "a significant increase in the frequency of urination in the 5-h period after the first dose. For all subjects, there was also a significant increase in the excretion ratio in the 5-h period after the second dose of extract. The third dose failed to change any of the measured parameters," although the study concluded that "*T. officinale* ethanolic extract shows promise as a diuretic in humans."[6] In laboratory studies, dandelion extracts exhibited anticarcinogenic and hepatoprotective properties.[4,7–9] In animal studies, taraxasterol was chemopreventative.[4]

bioactive dose

Not known.

safety

Presumed safe when consumed in normal dietary quantities by non-allergic adults. No negative effects have been reported of consuming dandelion during pregnancy or lactation, in children, or in combination with pharmaceutical drugs; however, dandelion impaired the absorption of ciprofloxacin.[5]

Date (Phoenix dactylifera)

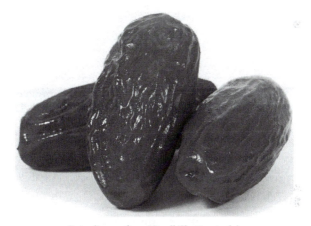

Date. (Image from Ninell/Shutterstock.)

definition

Small, intensely sweet cylindrical fruit covered by a leathery, fibrous skin that is brown when ripe. A 1/4-cup of medjool dates, a common type eaten as a snack and used for baking, supplies approximately 105 cal, 27 g of carbohydrate (23 g of sugar and 3 g of fiber), and 7% DV of potassium.[10] Dates have the highest total polyphenol content among commonly eaten fruits and vegetables.[11]

scientific findings

Dates exhibited antioxidant activity in laboratory research.[12,13]

bioactive dose

Not known.

safety

Presumed safe when consumed in normal dietary amounts by nonallergic individuals.

Dihydrocapsiate

definition

A major capsaicinoid, the other being capsaicin, found in *Capsicum frutescens* (chili pepper).

scientific findings

Dihydrocapsiate nominally increased thermogenesis in two clinical trials. In a double-blind, parallel-arm trial (n = 78), healthy subjects were randomly assigned to receive either 0 (placebo), or 3 or 9 mg dihydrocapsiate/day for 28 days. After a 10-h overnight fast, resting metabolic rate was measured by indirect calorimetry for 30 min before and 120 min after ingestion of dihydrocapsiate. Dihydrocapsiate had a small, thermogenic effect of ≈50 kcal/day, which was significant compared to placebo, but that is within the range of day-to-day resting metabolic rate variability.[14] In a second study, outpatients (n = 33) following a very low calorie diet (800 kcal/day providing 120 g/day protein) over 4 weeks were randomly assigned to receive either dihydrocapsiate capsules three times per day (3 mg or 9 mg) or placebo. In the treatment group, postprandial increases in thermogenesis and fat oxidation secondary to administration of dihydrocapsiate occurred.[15] In an experimental study, dihydrocapsiate was chemopreventive in tumor cells.[16]

bioactive dose

Not known.

safety

Presumed safe when consumed in normal dietary quantities by nonallergic individuals.

Dill (Anethum graveolens)

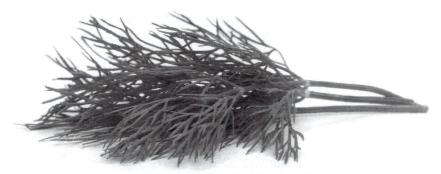

Dill. (Image fron photolinc/Shutterstock.)

definition

Aromatic herb with very fine, fern-like, feathery leaves whose distinctive taste is used to flavor pickles; also used to garnish foods such as potato salad, Greek yogurt, and borscht. Dill contains numerous phytochemicals including quercetin and limonene.[17] Dill has been used to increase menstrual flow.[18]

scientific findings

Laboratory studies have shown essential oil of dill to have antibiotic and antifungal properties.[19,20] There is insufficient reliable information available about the effectiveness of dill for any physiological use.[18]

bioactive dose

Not known.

safety

Presumed safe when consumed in normal dietary amounts by nonallergic individuals. The essential oil of dill herb and seed was shown to be genotoxic in a laboratory study.[21]

Docosahexaenoic acid (DHA)

definition

An omega-3 polyunsaturated fatty acid that is synthesized in limited amounts by the body through the conversion of α-linolenic acid to eicosapentaenoic acid (EPA) and then to docosahexaenoic acid (DHA). DHA is abundant in the brain and retina. Fatty fish, including kippers, mackerel, trout, salmon, sardines, anchovies, herrings, and tuna are good sources of naturally occurring DHA. Human milk is a source of DHA.[1]

scientific findings

DHA is essential for normal growth and neurological function.[22] DHA deficiency has been linked to a decline in cognitive ability, and low DHA levels are associated with an increase in neural cell death.[23] It is also absent in the cerebral cortex of individuals with extreme depression.[24] Increased dietary consumption of DHA is associated with a decreased risk of age-related macular degeneration.[18] Increased dietary consumption of DHA may reduce the risk of death in patients with coronary artery disease.[18]

bioactive dose

The current mean intake for DHA and EPA in the United States is approximately 100 mg/day, an amount that is suboptimal according to experts.[25] An RDA has not been established for DHA, but an AI has been set for its precursor, linolenic acid (also called omega-3-fatty acid). See also omega-3-fatty acid. Prenatal ingestion of at least 200 mg of DHA daily has been suggested as adequate for normal fetal growth and development.[18,26]

safety

Presumed safe when consumed in normal dietary quantities by non-allergic individuals. Doses greater than 3 g daily might decrease platelet aggregation and increase the risk of bleeding.[18]

References

1. Whitney ER, Rolfes SR. *Understanding Nutrition*, 12th edn. Belmont CA: Wadsworth Cengage; 2011.
2. US Department of Agriculture. Choose My Plate.gov. http://www.choosemyplate.gov/food-groups/dairy-why.html. Accessed June 9, 2013.
3. US Department of Agriculture. Agricultural Research Service. Nutrient Data Laboratory. Dandelion greens, raw. http://ndb.nal.usda.gov/ndb/foods/show/2946?fg=&man=&lfacet=&format=&count=&max=25&offset=&sort=&qlookup=dandelion. Accessed June 9, 2013.
4. Chatterjee SJ, Ovadje P, Mousa M, Hamm C, Pandey S. The efficacy of dandelion root extract in inducing apoptosis in drug-resistant human melanoma cells. *Evid Based Complementary Altern Med.* 2011;2011:129045. doi: 10.1155/2011/129045. Epub 2010 December 30.

5. Yarnell E, Abascal K. Dandelion (*Taraxacum officinale* and *T. mongolicum*). *Integr Med Clin J*. 2009;8(2):34–38.

6. Clare BA, Conroy RS, Spelman K. The diuretic effect in human subjects of an extract of *Taraxacum officinale* folium over a single day. *J Altern Complementary Med*. 2009;15(8):929–934. doi:10.1089/acm.2008.0152.

7. Sigstedt SC, Hooten CJ, Callewaert MC, Jenkins AR, Romero AE, Pullin MJ, Kornienko A et al. Evaluation of aqueous extracts of *Taraxacum officinale* on growth and invasion of breast and prostate cancer cells. *Int J Oncol*. 2008;32:1085–1090.

8. You Y, Soonam Y, Ho-Geun Y, Jeongjin P, Yoo-Hyun L, Sunoh K, Kyung-Taek O et al. *In vitro* and *in vivo* hepatoprotective effects of the aqueous extract from *Taraxacum officinale* (dandelion) root against alcohol-induced oxidative stress. *Food Chem Toxicol*. 2010;48(6):1632–1637.

9. Park J-Y, Kim J-J, Park C-M, Noh K-H, Song Y-S. Hepatoprotective activity of *Taraxacum officinale* water extract against D-galactosamine-induced hepatitis in rats. *FASEB J* [serial online]. 2007;21(6):A1088.

10. US Department of Agriculture. National Nutrient Database. Medjool dates. http://ndb.nal.usda.gov/ndb/foods/show/2468?fgcd=&manu=&lfacet=&format=&count=&max=35&offset=&sort=&qlookup=medjool+dates. Accessed March 1, 2015.

11. Fruit and Veggies More Matters. Dates. http://www.fruitsandveggiesmorematters.org/dates. Accessed March 27, 2015.

12. Abdelhak M, Embarek G, Kokkalou E, Kefalas P. Phenolic profile and antioxidant activity of the Algerian ripe date palm fruit (*Phoenix dactylifera*). *Food Chem*. 2005;89(3):411–420.

13. Biglari F, AlKarkhi AFM, Mat Easa A. Antioxidant activity and phenolic content of various date palm (*Phoenix dactylifera*) fruits from Iran. *Food Chem*. 2008;107(4):1636–1641.

14. Galgani JE, Ravussin E. Effect of dihydrocapsiate on resting metabolic rate in humans. *J Clin Nutr*. 2010;92(5):1089–1093. Epub 2010 September 8.

15. Lee TA, Li Z, Zerlin A, Heber D. Effects of dihydrocapsiate on adaptive and diet-induced thermogenesis with a high protein very low calorie diet: A randomized control trial. *Nutr Metab (London)*. 2010;7:78.

16. Macho A, Lucena C, Sancho R, Daddario N, Minassi A, Muñoz E, Appendino G. Non-pungent capsaicinoids from sweet pepper synthesis and evaluation of the chemopreventive and anticancer potential. *Eur J Nutr*. 2003;42(1):2–9.

17. US Department of Agriculture. Agricultural Research Service. Medicinal Foods Database. *Anethum graveolens*. http://www.pl.barc.usda.gov/usda_rrcp/rrecipe_detail.cfm?code=31410620&id=144&ThisName=sd1. Accessed December 23, 2011.

18. Jellin JM, Gregory PJ. Natural Medicine Comprehensive Database. Therapeutic Research Faculty. 2013. http://www.naturaldatabase.com. Accessed July 11, 2012.

19. Zeng H, Tian J, Zheng Y, Ban X, Zeng J, Mao Y, Wang Y. *In vitro* and *in vivo* activities of essential oil from the seed of *anethum graveolens* L. against *Candida* spp. 2011;2011:659704. doi: 10.1155/2011/659704. Epub 2011 May 11.

20. Kaur GJ, Arora DS. Antibacterial and phytochemical screening of *Anethum graveolens*, *Foeniculum vulgare* and *Trachyspermum ammi*. *BMC Complementary Altern Med*. 2009;9:30. doi:10.1186/1472-6882-9-30.

D

21. Lazutka JR, Mierauskien J, Slapšyt G, Dedonyt V. Genotoxicity of dill (*Anethum graveolens* L.), peppermint (*Mentha × piperita* L.) and pine (*Pinus sylvestris* L.) essential oils in human lymphocytes and *Drosophila melanogaster*. *Food Chem Toxicol*. 2001;39(5):485–492. doi:10.1016/S0278-6915(00)00157-5.

22. Huffman SL, Harika RK, Eilander A, Osendarp SJ. Essential fats: How do they affect growth and development of infants and young children in developing countries? A literature review. *Matern Child Nutr*. 2011;7(Suppl 3):44–65.

23. Lukiw WJ, Cui JG, Marcheselli VL, Bodker M, Botkjaer A, Gotlinger K, Serhan CN, Bazan NG. A role for docosahexaenoic acid-derived neuroprotectin D1 in neural cell survival and Alzheimer disease. *J Clin Invest*. 2005; 115(10):2774–2783.

24. McNamara RK, Hahn CG, Jandacek R, Rider T, Tso P, Stanford KE, Richtand NM. Selective deficits in the omega-3 fatty acid docosahexaenoic acid in the postmortem orbitofrontal cortex of patients with major depressive disorder. *Biol Psychiatry*. 2007;62(1):17–24.

25. Kris-Etherton PM, Grieger JA, Etherton TD. Dietary reference intakes for DHA and EPA. *Prostaglandins Leukotrienes Essent Fatty Acids*. 2009; 81(2–3):99–104.

26. Jia X, Pakseresht M, Wattar N, Wildgrube J, Sontag S, Andrews M, Subhan FB, McCargar L, Field CJ, APrON Study Team. Women who take n-3 long-chain polyunsaturated fatty acid supplements during pregnancy and lactation meet the recommended intake. *Appl Physiol Nutr Metab*. 2015;40(5):1–4.

D

E

Egg

definition

Low-fat, high-protein food and source of vitamins A, D, E, and choline, as well as phytochemicals lutein and xeaxanthin.[1] A large egg supplies approximately 215–250 mg of cholesterol.[2] The American Heart
Association (AHA) recommends a limit of 300 mg of cholesterol per day
for people whose LDL (low-density lipoprotein) cholesterol level is normal (and a limit of 200 mg of cholesterol per day for people who have
high LDL cholesterol or heart disease),[3] and according to AHA, eggs can
be part of one's recommended level of dietary cholesterol intake. Eggs
enriched with omega-3-fatty-acid supply 115 mg of omega-3-fatty acid per
large egg depending on the commercial brand.[4] Eggs are a versatile food
that can be prepared in a variety of ways and are used as an emulsifying
ingredient in baked products and salad dressings.

scientific findings

According to reviews examining the evidence of egg consumption and
plasma cholesterol, extensive research and epidemiologic literature has
not clearly established a link between egg consumption and risk for coronary heart disease.[5,6]

bioactive dose

Not applicable.

safety

Presumed safe when consumed in normal dietary quantities by non-
allergic individuals. USDA (United States Department of Agriculture) recommends children younger than 1-year old not be given egg whites due
to the potential for allergic reaction.[7] Raw egg consumption is not recommended due to potential *Salmonella* contamination.

Eggplant (Solanum melongena)

definition

White, spongy-fleshed vegetable with purple, shiny skin that is cooked and used to make dishes such as eggplant parmesan (Italian cooking), baba ghanoush (Middle Eastern cooking), ratatouille (French cooking), and stir-fried eggplant (Asian cooking). Eggplant is a good source of fiber[8] and contains anthocyanins, phenolics, saponins, terpenoids, and steroidal alkaloids.[9]

scientific findings

Dried powdered fruits of eggplant provided as capsules containing 450 mg of *Solanum melongena* (SM) or placebo (450 mg) twice daily reduced serum lipids in a small (n = 41 subjects with hyperlipidemia), randomized, placebo-controlled clinical trial.[10] After 3 months, serum total cholesterol, LDL, and LDL/HDL decreased in the eggplant-treated group.[10] To compare eggplant to lovastatin, a small, placebo-controlled study (n = 21 individuals with total cholesterol >200 mg/dL) divided participants into three groups each having similar baseline cholesterol levels: (1) a group that consumed eggplant extract; (2) a group that received 20 mg of lovastatin; and (3) a control group. After 6 weeks, a significant reduction in total cholesterol levels and in LDL-cholesterol levels was seen in the statin-treated group, but not in the eggplant-treated group.[11]

bioactive dose

Not applicable.

safety

Presumed safe when consumed in normal dietary quantities by non-allergic individuals.

Eicosapentaenoic acid

definition

One of the two predominant omega-3 fatty acids, the other being DHA. Eicosapentaenoic acid (EPA) and docosahexaenoic acid (DHA) are synthesized in limited amounts in the body from linolenic acid.[12] EPA is found in the eyes and the brain and is necessary for growth and cognition.[12] Good sources of EPA include mullet, which provides 150 mg of EPA per three ounces,[13] and other fatty fish, including mackerel, salmon, bluefish, sable-fish, menhaden, anchovy, sardines, herring, tuna, and lake trout. Human milk is also a source of EPA.

scientific findings

Current mean intake for DHA and EPA in the United States is approximately 100 mg/day, an amount that is suboptimal according to experts.[14] EFAs may be altered in obesity, hypertension, diabetes mellitus, coronary heart disease, alcoholism, schizophrenia, Alzheimer's disease, atherosclerosis, and cancer.[15] Whether the EFA alteration is a cause of or an effect of these conditions was not elucidated.[15]

bioactive dose

Although there is no specific RDA (recommended dietary allowance) for EPA, an RDA has been established for its precursor, linolenic acid. The adult RDA for linolenic acid is 1.1 g.

safety

Presumed safe when consumed in normal dietary quantities by non-allergic individuals.

Ellagic acid

definition

Polyphenolic antioxidant found in a wide variety of fruits including black-berries and strawberries.

scientific findings

In laboratory studies, ellagic acid reduced oxidative stress.[16,17]

bioactive dose

Not known.

safety

Presumed safe when consumed as part of a food and consumed in normal dietary quantities in foods by nonallergic individuals.

Endive (Cichorium intybus)

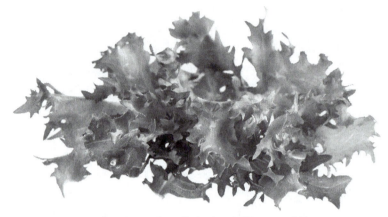

Endive. (Image from Slavko Sereda/Shutterstock.)

definition

Hardy, curled lettuce common in Mediterranean cooking. It can be eaten blanched, used in salads, and as a garnish.[18] One-half cup of endive provides 35 μg of folate (8% DV [daily value]), 540 IU of vitamin A (10% DV), and 55 μg of vitamin K (70% DV), and is a source of kaempferol. A red cultivar of endive (*Cichorium intybus* L. cultivar) is a source of antioxidant anthocyanins.[19]

scientific findings

In laboratory studies, *C. intybus* inhibited free radical-mediated DNA damage,[20] and exerted cytoprotective and antiproliferative effects in cells.[19]

bioactive dose

Not known.

safety

Presumed safe when consumed as part of a food and consumed in normal dietary quantities by nonallergic individuals.

Endive, Belgian (Cichorium endivia)

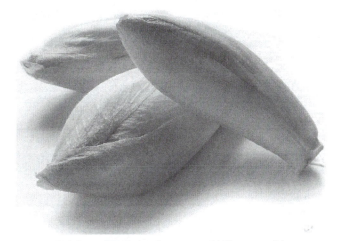

Belgian endive (Image from marmo81/Shutterstock.)

definition

Pale yellow-green, mild-tasting lettuce that grows in small, tight, cylindrical heads, differentiating it from curly endive, which has a bitter flavor and loose, lacy appearance. It may be eaten as a salad vegetable or steamed and consumed. Belgian endive is a source of potassium, vitamin C, and phytochemicals such as phenolics.[21,22] *Cichorium endivia* has been used in folk medicine for its anti-inflammatory properties.[23]

scientific findings

An amino acid in *C. endivia* was shown to be cytotoxic to colorectal cancer cells in a laboratory study.[23]

bioactive dose

Not known.

safety

Presumed safe when consumed in normal dietary quantities by non-allergic individuals.

Ethanol

definition

Also called ethyl alcohol and alcohol, a molecule formed during anaerobic fermentation of carbohydrate, such as sugars in berries or grains. It is a psychoactive compound and central nervous system depressant.[24] Alcohol from beer, wine, and distilled liquor supplies 7 kcal/g. Alcoholic beverages are a major calorie source that should be reduced for many U.S. adults.

scientific findings

Alcohol consumption can have beneficial or harmful effects, depending on the amount consumed, age, and other characteristics of the person consuming the alcohol.[25] Alcohol consumption may have beneficial effects when consumed in moderation.[25] Strong evidence from observational studies has shown that moderate alcohol consumption is associated with a lower risk of cardiovascular disease.[25] Moderate alcohol consumption is also associated with reduced risk of all-cause mortality among middle-aged and older adults and may help to keep cognitive function intact with age.[25] Beginning to drink alcohol or drinking more frequently on the basis of potential health benefits is not recommended, because even moderate alcohol intake is associated with certain health risks such as increased risk of breast cancer, involvement in violence, drowning, and injuries from falls and motor vehicle accidents.[25] Light-to-moderate alcohol intake is associated with reduced incidence of ischemic cardiovascular events, whereas heavy alcohol intake can predispose individuals to stroke.[26] Heavier than moderate consumption of alcohol over time is associated with weight gain.[25] Excess alcohol consumption increases blood pressure.[25] Alcohol aggravates many conditions, for example, it increases symptoms of gastrointestinal reflux disease. Ethanol increases oxidative stress.[27] Ethanol metabolism can produce free radicals and reduce the levels of glutathione, the major cellular protection against oxidative stress, and alcohol consumption has been identified as one of the top 10 risks contributing to the worldwide burden of disease.[27] The International Agency for Research on Cancer has classified ethanol as carcinogenic to humans.[28]

bioactive dose

If alcohol is consumed, it should be consumed in moderation. Moderate consumption of alcohol is defined as one drink per day for women, no more than two drinks per day for men. A drink has been defined as 12 fluid ounces of regular beer (5% alcohol), 5 fluid ounces of wine (12% alcohol), or 1.5 fluid ounces of 80 proof distilled spirits (40% alcohol), each of which contains about 0.6 fluid ounces of alcohol.[25]

safety

Presumed safe when consumed in normal dietary quantities by non-allergic individuals. Safety can vary by individual, gender, and other factors; therefore, following the Dietary Guidelines for Americans 2010 may be warranted for most people. Ethanol should not be consumed at all by certain individuals including pregnant women, people with a history of alcoholism, individuals taking certain medications, and people not of legal drinking age. More than 24 oz/day can cause significant adverse health effects.[29]

Eugenol

definition

Constituent of clove, nutmeg, cinnamon, basil, bay leaves, and other plant foods. It (and clove) has long been used topically for toothache pain.[30]

scientific findings

A review on eugenol states that eugenol has analgesic properties.[31] However, eugenol's effect on toothache has not been adequately clinically studied; therefore, there is insufficient evidence to support the use of topical eugenol to prevent toothache pain, according to FDA (Food and Drug Administration).[32] Experimental research in dental cells has shown eugenol to have anti-inflammatory properties in pulp cells but not in gingival cells.[33] In experimental research, eugenol demonstrated anticancer and anti-inflammatory activity in human cervical cancer cells[31] and had selective antiproliferative and antitumor properties on human cancer cells and their animal models.[34]

bioactive dose

Not known.

safety

Presumed safe when consumed in normal dietary quantities by non-allergic individuals. Eugenol is cytotoxic in large doses,[35] that is, in quantities greater than are normally eaten in the diet.

References

1. Hasler CM. The changing face of functional foods. *J Am Coll Nutr.* 2000;19(5 Suppl):499S–506S.
2. Institute of Medicine. *Dietary Reference Intakes for Energy, Carbohydrate, Fiber, Fat, Fatty Acids, Cholesterol, Protein and Amino Acids.* Washington, DC: National Academy Press; 2005.
3. The American Heart Association. Common Misconceptions about Cholesterol. http://www.heart.org/HEARTORG/Conditions/Cholesterol/PreventionTreatmentofHighCholesterol/Common-Misconceptions-about-Cholesterol_UCM_305638_Article.jsp. Accessed June 12, 2013.
4. Egglands Best Nutrition Information. http://www.egglandsbest.com/nutrition/nutrition-facts.aspx. Accessed December 20, 2011.
5. Fernandez ML. Effects of eggs on plasma lipoproteins in healthy populations. *Food Funct.* 2010;1(2):156–160. Epub 2010 October 19.
6. Kritchevsky SB. A review of scientific research and recommendations regarding eggs. *J Am Coll Nutr.* 2004;23(6):596S–600S.
7. Pennsylvania State University College of Agricultural Sciences Cooperative Extension Service. Upside Down Lunch. http://betterkidcare.psu.edu/BKCKitLunch/Lunches103.pdf. Accessed December 25, 2011.
8. US Department of Agriculture. Agricultural Research Service. Nutrient Data Laboratory. Eggplant, boiled. http://ndb.nal.usda.gov/ndb/foods/show/3383?fg=&man=&lfacet=&format=&count=&max=25&offset=&sort=&qlookup=eggplant. Accessed June 12, 2013.
9. US Department of Agriculture. Agricultural Research Service. Phytochemical Database. Eggplant. http://www.pl.barc.usda.gov/usda_rrcp/rrecipe_detail.cfm?code=69685564&id=98&ThisName=sd1. Accessed December 25, 2011.
10. Silva GE, Takahashi MH, Eik Filho W, Albino CC, Tasim GE, Serri Lde A, Assef AH, Cortez DA, Bazotte RB. Absence of hypolipidemic effect of *Solanum melongena* L. (eggplant) on hyperlipidemic patients. *Arq Bras Endocrinol Metabol.* 2004;48(3):368–373.
11. Praca JM, Thomaz A, Caramelli B. Eggplant (*Solanum melongena*) extract does not alter serum lipid levels. *Arq Bras Cardiol.* 2004;82(3):269–276. Epub 2004 April 5.
12. Whitney ER, Rolfes SR. *Understanding Nutrition*, 12th edn. Belmont, CA: Wadsworth Cengage; 2011.
13. US Department of Agriculture. Agricultural Research Service. Nutrient Data Laboratory. Mullet. http://www.nal.usda.gov/fnic/foodcomp/cgi-bin/list_nut_edit.pl. Accessed March 11, 2011.
14. Kris-Etherton PM, Grieger JA, Etherton TD. Dietary reference intakes for DHA and EPA. *Prostaglandins Leukotrienes Essent Fatty Acids.* 2009;81(2–3):99–104.
15. Das UN. Essential fatty acids—A review. *Curr Pharm Biotechnol.* 2006;7(6):467–482.
16. Kannan MM, Quine SD. Ellagic acid ameliorates isoproterenol induced oxidative stress: Evidence from electrocardiological, biochemical and histological study. *Eur J Pharmacol.* 2011;659(1):45–52. Epub 2011 March 5.

17. Uzar E, Alp H, Cevik MU, Fırat U, Evliyaoglu O, Tufek A, Altun Y. Ellagic acid attenuates oxidative stress on brain and sciatic nerve and improves histopathology of brain in streptozotocin-induced diabetic rats. *Neurol Sci.* 2012;33(3):567–574. Epub 2011 September 16.

18. University of Arkansas Cooperative Extension. Endive-Escarole. http://www.uaex.edu/publications/pdf/FSA-6068.pdf. Accessed March 13, 2015.

19. D'evoli L, Morroni F, Lombardi-Boccia G, Lucarini M, Hrelia P, Cantelli-Fort G, Tarozzi A. Red chicory (*Cichorium intybus* L. cultivar) as a potential source of antioxidant anthocyanins for intestinal health. *Oxid Med Cell Longevity.* 2013:704310. doi: 10.1155/2013/704310. Epub 2013 August 27.

20. Sultana S, Perwaiz S, Iqbal M, Athar M. Crude extracts of hepatoprotective plants, *Solanum nigrum* and *Cichorium intybus* inhibit free radical-mediated DNA damage. *J Ethnopharmacol.* 1995;45(3):189–192.

21. Koudela M, Petříková K. Nutritional composition and yield of endive cultivars *Cichorium endivia.* *Hort Sci.* 2007;34(1):6–10.

22. Innocenti M, Gallori S, Giaccherini C, Ieri F, Vincieri FF, Mulinacci N. Evaluation of the phenolic content in the aerial parts of different varieties of *Cichorium intybus* L. *J Agric Food Chem.* 2005;53(16):6497–6502.

23. Wang FX, Deng AJ, Li M, Wei JF, Qin HL, Wang AP. (3S)-1,2,3,4-Tetrahydro-β-carboline-3-carboxylic acid from *Cichorium endivia.* L induces apoptosis of human colorectal cancer HCT-8 cells. *Molecules.* 2012;18(1):418–429.

24. National Institutes of Health. Alcohol. *MedlinePlus Encyclopedia.* http://vsearch.nlm.nih.gov/vivisimo/cgi-bin/query-meta?v%3Aproject=medlineplus&query=alcohol. Accessed March 11, 2011.

25. US Department of Agriculture. US Department of Health and Human Services. *Dietary Guidelines for Americans,* 2010, 7th ed. Washington, DC: U.S. Government Printing Office, December 2010.

26. Dimmitt SB, Rakic V, Puddey IB, Baker R, Oostryck R, Adams MJ, Chesterman CN, Burke V, Beilin LJ. The effects of alcohol on coagulation and fibrinolytic factors: A controlled trial. *Blood Coagulation Fibrinolysis.* 1998;9(1):39–45.

27. Ehrlich D, Humpel C. Effects of ethanol on aggregation, serotonin release, and amyloid precursor protein processing in rat and human platelets. *Platelets.* 2014;25(1):16–22. Epub 2013 February 12.

28. Arranz S, Chiva-Blanch G, Valderas-Martínez P, Medina-Remón A, Lamuela-Raventós RM, Estruch R. Wine, beer, alcohol and polyphenols on cardiovascular disease and cancer. *Nutrients.* 2012;4(7):759–781.

29. Jellin JM, Gregory PJ. *Natural Medicine Comprehensive Database.* Therapeutic Research Faculty. 2013. http://www.naturaldatabase.com. Accessed July 11, 2012.

30. Der Marderosian A, Beutler J, eds. *The Review of Natural Products,* 5th edn. St. Louis, MO: Wolters Kluwer Health; 2008.

31. Hussain A, Brahmbhatt K, Priyani A, Ahmed M, Rizvi TA, Sharma C. Eugenol enhances the chemotherapeutic potential of gemcitabine and induces anti-carcinogenic and anti-inflammatory activity in human cervical cancer cells. *Cancer Biother Radiopharm.* 2011;26(5):519–27. Epub 2011 September 22.

32. US National Library of Medicine. National Institutes of Health. Clove. *MedlinePlus Encyclopedia.* http://www.nlm.nih.gov/medlineplus/druginfo/natural/251.html#Effectiveness. Accessed November 8, 2011.

33. Koh T, Murakami Y, Tanaka S, Machino M, Sakagami H. Re-evaluation of anti-inflammatory potential of eugenol in IL-1β-stimulated gingival fibroblast and pulp cells. *In Vivo*. 2013;27(2):269–273.

34. Zhang L, Lokeshwar BL. Medicinal properties of the Jamaican pepper plant pimenta dioica and allspice. *Curr Drug Targets*. 2012;13(14):1900–1906. Epub 2012 November 6.

35. Zhang P, Zhang E, Xiao M, Chen C, Xu W. Study of anti-inflammatory activities of α-D-glucosylated eugenol. *Arch Pharmacal Res*. 2013;36(1):109–115. doi: 10.1007/s12272-013-0003-z.

E

F

Fatty fish

definition

Characteristically strong-flavored fish owing to concentration of fish oils concentration in flesh, as opposed to white fish that has a relatively low fish oil concentration in flesh. Fatty fish are generally excellent sources of protein, vitamin D, and omega-3 fatty acids,[1] and supply coenzyme q10.[2] Bluefish, herring, salmon, trout (both wild and farmed), mackerel, sardines, and tuna are fatty fish. Canned sardines with edible bones are excellent sources of calcium: 3 oz supplies 325 mg of calcium.[3] Marination and use of various seasonings before broiling or grilling can mask the fishy flavor.

scientific findings

Fish oil constituents DHA, EPA, and vitamin D are anti-inflammatory.[4–6] A meta-analysis of 14 randomized, controlled trials (n = 682; placebo, n = 641) found omega-3 fatty acid consumption improved insulin sensitivity.[7] Fish oil reduces triglycerides by 20%–50%.[8]

bioactive dose

The American Heart Association recommends eating two 3.5-oz servings of (ideally fatty) fish per week.[9]

safety

Presumed safe when consumed in normal dietary quantities by nonallergic individuals. Shark, swordfish, tilefish, and king mackerel (*Scomberomorus cavalla*), not to be confused with North Atlantic mackerel (*Scomber scombrus*), are considered high-methyl-mercury fish and therefore should be avoided by pregnant and lactating women; and in addition, pregnant and lactating women may eat no more than 6 oz of (white) albacore tuna per week.[10] According to a review: "The vast majority of epidemiological studies have proven that the benefits of fish intake exceed the potential risks [of … contaminated fish] with the exception of a few selected species in sensitive populations."[11]

Fennel (Foeniculum vulgare)

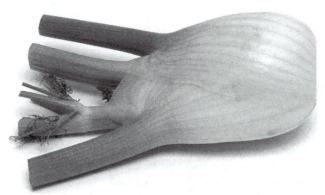

Fennel. (Image from Diana Taliun/Shutterstock.)

definition

Herb with a licorice-like flavor that contains the phenolic compound ane-thole.[12] Fennel leaves are used to season pork roasts, fennel seeds are used to flavor spicy sausages, and fennel stalks are used in preparing soups or mixed dishes.

scientific findings

Fennel experimentally improved hypertension[13] and glaucoma[14] in ani-mal models. Limited clinical trial data suggest fennel extracts may have the potential to treat infantile colic.[15]

bioactive dose

Not known.

safety

Presumed safe when consumed in normal dietary quantities by non-allergic individuals.

Fenugreek (Trigonella foenum-graecum)

definition

Plant whose leaves are used as an herb and seeds as a spice. Its seeds are also used to make flour. Fenugreek is a common flavor in Middle Eastern foods. It is commonly used to fortify the maple flavor in imitation maple syrup. Flour supplemented with fenugreek fiber has been used in the production of baked goods such as bread, pizza, muffins, and cakes. The first recorded use of fenugreek is described on an ancient Egyptian papyrus dated 1500BC.[16] Folkloric knowledge describes uses of fenugreek to induce childbirth and promote lactation.[17]

scientific findings

Fenugreek reduced serum glucose in diabetes in a few small clinical trials and animal studies.[16,18] The gum within the fenugreek seed fiber contains galactose and mannose, which are associated with reducing serum glucose and cholesterol.[18] There is not enough evidence to support its use as a galactogogue (to promote breast milk production in lactating women) or a pregnancy inducer.[19] Fenugreek fiber significantly increased satiety in a small, single-blind, randomized trial of healthy obese patients.[20]

bioactive dose

Not known. Trials in which fenugreek was employed to reduce glucose have used varying doses and delivery forms; for example, 1 g of fenugreek extract[21] or 100 g of fenugreek seed powder.[22] For hyperlipidemia, 0.6–2.5 g of fenugreek two times daily with meals has been used.[23]

safety

Presumed safe when consumed in normal dietary quantities by non-allergic individuals. Possible side effects of fenugreek when taken by mouth include gas, bloating, and diarrhea.[21] Since fenugreek has uterine stimulant activity, intake of amounts greater than those found in food should be avoided during pregnancy.[23] Since fenugreek has not been adequately studied during lactation for potential harmful effects to the infant or mother, it should be avoided during lactation.[23]

Ferulic acid

definition

Phytochemical found in seeds and leaves made from the metabolism of phenylalanine and tyrosine.[24] Found in high levels in vegetables, fruits, cereals, and coffee with the average intake estimated to be 150–250 mg/day.[25]

scientific findings

In laboratory studies, ferulic acid exhibited antioxidant, antimicrobial, anti-inflammatory, antithrombotic, anticancer, and increased sperm viability effects.[26,27]

bioactive dose

Not known.

F

safety

Presumed safe when consumed in normal dietary quantities by non-allergic individuals. Ferulic acid has a low toxicity potential.[27]

Fiber

definition

Nondigestible, structural material in plant foods that is generally categorized into soluble and insoluble types, each varying in water solubility, fermentability, and viscosity, characteristics responsible for distinct physiological effects and unique food characteristics. Soluble and insoluble fibers often occur together in foods. Particularly rich sources of soluble fiber include citrus fruits, apple pulp, apple pectin, infant banana flakes, green bananas, legumes, oat bran, oatmeal, barley, beans, okra, peas, rice bran, and strawberries.[28–30] Soluble fibers (also called viscous fibers), such as guar gum, pectin, psyllium, and certain hemicelluloses, retain water and form gels within the GI tract, thereby delaying gastric emptying and slowing the transit of food through the upper GI tract, slowing the absorption of nutrients from the small intestine, and entrapping bile salts and cholesterol in the large intestine; in addition, soluble fiber holds moisture in stools, softening them.[31] Rich sources of insoluble fibers include whole-wheat breads, wheat cereals, wheat bran, rye, brown rice, barley, most other grains, cabbage, beets, carrots, brussels sprouts, turnips, cauliflower, and apple skin.[30] Insoluble fibers, such as hemicellulose and cellulose, serve as bulk that increases fecal weight and promotes stool passage through the colon.[31] The food group that is highest in fiber as a group is legumes (8 g per 1/2 cup serving) followed by vegetables (3 g per 1/2 cup), nuts and seeds (3 g per 1 oz), fruits (2 g per 1/2 cup), and whole-grain products (1–2 g per 1 slice or 1/2 cup). The usual dietary fiber intake in the United States is 15 g/day[32] and should be increased by expanding variety in daily food patterns to include more and different types of plant foods.

scientific findings

Foods high in dietary fiber are generally low in calories. Dietary fiber intake from whole foods may lower blood pressure, improve serum lipids, and reduce indicators of inflammation.[33] Insoluble fibers help to prevent and alleviate constipation; reduce the risk of diverticulosis, hemorrhoids, and appendicitis; and promote satiety, which may aid in weight management.[31] Soluble fibers help to alleviate diarrhea; reduce fasting plasma cholesterol which is associated with reduced risk of heart disease; and reduce postprandial glycemia, which is associated with reduced risk of diabetes.[31,34] Soluble fibers may help to modestly reduce LDL cholesterol levels beyond that achieved by a diet low in cholesterol, saturated fat, and transfats alone.[30]

bioactive dose

The Dietary Reference Intakes recommend 14 g dietary fiber per 1000 kcal; the AI for adults aged 19–50 is 25 g/day for women and 38 g/day for men.[35] Due to the bulky nature of fibers, excess consumption is likely to be self-limiting.[35]

safety

There is no UL for fiber. Increasing dietary fiber too quickly can lead to gas, bloating, and cramps. Fiber binds to minerals and increases their excretion; therefore, excessive fiber intake may have adverse effects on mineral absorption. The World Health Organization recommends an upper limit of 40 g/day.[29]

Fig (Ficus carica)

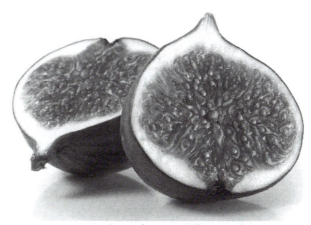

Fig. (Image from oriori/Shutterstock.)

definition

Purple snack fruit that is approximately the size of a ping-pong ball. It is mild in flavor and full of small edible seeds. Figs are a good source of fiber. Phytochemical components include phenolics, coumarins, flavonoids (e.g., anthocyanins, quercetin, luteolin), and terpenoids.[36] Consumed fresh, dried, as jam, and made into fruit filling for baked products. Used orally as a laxative, for diabetes, hyperlipidemia, eczema, psoriasis, and vitiligo, although there is no reliable evidence to evaluate the effectiveness of fig for any of these conditions.[23]

F

scientific findings

The equivalent of one small, fresh fig[37] produced a measurable increase in plasma antioxidant capacity in a small study (n = 10 healthy subjects).[38]

bioactive dose

Not known.

safety

Presumed safe when consumed in normal dietary quantities by non-allergic individuals. Fig can cause allergy, and in rare cases, anaphylaxis.[23]

Flavonoids

definition

Class of hundreds of structurally unique phytochemicals that are relatively common in the average American diet, and which "… are usually subdivided according to their substituents into: anthocyanidins, catechins, chalcones, flavones, flavonols, flavanones, and isoflavones."[39,40] "Flavonoids provide the bright orange, yellow, and red pigments of various foods, along with characteristic flavors, such as the hearty taste of whole-wheat foods or the bitter taste of red grapes."[41] Flavonoids are found in citrus fruits and citrus-based juices, other fruits, vegetables, grains, nuts, seeds, spices, flowers, tea, red wine, and products made from soy and cocoa beans.[39,41,42] Plants and spices containing flavonoids have been used for thousands of years in traditional Eastern medicine.[39] Flavonoids are transported in serum by albumin, thus, theoretically, protein malnutrition may reduce serum circulating levels of flavonoids.[43]

scientific findings

"Flavonols, flavanones, and flavones are subclasses of flavonoids that exert cardioprotective and anticarcinogenic properties *in vitro* and *in vivo*."[42] Some experimental evidence indicates that flavonoids could prevent prostate cancer.[44] Dietary flavonoid intake and black tea, a major source of flavonoids, were associated with a decreased risk of advanced stage prostate cancer in the Netherlands Cohort study (n = 58,279 men).[44]

bioactive dose

Not known.

safety

Presumed safe when consumed in normal dietary quantities by non-allergic individuals.

Flaxseed (Linum usitatissimum)

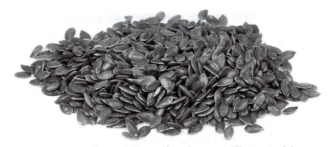

Flaxseed. (Image from hsagencia/Shutterstock.)

definition

Usitatissimum, or "most useful," is ascribed to flaxseed because it is a source of food products such as grains, seeds, and oil, and a source of fiber, which can be made into linen. Flaxseeds are a good source of iron and potassium with 1/4 cup supplying 341 mg of potassium (7% DV) and 2.4 mg of iron (13% DV),[45] omega-3 fatty acid, and β-sitosterol.[46] Flaxseeds, flaxseed cereals and breads, and flaxseed oil may require refrigeration to prevent rancidity; the oil should not be heated to high temperatures.

scientific findings

Flaxseed is an effective bulk-forming laxative.[47] According to a review, studies of flaxseed preparations used to reduce cholesterol levels have been inconclusive[47]; however, a review of six clinical trials found that those using various flaxseed preparations significantly reduced total cholesterol and LDL cholesterol in people with both normal and high cholesterol levels,[23] and flaxseed has additional LDL-lowering capabilities when used concomitantly with statin medications.[48] However, flaxseed does not improve triglyceride levels, and a certain type of flaxseed (defatted flaxseed with reduced linolenic acid content) may have raised triglycerides in a clinical trial.[23] Flaxseed lignan, a component of flaxseed but not flaxseed oil, had no effect on bone mineral density body composition, lipoproteins, glucose, or inflammation in a small, randomized, placebo-controlled study (n = 100 adults aged ≥50).[49] β-sitosterol is "likely effective" for symptoms of enlarged prostate, and improved urinary symptoms, increased maximum urinary flow, and decreased postvoid residual urine volume; however, it did not affect prostate size in clinical trials according to a review.[23] Taking flaxseed improved renal function in patients with systemic lupus erythematosus nephritis in two clinical trials.[23] Study results are mixed on whether flaxseed decreases hot flashes.[47]

bioactive dose

A dose of 3–50 g (1 teaspoon–5 Tablespoons)[50] of flaxseed daily reduced total cholesterol by 5%–9% and LDL cholesterol by 8%–18% in the majority of clinical trials performed.[23]

safety

Presumed safe when consumed in normal dietary quantities by non-allergic individuals; however, severe allergic reactions have been reported to flaxseed and flaxseed oil, and those with known allergy to any member of the *Linum* genus should avoid flaxseed products.[23] Flaxseed may stimulate menstruation and animal studies have shown possible harmful effects during pregnancy; therefore, the use of flaxseed or flaxseed oil during pregnancy and breastfeeding is not recommended.[51]

Folate

definition

Water soluble vitamin involved in the manufacture of DNA necessary for cell division and tissue growth. Folate requires vitamin B12 to be converted to a form necessary to manufacture DNA.[52] Synthetic folic acid is more bioavailable than naturally occurring folate. The quantity of this vitamin in the diet, though measured in micrograms, may be expressed in Dietary Folate Equivalents to encompass the absorption difference between the synthetic form, found in commercial grain products, and the natural form found in fruits, vegetables, and "foliage" such as spinach, in addition to legumes, beets, and orange juice.

scientific findings

To reduce the risk of in utero neural tube defects, women of reproductive age should consume 400 µg of folate/folic acid daily beginning before pregnancy, and 600 µg of folate/folic acid throughout gestation.[53] High dietary intake of vegetables during pregnancy reduces the risk of folate deficiency.[23] Folate deficiency impairs cell division and protein synthesis, and can cause megaloblastic anemia. Several, but not all, epidemiologic studies provide evidence of an inverse relationship between folate intake and the risk of pancreatic cancer.[54] Observational studies suggest that low folate status, particularly in women, is associated with depression.[23] A diet rich in folate may reduce the risk of stroke in male smokers, according to a large observational trial (n = 26,556 male Finnish smokers, aged 50–69 years).[55] "Dietary intake of folate greater than 249 µg daily in men and 400 µg in women is associated with a reduced risk of colon cancer, especially in women with a family history of the disease".[23]

bioactive dose

The RDA for folic acid/folate is 400 µg for adults; 600 µg for pregnant women; and 500 µg for lactating women.

safety

The UL for folic acid is 1000 µg. Patients should avoid exceeding the folate UL because folate can mask megaloblastic anemia caused by vitamin B12 deficiency.

Fructan

definition

Naturally occurring polymer of fructose molecules such as inulin. Fructooligosaccharides are a type of fructan. Found in asparagus, jerusalem artichokes, chicory, bananas, garlic, and onion.[56–59]

scientific findings

Fructans are natural sweeteners that have a low caloric value, do not lead to a rise in serum glucose, do not stimulate insulin secretion, promote the growth of intestinal bifidobacteria, and may improve the absorption of certain minerals.[59,60] Taking fructans orally does not seem to reduce the incidence of traveler's diarrhea; some evidence suggests that fructans may relieve constipation by increasing fecal mass.[23]

bioactive dose

Not known. For prebiotic effect (to increase fecal bifidobacteria), the typical dose is 4–10 g/day.[23]

safety

Presumed safe when consumed in normal dietary quantities by non-allergic individuals.

Fruit foods group

definition

Underconsumed food group that is a good source of folate, vitamins C and A, and underconsumed potassium.[61] Fruit phytochemicals may vary by color, where generally blue/purple plant foods contain anthocyanidins, flavonols, flavan-3-ols, proanthocyanidins, ellagic acid, and resveratrol; green plant foods typically contain flavones, flavanones, flavonols, β-carotene, lutein, xeaxathin, indoles, isothiocyanates, and organosulfur compounds; white plant foods typically contain flavonols, flavanones, indoles, isothiocyanates, and organosulfur compounds; yellow plant foods typically contain flavonols, flavanones, α-carotene, β-carotene, β-cryptoxanthin, and xeaxanthin; and red plant foods typically contain anthocyanins, flavonols, flavones, flavan-3-ols, flavanones, proanthocyanidins, lycopene, ellagic acid, and resveratrol.[62]

scientific findings

"People whose diets are rich in plant foods such as fruits and vegetables have a lower risk of getting cancers of the mouth, pharynx, larynx, esophagus, stomach, and lung, and some evidence suggests that maintaining a diet rich in plant foods also lowers the risk of cancers of the colon, pancreas, and prostate. This diet also reduces the risk of diabetes, heart disease, and hypertension, helps to reduce calorie intake, and may help to control weight."[63] Consuming a diet containing high amounts of fruits is associated with fewer age-related diseases such as Alzheimer disease.[64]

bioactive dose

One cup for children aged 2–3 years, to 1 1/2 to 2 cups daily for people aged 19–50 for general health.[65] One to 2.5 cups of fruits daily, depending on age and calorie needs, where 0.9 daily cup equivalents of fruit per 1000 cal is recommended to help prevent the cancers cited in Scientific Findings.[65]

F

safety

Presumed safe when consumed in normal dietary quantities by non-allergic individuals. Allergies to different fruits have been reported.

References

1. US Department of Agriculture. Agricultural Research Service. National Nutrient Database. Fish, mackerel, Atlantic, raw. http://ndb.nal.usda.gov/ndb/foods/show/4509?fg=&man=&lfacet=&format=&count=&max=25&offset=&sort=&qlookup=mackerel. Accessed May 7, 2014.

2. Kamei M, Fujita T, Kanbe T, Sasaki K, Oshiba K, Otani S, Matsui-Yuasa I, Morisawa S. The distribution and content of ubiquinone in foods. *Int J Vit Nutr Res.* 1986;56:57–63.

3. US Department of Agriculture. Agricultural Research Service. Nutrient Data Laboratory. Fish, sardine, Atlantic, canned in oil, drained solids with bone. http://ndb.nal.usda.gov/ndb/foods/show/4445?fg=&man=&lfacet=&format=&count=&max=25&offset=&sort=&qlookup=canned+sardines+with+bones. Accessed July 29, 2013.

4. Bittiner SB, Cartwright I, Tucker WFG, Bleehen SS. A double-blind, randomised, placebo-controlled trial of fish oil in psoriasis. *Lancet.* 1988;331(8582):378–380.

5. Lips P. Vitamin D physiology. *Prog Biophys Mol Biol.* 2006;92(1):4–8. Epub 2006 February 28.

6. Berger MM, Delodder F, Liaudet L, Tozzi P, Schlaepfer J, Chiolero RL, Tappy L. Three short perioperative infusions of n-3 PUFAs reduce systemic inflammation induced by cardiopulmonary bypass surgery: A randomized controlled trial. *Am J Clin Nutr.* 2013;97(2):246–254. doi: 10.3945/ajcn.112.046573. Epub 2012 December 26.

7. Wu JH, Cahill LE, Mozaffarian D. Effect of fish oil on circulating adiponectin: A systematic review and meta-analysis of randomized controlled trials. *J Clin Endocrinol Metab.* 2013;98(6):2451–2459. doi: 10.1210/jc.2012-3899. Epub 2013 May 23.

8. NIH Medline Plus. Fish oil. http://www.nlm.nih.gov/medlineplus/druginfo/natural/993.html. Accessed March 1, 2014.

9. American Heart Association. Fish and Omega-3 Fatty Acids. http://www.heart.org/HEARTORG/GettingHealthy/NutritionCenter/Healthy DietGoals/Fish-and-Omega-3-Fatty-Acids_UCM_303248_Article.jsp. Accessed August 29, 2013.

10. US Food and Drug Administration. What You Need to Know About Mercury in Fish and Shellfish. http://www.fda.gov/Food/ResourcesForYou/Consumers/ucm110591.htm. Accessed April 15, 2015.

11. Gil A, Gil F. Fish. A mediterranean source of n-3 PUFA: Benefits do not justify limiting consumption. *Br J Nutr.* 2015;113 Suppl 2:S58–67. doi: 10.1017/S0007114514003742.

12. Albert-Puleo M. Fennel and anise as estrogenic agents. *J Ethnopharmacol.* 1980;2(4):337–344.

13. El Bardai S, Lyoussi B, Wibo M, Morel N. Pharmacological evidence of hypotensive activity of *Marrubium vulgare* and *Foeniculum vulgare* in spontaneously hypertensive rat. *Clin Exp Hypertens.* 2001;23(4):329–343.

14. Agarwal R, Gupta SK, Agrawal SS, Srivastava S, Saxena R. Oculohypotensive effects of *Foeniculum vulgare* in experimental models of glaucoma. *Indian J Physiol Pharmacol.* 2008;52(1):77–83.

15. Perry R, Hunt K, Ernst E. Nutritional supplements and other complementary medicines for infantile colic: A systematic review. *Pediatrics.* 2011;127(4): 720–733.

16. National Institutes of Health. National Center for Complementary and Alternative Medicine. Fenugreek. http://nccam.nih.gov/health/fenugreek/. Accessed December 30, 2011.

17. Basch E, Ulbricht C, Kuo G, Szapary P, Smith M. Therapeutic applications of fenugreek. *Altern Med Rev.* 2003;8(1):20–27.

18. Roberts KT. The potential of fenugreek (*Trigonella foenum-graecum*) as a functional food and nutraceutical and its effects on glycemia and lipidemia. *J Med Food.* 2011;14(12):1485–1489. Epub 2011 August 23.

19. Chantry CJ, Howard CR, Montgomery A, Wight N. Use of galactogogues in initiating or augmenting maternal milk supply. ABM protocols, Protocol#9. The Academy of Breastfeeding Medicine; 2004.

20. Mathern JR, Raatz SK, Thomas W, Slavin JL. Effect of fenugreek fiber on satiety, blood glucose and insulin response and energy intake in obese subjects. *Phytother Res.* 2009;23(11):1543–1548.

21. Gupta A, Gupta R, Lal B. Effect of *Trigonella foenum-graecum* (fenugreek) seeds on glycaemic control and insulin resistance in type 2 diabetes mellitus: A double blind placebo controlled study. *J Assoc Physicians India.* 2001;49:1057–1061.

22. Sharma RD, Raghuram TC, Rao NS. Effect of fenugreek seeds on blood glucose and serum lipids in type I diabetes. *Eur J Clin Nutr.* 1990;44(4):301–306.

23. Jellin JM, Gregory PJ. et al. *Natural Medicine Comprehensive Database.* Therapeutic Research Faculty; 2013. http://www.naturaldatabase.com. Accessed July 11, 2012.

24. Graf E. Antioxidant potential of ferulic acid. *Free Radical Bio Med.* 1992;13(4): 435–448.

25. Zhao Z, Moghadasian MH. Chemistry, natural sources, dietary intake and pharmacokinetic properties of ferulic acid: A review. *Food Chem.* 2008;109(4):691–702.

26. Huang M-T, Smart RD, Wong C-Q, Conney AH. Inhibitory effect of curcumin, chlorogenic acid, caffeic acid, and ferulic acid on tumor promotion in mouse skin by 12-O-tetradecanoylphorbol-13-acetate. *Cancer Res.* 1988;48(21):5941–5946.

27. Ou S, Kwok K-C. Ferulic acid: Pharmaceutical functions, preparation and applications in foods. *J Sci Food Agric.* 2004;84(11):1261–1269(9).

28. University of Maryland Medical Center. Hypercholesterolemia. http://www.umm.edu/altmed/articles/hypercholesterolemia-000084.htm. Accessed June 16, 2011.

29. Whitney ER, Rolfes SR. *Understanding Nutrition*, 12th edn. Belmont, CA: Wadsworth Cengage; 2011.

30. The American Heart Association. About cholesterol. http://www.heart.org/HEARTORG/GettingHealthy/NutritionCenter/HealthyDietGoals/Whole-Grains-and-Fiber_UCM_303249_Article.jsp. Accessed December 31, 2011.

31. DeBruyne LK, Pinna K. *Nutrition for Health and Healthcare*, 5th edn. Belmont, CA: Wadsworth Cengage Learning; 2014.

32. Slavin JL. Position of the American Dietetic Association: Health implications of dietary fiber. *J Am Diet Assoc.* 2008;108(10):1716–1731.

33. Academy of Nutrition and Dietetics Evidence Analysis Library. What is the evidence that dietary fiber from whole foods and dietary supplements is beneficial in cardiovascular disease? http://andevidencelibrary.com/conclusion.cfm?conclusion_statement_id=250904. Accessed July 20, 2013.

34. Wang Q, Ellis PR. Oat β-glucan: Physico-chemical characteristics in relation to its blood-glucose and cholesterol-lowering properties. *Br J Nutr.* 2014;112(Suppl 2):S4–S13. doi: 10.1017/S0007114514002256.

35. Institute of Medicine. Dietary Reference Intakes: Macronutrients. http://www.iom.edu/Global/News%20Announcements/~/media/C5CD2DD7840544979A549EC47E56A02B.ashx. Accessed December 30, 2011.

36. US Department of Agriculture. Agricultural Research Service. Phytochemical Database. Ficus carica. http://www.pl.barc.usda.gov/usda_rrcp/rrecipe_detail.cfm?code=69685564&id=75&ThisName=sd1. Accessed December 31, 2011.

37. US Department of Agriculture. Agricultural Research Service. National Nutrient Database. Fig, raw. http://ndb.nal.usda.gov/ndb/foods/show/2250?fgcd=&manu=&lfacet=&format=&count=&max=35&offset=&sort=&qlookup=fig%2C+raw Accessed August 29, 2015.

38. Vinson JA, Zubik L, Bose P, Samman N, Proch J. Dried fruits: Excellent *in vitro* and *in vivo* antioxidants. *J Am Coll Nutr.* 2005;24(1):44–50.

39. Middleton Jr. E, Kandaswami C, Theoharides TC. The effects of plant flavonoids on mammalian cells: Implications for inflammation, heart disease, and cancer. *Pharmacol. Rev.* 2011;52(4):1–79.

40. Kocic B, Kitic D, Brankovic S. Dietary flavonoid intake and colorectal cancer risk: Evidence from human population studies. *J BUON.* 2013;18(1):34–43.

41. Whitney E, DeBruyne LK, Pinna K, Rolfes SR. *Nutrition for Health and Health Care*, 4th ed. Belmont, CA: Wadsworth Cengage Learning; 2011.

42. Zamora-Ros R, Knaze V. et al. Estimated dietary intakes of flavonols, flavanones and flavones in the European prospective investigation into cancer and nutrition (EPIC) 24 hour dietary recall cohort. *Br J Nutr.* 2011;106(12):1915–1925. Epub 2011 June 17.

43. Pal S, Saha C. A review on structure-affinity relationship of dietary flavonoids with serum albumins. *J Biomol Struct Dyn*. 2014;32(7):1132–1147. Epub 2013 July 1.

44. Geybels MS, Verhage BA, Arts IC, van Schooten FJ, Goldbohm RA, van den Brandt PA. Dietary flavonoid intake, black tea consumption, and risk of overall and advanced stage prostate cancer. *Am J Epidemiol*. 2013;177(12):1388–1398. doi: 10.1093/aje/kws419. Epub 2013 May 30.

45. US Department of Agriculture. National Nutrient Database. Flaxseed. http://ndb.nal.usda.gov/ndb/foods/show/3745?fgcd=&manu=&lfacet=&format=&count=&max=35&offset=&sort=&qlookup=flaxseed. Accessed April 6, 2015.

46. Herchi W, Harrabi S, Sebei K, Rochut S, Boukhchina S, Pepe C, Kallel H. Phytosterols accumulation in the seeds of *Linum usitatissimum* L. *Plant Physiol Biochem*. 2009;47(10):880–885.

47. The National Institutes of Health. National Center for Complementary and Alternative Medicine. Herbs at a Glance Flaxseed. Flaxseed and flaxseed oil. http://nccam.nih.gov/health/flaxseed/ataglance.htm. Accessed July 18, 2010.

48. Edel AL, Rodriguez-Leyva D, Maddaford TG, Caligiuri SP, Austria JA, Weighell W, Guzman R, Aliani M, Pierce GN. Dietary flaxseed independently lowers circulating cholesterol and lowers it beyond the effects of cholesterol-lowering medications alone in patients with peripheral artery disease. *J Nutr*. 2015;145(4):749–57. doi: 10.3945/jn.114.204594. Epub 2015 February 18.

49. Cornish SM, Chilibeck PD, Paus-Jennsen L, Biem HJ, Khozani T, Senanyake V, Vatanparast H, Little JP, Whiting SJ, Pahwa P. A randomized controlled trial of the effects of flaxseed lignan complex on metabolic syndrome composite score and bone mineral in older adults. *Appl Physiol Nutr Metab*. 2009;34(2):89–98. doi: 10.1139/H08-142.

50. US Department of Agriculture. Agricultural Research Service. National Nutrient Database. Flaxseed. http://ndb.nal.usda.gov/ndb/foods/show/3745?man=&lfacet=&count=&max=35&qlookup=Seeds%2C+flaxseed&offset=&sort=&format=Abridged&reportfmt=other&rptfrm=&ndbno=&nutrient1=&nutrient2=&nutrient3=&subset=&totCount=&measureby=&_action_show=Apply+Changes&Qv=1&Q7044=1&Q7045=0.33&Q7046=1&Q7047=7&Q7048=1 Accessed August 29, 2015.

51. The Natural Standard Research Collaboration. Flaxseed, Flaxseed Oil. www.naturalstandard.com/databases/flaxseed. Accessed December 29, 2011.

52. Herbert V, Subak-Sharpe GJ. *Total Nutrition*. New York, NY: St. Martin's Press; 1995.

53. March of Dimes. Statement on Folate Status of Women. http://www.marchofdimes.com/aboutus/791_1869.asp. Accessed September 2, 2010.

54. Sanchez GV, Weinstein SJ, Stolzenberg-Solomon RZ. Is dietary fat, vitamin D, or folate associated with pancreatic cancer? *Mol Carcinogen*. 2012;51(1):119–127. doi: 10.1002/mc.20833.

55. Larsson SC, Mannisto S, Virtanen MJ, Kontto J, Albanes D, Virtamo J. Folate, vitamin B6, vitamin B12, and methionine intakes and risk of stroke subtypes in male smokers. *Am J Epidemiol*. 2008;167(8):954–961. Epub 2008 February 12.

F

56. Ramnani P, Gaudier E, Bingham M, van Bruggen P, Tuohy KM, Gibson GR. Prebiotic effect of fruit and vegetable shots containing Jerusalem artichoke inulin: A human intervention study. *Br J Nutr.* 2010;104(2):233–240. Epub 2010 March 1.

57. Chandrashekar PM, Venkatesh YP. Fructans from aged garlic extract produce a delayed immunoadjuvant response to ovalbumin antigen in BALB/c mice. *Immunopharmacol Immunotoxicol.* 2012;34(1):163–169. Epub 2011 June 2.

58. Roberfroid MB. Introducing inulin-type fructans. *Br J Nutr.* 2005;93(Suppl 1):S13–25.

59. Sabater-Molina M, Larqué E, Torrella F, Zamora S. Dietary fructooligosaccharides and potential benefits on health. *J Physiol Biochem.* 2009;65(3):315–328.

60. Niness KR. Inulin and oligofructose: What are they? *J Nutr.* 1999;129 (7 Suppl):1402S–1406S.

61. U.S. Department of Agriculture and U.S. Department of Health and Human Services. *Dietary Guidelines for Americans, 2010.* 7th Edition, Washington, DC: U.S. Government Printing Office, December 2010.

62. Produce for Better Health. Fruit and Veggies More Matters Phytochemical List. http://www.pbhfoundation.org/about/res/pic/phytolist/. Accessed July 21, 2013.

63. National Cancer Institute. Cancer Progress Trends Report. http://progress-report.cancer.gov/prevention/fruit_vegetable Accessed 6 February 2015.

64. Joseph JA, Shukitt-Hale B, Willis LM. Grape juice, berries, and walnuts affect brain aging and behavior. *J. Nutr.* 2009;139(9):1813S–1817S.

65. ChooseMyPlate.gov. How much fruit is needed daily? http://www.choosemyplate.gov/food-groups/fruits-amount.pdf. Accessed February 6, 2015.

F

G

Garbanzo bean (Cicer arietinum)

definition

Italian name for the legume commonly called chickpea in the United States. It is an excellent source of vitamin B6, riboflavin, fiber, and protein; and it is a source of flavonoid glycosides.[1,2] It is commonly found on salad bars and made into hummus, a puree of garbanzo beans, lemon, cumin, and tahini.

scientific findings

Garbanzo beans have a low glycemic index[3] and may be used as a cholesterol-free substitute for meat. One ounce of meat, poultry, or fish is nutritionally equivalent to 1/4 cup cooked of garbanzo beans, though the bioavailability of iron in legumes is lower than the bioavailability of heme iron in meat, poultry, or fish.

bioactive dose

Not known.

safety

Presumed safe when consumed in normal dietary quantities by non-allergic individuals.

Garlic (Allium sativum)

definition

Edible lily family bulb that is a common culinary ingredient. When cut or crushed, it produces allyl sulfur compounds such as allicin, methyl allyl trisulfide, and diallyl trisulfide, each of which may have unique health properties. Other phytochemical constituents include vanillic acid, flavonoids, and terpenoids. Garlic is among the oldest of all cultivated plants and has been used for culinary and medicinal purposes for thousands of years.[4] Allicin is partly responsible for the flavor and odor of cut garlic.[5]

Allicin was previously considered to be a key bioactive constituent of garlic but was found to be highly unstable when processed. It quickly transforms into a variety of other bioactive organosulfur compounds when processed; hence, freshly crushed garlic may contain only limited amounts of allicin and commercially available processed garlic preparations do not contain allicin.[5] The biological activity of garlic is likely due to several components, which may include organosulfur transformation products of allicin.

scientific findings

Although preliminary research demonstrated a relationship between garlic consumption and a slight reduction in blood cholesterol level and that garlic may slow the progression of atherosclerosis,[6] fresh garlic, dried powdered garlic tablets, and aged garlic extract tablets were all found to be ineffective at lowering serum cholesterol in a controlled trial,[6] and a meta-analysis representative of available evidence on the effects of garlic on serum cholesterol from randomized controlled trials found no beneficial effect of garlic on serum cholesterol.[7] The same meta-analyses found the methyl allyl trisulfide component of garlic may be antithrombotic.[6] Garlic may reduce cardiac arrhythmias.[8] Some evidence has suggested that garlic consumption may slightly reduce blood pressure, particularly in people with high blood pressure[6]; other evidence does not support an appreciable effect of garlic in reducing blood pressure in people with high blood pressure.[9] Taking low doses of garlic powder orally, 300 mg/day, lessened age-related decreases in aortic elasticity, while higher doses of 900 mg/day seemed to slow development of atherosclerosis in both aortic and femoral arteries when used over a 4-year period.[10] Laboratory studies support that garlic, and or some of its allyl sulfur compounds, suppress carcinogen formation, carcinogen bioactivation, and tumor proliferation.[11] Diallyl trisulfide exhibited chemoprotective properties experimentally.[12] However, a review on the effects of garlic consumption and various cancers found "no credible evidence to support a relation between garlic intake and a reduced risk of gastric, breast, lung, or endometrial cancer," and very limited evidence of a relationship between garlic consumption and a reduced risk of colon, prostate, esophageal, larynx, oral, ovary, or renal cell cancers.[13] According to the National Cancer Institute, "Preliminary studies suggest that garlic consumption may reduce the risk of developing several types of cancer, especially cancers of the gastrointestinal tract. Most of the studies evaluated different types of garlic preparations and used them in varying amounts."[14] Garlic's antifungal properties have been demonstrated in laboratory research.[15,16] In laboratory studies, aged garlic extract, but not fresh garlic extract, exhibited antioxidative activity.[17] Garlic components exhibited neuroprotective properties in experimental research.[18] In laboratory studies, allicin and compounds into which it transforms when processed, exhibited antimicrobial properties,[19] and treatment with allicin arrested human mammary cancer cells in a laboratory study.[20]

bioactive dose

Not known. A dose of fresh garlic 4 g (approximately one clove) once daily has been used to treat hyperlipidemia[10]; for hypertension, the dose of garlic powder 600–900 mg daily has been used.[10] If garlic consumption does reduce the risk of developing cancer, the amount needed to lower risk remains unknown.[14]

safety

Presumed safe when consumed in normal dietary quantities by non-allergic individuals. Raw garlic appears to be safe for most adults and its side effects are generally mild (most commonly, breath and body odor, heartburn, upset stomach, and allergic reactions). Garlic is also an anti-coagulant, and therefore, its intake should be considered when monitoring patients with bleeding disorders or on anticoagulants, during or after surgery (garlic use should be stopped 7–10 days in advance of surgery, or if dental work is planned).[21] In addition, garlic has been found to interfere with the effectiveness of saquinavir, a drug used to treat HIV (human immunodeficiency virus) infection.[6]

Ginger (Zingiber officinale)

definition

A rhizome, or underground stem similar to a root. Ginger contains niacin, phytosterols, berberine, zingerone, a phenolic alkanone[22] responsible for the pungency of ginger,[23] shogaol, and zingiberene.[24] Ginger has been used in Asian traditional medicine to alleviate stomach ache, nausea, and diarrhea. Ginger is also used to treat rheumatoid arthritis, osteoarthritis, and joint and muscle pain; however, evidence for these uses is lacking.[25] Though ginger products are commonly used to relieve nausea,[26] ginger ale may be artificially flavored or contain real ginger, so consumers should look for "made from real ginger."

scientific findings

Ginger promotes saliva production and gastric juice secretion and produces an increase in the tone and peristalsis of the intestine.[27] Studies are inconclusive on whether ginger is effective for nausea caused by motion, chemotherapy.[26] Though studies do suggest that the short-term use of ginger can safely relieve pregnancy-related nausea and vomiting, according to the National Institutes of Health.[26] A review of random-ized, controlled clinical trials examining various interventions, among them use of ginger for nausea, vomiting, and retching in early preg-nancy, found a lack of high-quality evidence.[28] In a meta-analysis of 12 randomized, controlled clinical trials (n = 1278 pregnant women), ginger significantly improved nausea in pregnant women compared to placebo but did not affect vomiting.[29] It is unclear whether ginger is effective in treating rheumatoid arthritis, osteoarthritis, joint pain, or muscle pain.[26] In an animal study, zingerone inhibited colonic motility via direct action on smooth muscles.[30]

bioactive dose

For morning sickness, a dose equivalent to 1 g of ginger (250 mg ginger four times daily, or 500 mg twice daily) was found to be effective in two clinical trials; 650 mg three times daily has also been used.[10]

safety

Presumed safe when consumed in normal dietary quantities by non-allergic individuals. However, the *Physician's Desk Reference for Herbal Medicines* contraindicates the use of ginger during pregnancy for morning sickness because ginger during pregnancy theoretically might affect fetal sex hormones, and a case report of spontaneous abortion during week 12 of pregnancy in a patient who used ginger for morning sickness has been published.[27] Other reviews state that short-term use of ginger can safely relieve nausea of pregnancy. They state that: "ginger can be used safely for morning sickness without harm to the fetus"[10]; and "short-term use can safely relieve nausea of pregnancy."[26] Ginger should not be taken by individuals suffering from gallstones, except after consultation with a medical professional, because it increases bile production.[10]

Glucosinolates

definition

Phytochemicals found widely in *Brassica* plants that undergo biotrans-formation into various active compounds including sulforaphane and indole-3-carbinol. When Brassica foods are prepared by boiling and blanching, glucosinolate content is significantly reduced, whereas when prepared by steaming, microwaving, or stir frying the glucosinolate con-tent is either retained or slightly reduced.[31] Sprouts of brassica vegetables typically contain significantly higher concentrations of glucosinolates than mature plants.[32]

scientific findings

Sulforaphane and indole-3-carbinol have demonstrated anticarcinogenic properties in laboratory studies.[33]

bioactive dose

Not known.

safety

Presumed safe when consumed in normal dietary quantities by nonallergic individuals. Glucosinolates are goitrogens; they impair thyroid uptake of iodine.[34]

Glutamine

definition

Nonessential amino acid that is abundant in the American diet. It is required for cell proliferation, immune function, and the maintenance of redox potential; as a respiratory fuel for rapidly proliferating cells; as a regulator of acid–base balance through the production of urinary ammonia; as a carrier of nitrogen; and as a precursor for nucleic acids, nucleotides, amino sugars, and proteins.[35-37] Glutamine is found in many protein foods such as flaxseed protein.[38]

scientific findings

Glutamine is considered to be conditionally essential during physiologic stress.[37]

bioactive dose

Not known.

safety

Presumed safe when consumed in normal dietary quantities by non-allergic individuals.

Glutathione

definition

Compound that is synthesized in the body and is a component of the antioxidant enzyme glutathione peroxidase. Fresh fruits, vegetables, and meats have moderate-to-high amounts of glutathione.[39] The spice cumin is also a source of glutathione.[40]

scientific findings

Glutathione is thought to prevent free radical formation in humans.[41]

bioactive dose

Not known.

safety

Presumed safe when consumed in normal dietary quantities by non-allergic individuals.

Glycosides

definition

Sugar derivatives produced biochemically in plants, such as garbanzo beans, blackberries,[1,42] and *Stevia rebaudiana*, are used to make the natural sweetener Stevia.[43]

scientific findings

Glycosides were shown to be antioxidants, suppress cancer cell growth, and exert antiatherogenic properties in laboratory studies.[42]

bioactive dose

Not known.

safety

Presumed to be safe when consumed in normal dietary quantities by non-allergic individuals, except amygdalin, found in nonconsumable portions of fruits (e.g., the inedible pits of peaches), which is a well-known toxic cyanogenic glycoside.

Grains

definition

Seed-like fruits found at the stem tops of various plants but particularly those plants belonging to the Poaceae (grass) family. Cereals, the edible grain produced by plants within the grass family, consist of the outer husk called the bran, which encloses the center endosperm and inner germ. The outer bran consists mostly of fibers, but also contains phytates. The endosperm consists mostly of starch and the inner germ contains high concentrations of fats, proteins, and vitamins such as vitamin E. When the bran and germ are removed during processing (refined) to increase shelf life and palatability, many nutrients are also removed including fiber, fat, protein, vitamins, and phytochemicals. "Enriched" refined grains (typically breads, cereals, and baked products containing the word "enriched flour" in their ingredient listing) are processed grain foods to which thiamin, riboflavin, niacin, folic acid, and iron have been added.

G

scientific findings

Although whole grains are recommended, consuming half of one's grain food intake as refined grains without high levels of added fat, sugar, or sodium, was not associated with an increased disease risk, according to a review of 135 studies of refined grains and health outcomes.[44] A case–control study (n = 384 pancreatic adenoma cases and 983 matched controls) found an increased association between pancreatic adenocarcinoma and intake of nonwhole grains, and an inverse association between pancreatic adenocarcinoma and intake of whole grains.[45]

bioactive dose

The recommended number of grain group foods one should consume daily varies according to calorie requirements; see also grains, whole.

safety

Presumed safe when consumed in normal dietary quantities by non-allergic individuals.

Grains, whole

definition

Grains with the bran, germ, and endosperm intact are "whole grains." Whole grains provide fiber and a wide variety of naturally occurring nutrients, depending upon the specific grain, but generally include B vitamins, vitamin E, selenium, zinc, copper, and magnesium, along with phytochemicals such as phenolic compounds,[46] antioxidants, and phytoestrogens. Examples include oats, popcorn, brown rice, and products whose first ingredient in the ingredient listing contains the word "whole," for example: Ingredients: Whole wheat.

scientific findings

Epidemiological studies have shown that whole grain intake is protective against cancer, cardiovascular disease, diabetes, and obesity.[47] The exact mechanisms linking whole grains to disease prevention are not known but may include gastrointestinal effects, antioxidant protection, and the intake of phytoestrogens.[46] A systematic review with meta-analysis of 11 cohort studies (n = 1,719,590 participants between 25 and 76 years of age) found consumption of whole grains was inversely associated with the risk of developing colorectal cancer.[48] A systematic review and meta-analysis of 25 prospective observational studies (n = >14,500 cases) found that a high intake of dietary fiber, in particular cereal fiber and whole grains, was associated with a reduced risk of colorectal cancer.[49] Possible mechanisms of action for a protective effect of dietary fiber and whole grain consumption and risk of colorectal cancer include diluting fecal carcinogens, decreasing transit time, thus reducing the contact between carcinogens and the lining of the colorectum, and the production of short-chain fatty acids by the fermentation of fiber, in addition to individual constituents of grains, such as antioxidants, vitamins, trace minerals, phytate, phenolic acids, lignans, phytoestrogens, and a high content of folate and magnesium, which have been associated with a reduced risk of colorectal cancer.[49] In a case–control study (n = 384 pancreatic adenoma cases and 983 matched controls), epidemiologic surveys and food frequency questionnaires showed that highest quintiles of whole grain intake were inversely associated with having pancreatic adenocarcinoma (for which several mechanisms associated with whole grains or fiber were postulated: decrease insulin resistance, decreased triglyceride levels, and/or elevated high density lipoprotein levels).[45]

bioactive dose

Depending upon calorie requirements, approximately three servings of whole grains is the daily minimum whole grain recommendation for men and woman aged 19 to 50, though the actual amount required may vary based on calorie needs. One "serving" varies with each food (e.g., one serving of oatmeal is 1/2 cup while one serving of a whole wheat bread is a 1-oz slice).

safety

Presumed safe when consumed in normal dietary quantities by non-allergic individuals.

Grape (Vitis vinifera)

definition

Marble-sized snack fruit that contains numerous phytochemicals, depending on variety, such as catechin, epicatechin, resveratrol, flavonoid proanthocyanidins, quercetin, and kaempferol.[50] Eaten fresh and made into other products such as juice, jam or jelly, raisins, and wine. Grape leaves are consumed in Middle Eastern cuisine and are an excellent source of vitamin K.[51] Concord grapes and its juice are violet in color and are a source of vitamin C and polyphenols.

G

scientific findings

Grape seed skins contain potent antioxidants that theoretically improve microcirculation and protect the vascular endothelium.[52] Grape seed extract, in doses of 360–720 mg, or its proanthocyanidin constituents, in doses of 150–300 mg/day, orally seemed to reduce subjective symptoms of chronic venous insufficiency and improve venous tone in patients with stage I and stage II chronic venous insufficiency, compared to placebo. Patients also reported significant decreases in subjective complaints such as tired or heavy legs, tension, and tingling and pain after 12 weeks of treatment.[10] Both the concord grape and its juice contain polyphenols, including anthocyanin and proanthocyanidin, which are associated in epidemiological studies with a decreased risk of cancer and heart disease, and a reduction in age-related motor and cognitive deficits.[53]

bioactive dose

Not known.

safety

Presumed safe when consumed in normal dietary quantities by non-allergic individuals. Grape seed extracts have been safely used for up to 8 weeks in clinical studies.[10]

Grapefruit (Citrus paradisi)

definition

Large yellow-, white-, red-, or pink-fleshed citrus fruit that is an excellent source of vitamin C and a source of folate and potassium, whether its juice or the whole fruit is consumed.[54]

scientific findings

A red grapefruit variety (*Citrus paradise* Macf.) exhibited antioxidant properties in a laboratory study.[55] Eating 1.5 grapefruit daily for 6 weeks did not significantly reduce markers of inflammation and oxidative stress in a small, controlled clinical trial of overweight/obese subjects (n = 69), though grapefruit consumption produced a favorable modulation of oxidative stress in overweight and obese adults with metabolic syndrome.[56] "Preliminary population research shows that consuming a quart or more per day of grapefruit juice is associated with a 25%–30% increased risk of breast cancer in postmenopausal women, a mechanism for which may be that grapefruit juice reduces estrogen metabolism resulting in increased endogenous estrogen levels; however, more evidence is needed to validate this finding.[10] Grapefruit juice produced a greater decrease in mean arterial blood pressure when compared with orange juice in an experimental study."[57]

bioactive dose

Not known.

safety

Presumed safe when consumed in normal dietary quantities by nonallergic individuals. Grapefruit juice has been found to increase the absorption of certain drugs, including simvastatin and lovastatin,[24] and to increase cortisol availability in patients with Addison disease[58]; therefore, people on these medications may be advised to avoid grapefruit juice.

Green leaf(y) vegetables

definition

Versatile family of leafy food plants, such as basil, arugula, and spinach, known for their antioxidant capacity. In particular, *Brassica* vegetables are sources of specific phytochemicals, such as flavonoids and glucosinolates. Generally, dark green leafy vegetables are noted for providing vitamin E, folate, magnesium, vitamin K, and chlorophyll. Tender leafy green vegetables are common salad vegetables; heartier leafy greens are cooked or can be thinly minced and added to cooked recipes. Herb-like leafy green vegetables, such as basil and arugula, are used for their pungent flavors, as seasonings, but can be made into main dishes, such as pesto, when combined with garlic and parmesan cheese.

scientific findings

Consumption of green leafy vegetables is associated with a reduced risk of several types of cancer and cardiovascular disease.[59] In a population-based case–control study (n = 348 cases and 470 controls) higher intake of green leafy vegetables and cruciferous vegetables was associated with a lower risk of non-Hodgkin's lymphoma.[60]

In a case–control study (n = 384 pancreatic adenoma cases and 983 matched controls) where dark green vegetable consumption was determined by epidemiologic survey and food frequency questionnaire, evidence was observed to support that higher vegetable consumption, including dark green vegetables and other plant foods, was significantly inversely associated with pancreatic adenocarcinoma.[45]

G

bioactive dose

Not known.

safety

Presumed safe when consumed in normal dietary quantities by non-allergic individuals.

Guava (Psidium guajava)

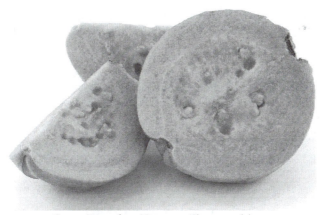

Guava. (Image from Nuttapong/Shutterstock.)

definition

Lemon-sized fruit whose skin may be yellow, red, or purple; whose flesh may be yellow, pink, or red, depending on the variety; and whose seeds are edible.[61] A uniquely flavored tropical fruit that contains polyphenol antioxidants and is a good source of fiber and vitamin A, and an excellent source of vitamin C.[61,62] Consumed fresh or as a juice or juice blend.

scientific findings

Vitamin C increases nonheme iron absorption. Guava juice added to schoolchildren's diets (n = 95 children aged 6–9), in order to prevent their high-phytate diet from diminishing iron absorption, was found to "marginally increase hemoglobin and plasma ferritin."[63] Preliminary research suggests guava lectin and galactose may have antidiarrheal properties.[64]

bioactive dose

Not known.

References

1. Bagri P, Ali M, Sultana S, Aeri V. A new flavonoid glycoside from the seeds of *Cicer arietinum* Linn. *Acta Pol Pharm.* 2011;68(4):605–608.
2. US Department of Agriculture. Agricultural Research Service. Nutrient Database. Chickpea. http://ndb.nal.usda.gov/ndb/foods/show/4673?fg=&man=&lfacet=&count=&max=25&qlookup=garbanzo + bean&offset=&sort=&format=Abridged&_action_show=Apply + Changes&Qv=1&Q8649=0.5&Q8650=1.0. Accessed June 16, 2013.
3. Panlasigui LN, Panlilio LM, Madrid JC. Glycaemic response in normal subjects to five different legumes commonly used in the Philippines. *Int J Food Sci Nutr.* 1995;46(2):155–160.
4. Gonen A, Harats D, Rabinkov A, Miron T, Mirelman D, Wilchek M, Weiner L et al. The antiatherogenic effect of allicin: Possible mode of action. *Pathobiology.* 2005;72(6):325–334.
5. Amagase H, Petesch BL, Matsuura H, Kasuga S, Itakura Y. Intake of garlic and its bioactive components. *J Nutr.* 2001;131:955S–962S.
6. National Institutes of Health. National Center for Complementary and Alternative Medicine. Herbs at a Glance. Garlic. National Center for Complementary and Alternative Medicine. http://nccam.nih.gov/health/garlic/ataglance.htm. Accessed June 29, 2010.
7. Khoo YS, Aziz Z. Garlic supplementation and serum cholesterol: A meta-analysis. *J Clin Pharm Ther.* 2009;34(2):133–145.
8. Martín N, Bardisa L, Pantoja C, Román R, Vargas M. Experimental cardiovascular depressant effects of garlic (*Allium sativum*) dialysate. *J Ethanopharmacol.* 1992;37:145–149.
9. Stabler SN, Tejani AM, Huynh F, Fowkes C. Garlic for the prevention of cardiovascular morbidity and mortality in hypertensive patients. *Cochrane Database Syst. Rev.* 2012;8:CD007653. doi: 10.1002/14651858.CD007653.pub2.
10. Jellin JM, Gregory PJ. *Natural Medicine Comprehensive Database.* Therapeutic Research Faculty; 2013. http://www.naturaldatabase.com. Accessed July 30, 2012.
11. Milner JA. A historical perspective on garlic and cancer. *J Nutr.* 2001;131(3s):1027S–1131S.

12. Toyohiko A, Taiichiro S. Antithrombotic and anticancer effects of garlic-derived sulfur compounds: A review. *Biofactors*. 2006;26(2):93–103.

13. Kim JY, Kwon O. Garlic intake and cancer risk: An analysis using the Food and Drug Administration's evidence-based review system for the scientific evaluation of health claims. *Am J Clin Nutr*. 2009;89(1):257–264.

14. National Cancer Institute. Garlic and Cancer Prevention. http://www.cancer.gov/cancertopics/causes-prevention/risk/diet/garlic-fact-sheet. Accessed March 22, 2015.

15. Benkeblia N. Antimicrobial activity of essential oil extracts of various onions (*Allium cepa*) and garlic (*Allium sativum*). *Food Sci Technol-LEB*. 2004;37(2):263–268. doi: 10.1016/j.lwt.2003.09.001.

16. Shams-Ghahfarokhia M, Shokoohamiria M-R, Amirrajaba N, Moghadasia B, Ghajarib A, Zeinic F, Sadeghid G, Razzaghi-Abyanehd M. *In vitro* antifungal activities of *Allium cepa*, *Allium sativum* and ketoconazole against some pathogenic yeasts and dermatophytes. *Fitoterapia*. 2006;77(4):321–323.

17. Thompson M, Ali M. Garlic [*Allium sativum*]: A review of its potential use as an anti-cancer agent. *Curr Cancer Drug Targets*. 2003;3(1):67–81(15).

18. Mathew B, Biju R. Neuroprotective effects of garlic: A review. *Libyan J Med*. 2008;3(1):23–33. doi: 10.4176/071110.

19. Leng BF, Qiu JZ, Dai XH, Dong J, Wang JF, Luo MJ, Li HE et al. Allicin reduces the production of α-toxin by *Staphylococcus aureus*. *Molecules*. 2011;16(9):7958–7968.

20. Powolny AA, Singh SV. Multitargeted prevention and therapy of cancer by diallyl trisulfide and related allium vegetable-derived organosulfur compounds. *Cancer Lett*. 2008;269(2):305–314.

21. Tattleman E. Health effects of garlic. *Am Fam Physician*. 2005;72:103–106.

22. Rao BN, Rao BS. Antagonistic effects of Zingerone, a phenolic alkanone against radiation-induced cytotoxicity, genotoxicity, apoptosis and oxidative stress in Chinese hamster lung fibroblast cells growing *in vitro*. *Mutagenesis*. 2010;25(6):577–587. Epub 2010 August 16.

23. Monge P, Scheline R, Solheim E. The metabolism of zingerone, a pungent principle of ginger. *Xenobiotica*. 1976;6(7):411–423.

24. DerMarderosian A, Beutler J. *The Review of Natural Products*, 5th edn. St. Louis: Wolters Kluwer Health; 2008.

25. University of Maryland Medical Center. Ginger. http://umm.edu/health/medical/altmed/herb/ginger. Accessed August 30, 2015.

26. National Institutes of Health. National Center for Complementary and Alternative Medicine. Herbs at a Glance. Ginger. http://nccam.nih.gov/health/ginger. Accessed January 12, 2011.

27. Gruenwald J, Brendler T, Jaenicke C, eds. *Physician's Desk Reference for Herbal Medicines*. Montvale, NJ: Medical Economics Company; 1998.

28. Matthews A, Dowswell T, Haas DM, Doyle M, O'Mathúna DP. Interventions for nausea and vomiting in early pregnancy. *Cochrane Database Syst. Rev*. 2010;(9):CD007575. doi: 10.1002/14651858.CD007575.pub2.

29. Viljoen E, Visser J, Koen N, Musekiwa A. A systematic review and meta-analysis of the effect and safety of ginger in the treatment of pregnancy-associated nausea and vomiting. *Nutr J*. 2014;13:20. doi: 10.1186/1475-2891-13-20.

30. Iwami M, Shiina T, Hirayama H, Shima T, Takewaki T, Shimizu Y. Inhibitory effects of zingerone, a pungent component of *Zingiber officinale* Roscoe, on colonic motility in rats. *J Nat Med*. 2011;65(1):89–94. Epub 2010 August 27.

G

31. Nugrahedi PY1, Verkerk R, Widianarko B, Dekker M. A mechanistic perspective on process-induced changes in glucosinolate content in Brassica vegetables: A review. *Crit Rev Food Sci Nutr.* 2015;55(6):823–38. doi: 10.1080/10408398.2012.688076.

32. Dorland Biomedical. *Medical and Healthcare Marketplace Guide*, 16th edn. Vol. 1. Philadelphia, PA: Dorland Healthcare Information; 2000.

33. Keck A-S, Finley JW. Cruciferous vegetables: Cancer protective mechanisms of glucosinolate hydrolysis products and selenium. *Integr Cancer Ther.* 2004;3(1):5–12. doi: 10.1177/1534735403261831. Accessed June 30, 2011.

34. Mullin WJ, Sahas-Rabudhe MR. Glucosinolate content of cruciferous vegetable crops. *Can J Plant Sci.* 1977;57(4): 1227–1230.

35. Soeters PB, Grecu I. Have we enough glutamine and how does it work? A clinician's view. *Ann Nutr Metab.* 2011;60(1):17–26.

36. Kim H. Glutamine as an immunonutrient. *Yonsei Med J.* 2011;52(6):892–897. doi: 10.3349/ymj.2011.52.6.892.

37. Lacey JM, Wilmore DW. Is glutamine a conditionally essential amino acid? *Nutr Rev.* 1990;48(8):297–309.

38. Oomah BD. Flaxseed as a functional food source. *J Sci Food Agric.* 2001;81(9):889–894.

39. Jones DP, Coates RJ, Flagg EW, Eley JW, Block G, Greenberg RS, Gunter EW, Jackson B. Glutathione in foods listed in the national cancer institute's health habits and history food frequency questionnaire. *Nutr Cancer.* 1992;17(1):57–75.

40. Aruna K, Sivaramakrishnan VM. Plant products as protective agents against cancer. *Indian J Exp Biol.* 1990;28(11):1008–1011.

41. Whitney ER, Rolfes SR. *Understanding Nutrition*, 12th edn. Belmont, CA: Wadsworth Cengage Learning; 2011.

42. Kaume L, Howard LR, Devareddy L. The blackberry fruit: A review on its composition and chemistry, metabolism and bioavailability, and health benefits. *J Agric Food Chem.* 2012;60(23):5716–5727. Epub 2011 December 8.

43. Yadav SK, Guleria P. Steviol glycosides from Stevia: Biosynthesis pathway review and their application in foods and medicine. *Crit Rev Food Sci Nutr.* 2012;52(11):988–998.

44. Williams PG. Evaluation of the evidence between consumption of refined grains and health outcomes. *Nutr Rev.* 2012;70(2):80–99. Epub 2012 January 3.

45. Jansen RJ, Robinson DP, Stolzenberg-Solomon RZ, Bamlet WR, de Andrade M, Oberg AL, Hammer TJ et al. Fruit and vegetable consumption is inversely associated with having pancreatic cancer. *Cancer Causes Control.* 2011;22(12): 1613–1625. doi: 10.1111/j.1753-4887.2011.00452.x. Epub 2011 September 14.

46. Slavin JL, Jacobs D, Marquart L, Wiemer K. The role of whole grains in disease prevention. *J Am Diet Assoc.* 2001;101(7):780–785.

47. Slavin J. Why whole grains are protective: Biological mechanisms. *Proc Nutr Soc.* 2003;62(1):129–134.

48. Haas P, Machado MJ, Anton AA, Silva AS, de Francisco A. Effectiveness of whole grain consumption in the prevention of colorectal cancer: Meta-analysis of cohort studies. *Int J Food Sci Nutr.* 2009;60(Suppl 6):1–13.

49. Aune D, Chan DS, Lau R, Vieira R, Greenwood DC, Kampman E, Norat T. Dietary fibre, whole grains, and risk of colorectal cancer: Systematic review and dose–response meta-analysis of prospective studies. *BMJ.* 2011;343:d6617. doi: 10.1136/bmj.d6617.

50. US Department of Agriculture. Agricultural Research Service. Phytochemical Database. Grapes. http://www.pl.barc.usda.gov/usda_plant/plant_home. cfm. Accessed November 24, 2011.

51. US Department of Agriculture. Agricultural Research Service. Nutrient Database. Grape leaves. http://ndb.nal.usda.gov/ndb/foods/show/3565?f g=&man=&lfacet=&format=&count=&max=25&offset=&sort=&qlookup= grapes. Accessed June 16, 2013.

52. Werbach MR, Murray MT. *Botanical Influences on Illness*, 2nd edn. Tarzana, CA: Third Line Press, Inc.; 2000.

53. Joseph JA, Shukitt-Hale B, Willis LM. Grape juice, berries, and walnuts affect brain aging and behavior. *J Nutr*. 2009;139:1813S–1817S.

54. US Department of Agriculture. Agricultural Research Service. Nutrient Data Laboratory. Grapefruit, white, raw. http://ndb.nal.usda.gov/ndb/foods/sho w/2244?fg=&man=&lfacet=&format=&count=&max=25&offset=&sort=&ql ookup=grapefruit. Accessed August 9, 2013.

55. Jayaprakasha GK, Girennavar B, Patil BS. Radical scavenging activities of Rio Red grapefruits and Sour orange fruit extracts in different *in vitro* model systems. *Bioresour Technol*. 2008;99(10):4484–4494. Epub 2007 November 1.

56. Dow CA, Wertheim BC, Patil BS, Thomson CA. Daily consumption of grapefruit for 6 weeks reduces urine F2-isoprostanes in overweight adults with high baseline values but has no effect on plasma high-sensitivity c-reactive protein or soluble vascular cellular adhesion molecule 1. *J Nutr*. 2013;143(10):1586–1592. Epub 2013 July 31.

57. Díaz-Juárez JA1, Tenorio-López FA, Zarco-Olvera G, Valle-Mondragón LD, Torres-Narváez JC, Pastelín-Hernández G. Effect of *Citrus paradisi* extract and juice on arterial pressure both *in vitro* and *in vivo*. *Phytother Res*. 2009;23(7):948–54. doi: 10.1002/ptr.2680.

58. Methlie P, Husebye EE, Hustad S, Lien EA, Løvås K. Grapefruit juice and licorice increase cortisol availability in patients with Addison's disease. *Eur J Endocrinol*. 2011;165(5):761–769. Epub 2011 September 6.

59. Jin J, Koroleva OA, Gibson T, Swanston J, Magan J, Zhang Y, Rowland IR, Wagstaff C. Analysis of phytochemical composition and chemoprotective capacity of rocket (*Eruca sativa* and *Diplotaxis tenuifolia*) leafy salad following cultivation in different environments. *J Agric Food Chem*. 2009;57(12):5227–5234.

60. Chiu BC, Kwon S, Evens AM, Surawicz T, Smith SM, Weisenburger DD. Dietary intake of fruit and vegetables and risk of non-Hodgkin lymphoma. *Cancer Causes Control*. 2011;22(8):1183–1195. Epub 2011 June 22.

61. Produce for Better Health. Guava. http://www.fruitsandveggiesmoremat-ters.org/guava. Accessed June 16, 2013.

62. Jiménez-Escrig A, Rincón M, Pulido R, Saura-Calixto F. Guava fruit (*Psidium guajava* L.) as a new source of antioxidant dietary fiber. *J Agric Food Chem*. 2001;49(11):5489–5493.

63. Monárrez-Espino J, López-Alarcón M, Greiner T. Randomized placebo-controlled trial of guava juice as a source of ascorbic acid to reduce iron deficiency in Tarahumara indigenous schoolchildren of northern Mexico. *J Am Coll Nutr*. 2011;30(3):191–200.

64. Coutiño-Rodríguez R, Hernández-Cruz P, Giles-Ríos H. Lectins in fruits having gastrointestinal activity: Their participation in the hemagglutinating property of *Escherichia coli* O157:H7. *Arch Med Res*. 2001;32(4):251–257.

G

H

Hazelnut (Corylus avellana)

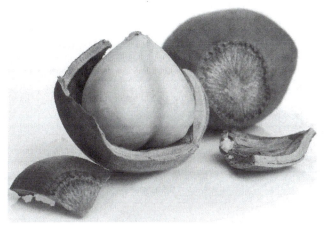

Hazelnut. (Image from Valentina Razumova/Shutterstock.)

definition

Marble-sized nut, also called filbert, which is a good source of protein, monounsaturated fatty acid, tocopherols, phytosterols,[1] and other phyto-chemicals. Hazelnuts and chocolate are used to make Nutella (Ferrero USA, Inc., Somerset, NJ 08873); dry-roasted hazelnuts add crunchiness to yogurt.

scientific findings

In a laboratory study, phenolic compounds of hazelnuts exerted antioxi-dant effects.[2] In a 4-week single intervention study (n = 21 normolipemic, healthy individuals), a hazelnut-enriched diet (1 g/kg/day) decreased the atherogenic tendency of LDL by reducing oxidized LDL levels and increasing vitamin E in LDL.[3]

bioactive dose

Not known.

safety

Presumed safe when consumed in normal dietary quantities by non-allergic individuals. Hazelnut allergy has been reported, and affected individuals must avoid hazelnut exposure.

Hemicellulose

definition

Type of dietary fiber that has characteristics of both insoluble and soluble fibers. It surrounds cellulose in plant cell walls.[4,5] Legumes, fruits, and vegetables (particularly younger or less mature vegetables), and grains are the main sources of hemicellulose in the diet.[6]

scientific findings

Fibers in the large intestine promote stool passage and are associated with lower rates of diverticular disease, hemorrhoids, and appendicitis.[4]

bioactive dose

Not known. The DRI for fiber (of all types) is 25–38 g daily for women and men aged 19–50 years, respectively.

safety

The World Health Organization recommends a dietary fiber upper limit of 40 g/day.[4] Fiber intake exceeding 40 g has been associated with decreased absorption of minerals.

Hesperidin

definition

Polyphenol compound classified as flavonoid and specifically a flavanone glycoside is found in lemons and sweet oranges.[7] Hesperidin is a citrus by-product.[8] It is converted into hesperetin by GI microflora, absorbed, and circulates in plasma as hesperetin glucuronide.[8]

scientific findings

A dietary deficiency of hesperidin has been associated with capillary fragility and extremity pain causing night leg cramps, according to a review of its pharmacologic properties.[8] Hesperidin exhibited anti-inflammatory, hypolipidemic, and vasoprotective properties in experimental studies and several small clinical trials.[8] Hesperidin may improve venous diseases such as hemorrhoids[9] and venous stasis[10] possibly by reducing capillary permeability.[11]

bioactive dose

Not known.

safety

Presumed safe when consumed in normal dietary quantities by non-allergic individuals. No signs of toxicity have been observed with the normal intake of hesperidin or related compounds.[12] Hesperidin appears to be safe when used up to 6 months by nonpregnant, nonlactating individuals.[13]

Honey

definition

Intensely sweet yellow–orange viscous carbohydrate liquid produced by bees from flower nectar. Flavors of honey vary depending upon the flower source. Honey is a concentrated source of the monosaccharides, glucose, and fructose, the same two monosaccharides that comprise sucrose.

scientific findings

Honey has topical healing properties.[14] It contains the antibacterial protein royalisin.[14] Four different varieties of honey exerted antimicrobial effects against *Staphylococcus aureus* in a laboratory study.[15] Some clinical research in children with upper respiratory infections has shown that taking 2.5–10 mL (0.5–2 teaspoons) of honey at bedtime can significantly reduce nighttime cough frequency and severity and improve sleep compared to placebo.[13] Honey appears to be as, or more, effective than the over-the-counter cough suppressant dextromethorphan and the antihistamine diphenhydramine.[13]

bioactive dose

Not known. For cough, 2.5–10 mL (0.5–2 teaspoons) of honey at bedtime has been used.[13]

safety

Fetal and infant exposure should be avoided because honey could contain potentially harmful pyrrolizidine alkaloids. Honey sourced from pyrrolizidine alkaloid-containing plants represents a significant source of honey worldwide.[16] Regarding botulism, honey consumption is safe in children over 1 year of age.[13]

Honeydew melon (*Cucumis melo* L. var. *inodorus* Naud)

definition

Considered to be the sweetest commercially available melon and one of the 10 most consumed melons in the United States, honeydew melon has pale green, juicy flesh and its ripeness is reflected by its creamy yellow, inedible rind. One-half cup of honeydew supplies 200 mg of potassium, is an excellent source of vitamin C and folate,[18] and supplies the phytochemical cucurbitacin-β.[17]

scientific findings

Cucurbitacin-β has exhibited antihepatotoxic, anti-inflammatory, and anticancer properties in laboratory studies.[17]

bioactive dose

Not known.

safety

Presumed safe when consumed in normal dietary quantities by non-allergic individuals.

Hops (*Humulus lupulus* L.)

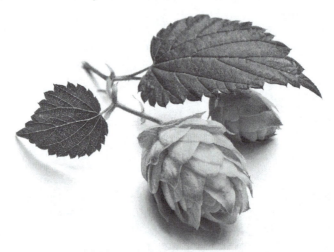

Hops. (Image from Zhukov Oleg/Shutterstock.)

H

definition

Flower of the hop plant. It contains phytoestrogens and chalcones. The major bitter flavoring in beer, it is also used as a food preservative. Traditional uses of hops include as a sleep aid, stomachic (an agent beneficial to digestion or to the stomach), antibacterial, and antifungal agent.[14,19]

scientific findings

Neuropharmacological effects of hops have been observed in laboratory animals.[19] *In vivo* and *in vitro* studies have demonstrated stomachic, antibacterial, antifungal, and cancer preventative properties.[19]

bioactive dose

Not known.

safety

Presumed safe when consumed in normal dietary quantities by non-allergic individuals. The phytoestrogen 8-prenylnaringenin was strongly estrogenic in a laboratory study and hops exposure has been attributed to menstrual abnormalities in female beer industry workers.[20]

Horseradish (*Armoracia rusticana, Cochlearia armoracia*)

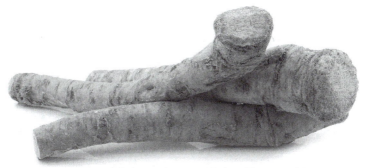

Horseradish. (Image from Peter Zijlstra/Shutterstock.)

definition

Thick, woody root vegetable belonging to the Brassicaceae family that is a source of potassium and phytochemicals such as lutein, xeaxanthin, cochlearine, and glucosinolates.[21–23] It is ground and processed into

H

prepared horseradish that is mixed with other ingredients, such as vinegar, and used as a condiment. Its major flavoring constituent, allyl isthiocyanate, causes a burning sensation when it comes in contact with the mouth. Green-colored horseradish is frequently substituted for wasabi, the sushi condiment, in the United States. Horseradish has been used to cure scurvy due to its high vitamin C content,[24] an effect that would be contingent upon amount consumed.

scientific findings

Horseradish exhibited antibacterial properties in an *in vitro* study.[23] In a placebo-controlled clinical trial, horseradish also helped prevent urinary tract infections.[25] The German Commission E has approved horseradish for oral use as "supportive therapy for infections of the urinary tract."[26]

bioactive dose

Not known.

safety

Presumed safe when consumed in normal dietary quantities by non-allergic individuals. It has a strong and irritating odor and contact with the mouth causes burning sensation.

References

1. Maguire LS, O'Sullivan SM, Galvin K, O'Connor TP, O'Brien NM. Fatty acid profile, tocopherol, squalene and phytosterol content of walnuts, almonds, peanuts, hazelnuts and the macadamia nut. *Int J Food Sci Nutr.* 2004;55(3):171–178.
2. Shahidi F, Alasalvar C, Liyana-Pathirana CM. Antioxidant phytochemicals in hazelnut kernel (*Corylus avellana* L.) and hazelnut byproducts. *J Agric Food Chem.* 2007;55(4):1212–1220. doi: 10.1021/jf062472o.
3. Yücesan FB, Orem A, Kural BV, Orem C, Turan I. Hazelnut consumption decreases the susceptibility of LDL to oxidation, plasma oxidized LDL level and increases the ratio of large/small LDL in normolipidemic healthy subjects. *Anadolu Kardiyol Derg.* 2010;10(1):28–35.
4. Whitney E, DeBruyne LK, Pinna K, Rolfes SR. *Nutrition for Health and Health Care*, 4th edn. Belmont CA: Cengage Learning; 2011.
5. Institute of Medicine. *Dietary Reference Intakes for Energy, Carbohydrate, Fiber, Fat, Fatty Acids, Cholesterol, Protein, and Amino Acids.* Washington DC: National Academy Press; 2002.
6. Dhingra D, Michael M, Rajput H, Patil RT. Dietary fibre in foods: A review. *J Food Sci Technol.* 2012;49(3):255–266.

7. US Department of Agriculture. Agricultural Research Service. Phytochemical Database. http://www.pl.barc.usda.gov/usda_chem/achem_detail.cfm?code= 69685564&chemical_id=492&ThisName=sd1. Hesperidin. http://www.pl. barc.usda.gov/usda_chem/achem_detail.cfm?code=69685564&chemical_ id=492&ThisName=sd1. Accessed January 10, 2012.

8. Rizza S, Muniyappa R et al. Citrus polyphenol hesperidin stimulates production of nitric oxide in endothelial cells while improving endothelial function and reducing inflammatory markers in patients with metabolic syndrome. *J Clin Endocrinol Metab.* 2011;96(5):E782–E792.

9. Cospite M. Double-blind, placebo-controlled evaluation of clinical activity and safety of Daflon 500 mg in the treatment of acute hemorrhoids. *Angiology.* 1994;45(6 Pt 2):566–573.

10. Ramelet AA. Clinical benefits of Daflon 500 mg in the most severe stages of chronic venous insufficiency. *Angiology.* 2000;52(Suppl 1):S49–S56.

11. Struckmann JR, Nicolaides AN. Flavonoids. A review of the pharmacology and therapeutic efficacy of Daflon 500 mg in patients with chronic venous insufficiency and related disorders. *Angiology.* 1994;45(6):419–428.

12. Garg A, Garg S, Zaneveld LJ, Singla AK. Chemistry and pharmacology of the Citrus bioflavonoid hesperidin. *Phytother Res.* 2001;15(8):655–669.

13. Jellin JM, Gregory PJ et al. *Natural Medicine Comprehensive Database.* Therapeutic Research Faculty. 2013. http://www.naturaldatabase.com. Accessed July 11, 2012.

14. DerMarderosian A, Beutler J. *The Review of Natural Products,* 5th edn. St. Louis, MO: Wolters Kluwer; 2008.

15. Boukraâ L, Niar A, Benbarek H, Benhanifia M. Additive action of royal jelly and honey against *Staphylococcus aureus. J Med Food.* 2008;11(1):190–192. doi: 10.1089/jmf.2007.567.

16. Edgar JA, Roeder E, Molyneux RJ. Honey from plants containing pyrrolizidine alkaloids: A potential threat to health. *J Agric Food Chem.* 2002;50(10):2719–2730.

17. Lester G. Melon (*Cucumis melo* L.). Fruit nutritional quality and health functionality. *Hort Technology.* 1997;7(3):222–227.

18. US Department of Agriculture. Agricultural Research Service. National Nutrient Database. Melon, honeydew, raw. http://www.nal.usda.gov/fnic/ foodcomp/cgi-bin/list_nut_edit.pl. Accessed April 12, 2011.

19. Zanoli P, Zavatti M. Pharmacognostic and pharmacological profile of *Humulus lupulus* L. *J Ethnopharmacol.* 2008;116(3):383–396. Epub 2008 January 20.

20. Milligan SR, Kalita JC, Heyerick A, Rong H, De Cooman SL, De Keukeleire D. Identification of a potent phytoestrogen in hops (*Humulus lupulus* L.) and beer. *J Clin Endocrinol Metab.* 1999;84(6):2249–2252.

21. US Department of Agriculture. Agricultural Research Service. National Nutrient Database. Horseradish, prepared. http://ndb.nal.usda.gov/ndb/ foods/show/274. Accessed January 11, 2012.

22. US Department of Agriculture. Agricultural Research Service. Phytochemical Database. *Cochlearia armoracia.* http://www.pl.barc.usda.gov/usda_plant/ plant_detail.cfm?code=69685564&plant_id=100&y1s27=&ThisName=ps721. Accessed January 10, 2012.

23. Mucete D, Borozan A, Radu R, Jianu I. Antibacterial activity of isothiocyanates, active principles in *Armoracia rusticana. J Agroaliment Processes Technol.* 2006;12(2):443–452.

H

24. Wedelsbäck Bladh K, Olsson KM. Introduction and use of horseradish (*Armoracia rusticana*) as food and medicine from antiquity to the present: Emphasis on the Nordic countries. *J Herbs, Spices Med Plants* 2011;17(3):197–213.

25. Albrecht U, Goos KH, Schneider B. A randomised, double-blind, placebo-controlled trial of a herbal medicinal product containing *Tropaeoli majoris herba* (nasturtium) and *Armoraciae rusticanae* radix (horseradish) for the prophylactic treatment of patients with chronically recurrent lower urinary tract infections. *Curr Med Res Opin.* 2007;23(10):2415–2422.

26. Gruenwald J, ed. *The PDR for Herbal Medicines*, 1st edn. Montvale NJ: Medical Economics; 1998.

H

I

Indole

definition

Phytochemicals, such as indole-3-carbinol and brassinin, that are formed from the hydrolysis of indoleglucosinolates in *Brassica* vegetables.[1]

scientific findings

The chemoprotective properties of indole-3-carbinol include the induction of phase II enzymes.[2] In animal studies, indole-3-carbinol exhibited chemopreventive properties.[3,4] Laboratory research found that brassinin demonstrated antiproliferative effects against cancer in both *in vivo* and *in vitro* models.[5]

bioactive dose

Not known.

safety

Presumed safe when consumed in normal dietary quantities by non-allergic individuals.

Inulin

definition

Type of carbohydrate that is fermented in the large intestine. Found in plant foods, such as asparagus, bananas, chicory, dandelion, garlic, Globe artichoke, Jerusalem artichoke, leeks, onions, wheat bran, and wheat flour.[6] The average inulin intake in the American diet has been estimated to be 2.6 g/day.[7]

scientific findings

Inulin improves laxation by increasing stool bulk and stool water content, and increases fecal bacteria,[8,9] and may improve stool frequency particularly in slightly constipated individuals.[9] Inulin may strengthen the intestinal epithelium and reduce the risk of gastrointestinal diseases.[9]

bioactive dose

Not known. For hypertriglyceridemia, the typical dose of inulin is 10–14 g daily; for treatment of hypercholesterolemia, inulin 6 g three times daily has been used for up to 6 weeks; for treatment of constipation in elderly, 20–40 g/day for 19 days has been used.[10]

safety

Presumed safe when consumed in normal dietary quantities by non-allergic individuals.

Iodine

definition

Trace mineral that functions as part of the thyroid hormones triodothyronine (T3) and thyroxine (T4) that regulate basal metabolism, growth, and body temperature.[11] Good sources of iodine include foods sourced from seawater including ocean fish, such as haddock, and seaweed; also iodized salt and processed foods to which additives, such as calcium iodate, potassium iodate, potassium iodide, and cuprous iodide, have been added. Dairy products may be sources of incidental iodine by way of feed additives given to dairy cows. The dairy farm and bakery industries may also use iodine-containing disinfectants, although this practice has been largely discontinued in the dairy industry.[12] Iodine may be absorbed transcutaneously via exposure to ocean mist, exhaust from the combustion of organic fuels, and topical exposure to iodine preparations, such as iodine antiseptics.[12] One-third of the world's population consumes insufficient iodine.[13] The average U.S. adult consumes more iodine than the RDA (between 210 and 300 µg daily).[11]

scientific findings

Iodine deficiency and iodine excess in otherwise healthy individuals can compromise thyroid function.[12] During pregnancy, insufficient maternal iodine intake causes maternal and neonatal hypothyroidism and increases the risk of neurological damage and cretinism, a form of preventable mental retardation and deafness in the baby.[11]

bioactive dose

The adult RDA for iodine is 150 µg.

safety

The UL for iodine for adults aged 19–50 years is 1100 µg. Excessive intake of iodine from food, water, and supplements has been associated with adverse effects such as thyroiditis, goiter, hypothyroidism, and hyperthyroidism.[11]

Iron

definition

Trace mineral found in the hemoglobin portion of red blood cells that binds to and transports oxygen to cells for energy metabolism. Heme iron occurs bound to hemoglobin or myoglobin in animal flesh and sources include meat, poultry, fish, and seafood, but not nonflesh animal foods such as eggs. Nonheme iron is found in legumes, beans, peas, processed soy products, and iron-fortified and enriched cereals. Heme iron is well absorbed (approximately 23%) compared to nonheme iron (2%–20%).[14] Hemoglobin concentrations lower than 12 g/dL in women and 13 g/dL in men indicate the presence of iron deficiency anemia.[15]

scientific findings

Insufficient iron intake during pregnancy increases the infant's risk of low birthweight, premature birth, low iron stores, and impaired cognitive and behavioral development, as well as increases the mother's risk for developing iron deficiency anemia.[15] Iron deficiency anemia affects approximately 10% of Americans and is especially common in toddlers, children, adolescents, and reproductive-aged women. A child with iron deficiency or iron deficiency anemia may exhibit fatigue on physical exertion and poor exercise tolerance; impaired energy metabolism, decreased mental productivity and aptitude; decreased neurotransmitter synthesis; and irritability, apathy, or restlessness.[16] Children who had iron deficiency anemia as infants may perform poorly as they grow older, even if their iron status improves.[16]

bioactive dose

The RDA for adults aged 19–50 is 18 mg for women and 8 mg for men. Since it is unlikely that the amount of iron required during pregnancy will be met by diet alone, iron-replete pregnant women require a daily dietary supplement to meet their iron RDA of 27 mg.[16] Women who are iron deficient going into pregnancy will require more than the RDA of 27 mg of iron to correct their deficiency.

safety

The UL for adults aged 19 and older is 45 mg. Excess iron may cause iron-induced oxidative stress.[17]

Isoflavone

definition

Phytoestrogen and type of flavonoid[18] whose chemical structure is similar to estrogen.[19] Daidzen, genistein, and glycitein are three major types of isoflavones found in certain fruits, vegetables, breads and cereals, meats, nuts, seeds, legumes, tofu, and tempeh.[20] Soybeans and soybean products are a major source of isoflavones.[22] In the U.S., intake of isoflavones has been estimated to be 1.13 mg/day,[21] whereas typical Japanese intake is 30–50 mg/day.[22] Soybean isoflavones exert estrogenic and nonestrogenic properties that may reduce risk of certain chronic diseases,[22] such as coronary heart disease, osteoporosis, and certain cancers, and alleviate symptoms of menopause.[24]

scientific findings

Meta-analyses have shown nonsignificant effects of soy isoflavones on total and LDL cholesterol[23]; cholesterol-lowering effects of soy isoflavones when consumed concurrently with soy protein[23]; no effect of soy isoflavones on lowering cholesterol levels[24]; and a significant effect of soy isoflavones on reducing serum total and LDL cholesterol.[25] Soy isoflavones may reduce LDL cholesterol oxidation.[26] Data on whether soy isoflavones or isoflavone-rich soy protein improve bone mineral density in younger postmenopausal women are inconsistent.[27] Limited "epidemiologic data generally show that among Asian populations, isoflavone intake is associated with higher bone mineral density."[29] Isoflavones did not affect serum prostate-specific antigen levels in healthy subjects, but "significantly favorably affected prostate-specific antigen in 4 of 8 clinical trials involving prostate cancer patients, while in no studies was there an absolute decrease in PSA concentrations."[24] "Soy isoflavones may mimic the actions and functions of estrogens on brain, and they have been shown to have positive effects on cognitive function in females; however, studies on their effects on spatial memory have not provided consistent results in males."[28] Soy isoflavones may help prevent or treat diabetic nephropathy.[24] Laboratory data show isoflavones exert chemopreventive properties, including cell cycle arrest and cell apoptosis.[22] Some trials reported a slight reduction in hot flashes and night sweats with phytoestrogen-based (isoflavone-based) treatment[29]; however, not all research has found soy extracts containing phytoestrogens to significantly reduce hot flashes leading researchers to conclude that "Isoflavones hold limited promise for the treatment of menopausal vasomotor symptoms."[30]

bioactive dose

The dose of soy isoflavones needed to achieve significant decreases in total or LDL cholesterol or triglycerides has not been established.[31] Doses used to reduce blood lipids in studies have ranged from 40 to 318 mg/day of isoflavones.[10] Forty milligrams is approximately the amount found in 100 g of tofu (depending on the brand name) and 318 mg would be supplied by two 100-g servings of dry roasted soybeans.[32] Clinical trial data suggest that approximately 80 mg/day isoflavones are needed to achieve improved bone–mineral density, whereas the epidemiologic data suggest lower amounts are efficacious.[27] The dose of isoflavones in the prostate clinical trials (supplied by dietary supplements) ranged from 60 to 900 mg/day.[24] A dose range of 34 to 76 mg isoflavones seemed to modestly reduce the frequency and severity of hot flashes in some menopausal women.[34]

safety

Presumed safe when consumed in normal dietary quantities by non-allergic individuals. The soy isoflavone genistein is goitrogenic.[33]

Isoprenoids

definition

Phytochemicals that impart flavors and fragrances, such as menthol from peppermint oil, citral from lemongrass oil, and limonene from citrus rinds. Fruits, vegetables, and cereal grains contain a variety of isoprenoid compounds.[34]

scientific findings

Isoprenoids have demonstrated anticancer activity in laboratory research.[35]

bioactive dose

Not known.

safety

Presumed safe when consumed in normal dietary quantities by non-allergic individuals.

Isothiocyanates

definition

Phytochemicals formed from the breakdown of glucosinolates[36] that are found in mustard seed and *Brassica* vegetables such as watercress and broccoli sprouts.[37]

scientific findings

Isothiocyanates have exerted antimicrobial and chemoprotective properties in experimental studies.[38,39] A review of epidemiological studies that examined associations between phytochemicals and cancer risk found mostly null associations between individual phytochemicals and cancer risk at various sites, and in those studies showing effect, "consistent protective effects were observed for higher levels—dietary intake, serum, plasma, or urinary metabolites—of ... isothiocyanates and lung cancer, [and] isothiocyanates and gastrointestinal cancer," among other effects.[40] Isothiocyanate has exhibited antimicrobial activity against a wide spectrum of pathogens, and anticancer activity experimentally (in cell cultures of cancer cells and in animal models) according to a report, which also stated that its bioavailability is very high.[41]

bioactive dose

Not known.

safety

Presumed safe when consumed in normal dietary quantities by non-allergic individuals. Isothiocyanates are known to be genotoxic, and therefore, pose a potential risk at high levels of intake, the specific level of which is not known.[41]

References

1. Mithen RF, Dekker M, Verkerk R, Rabot S, Johnson IT. The nutritional significance, biosynthesis and bioavailability of glucosinolates in human foods. *J Sci Food Agric.* 2000;80:967–984. doi: 10.1002/(SICI)1097-0010(20000515)80:7<967::AID-JSFA597>3.0.CO;2-V.

2. Potter JD, Steinmetz K. Vegetables, fruit and phytoestrogens as preventive agents. *IARC Sci Publ.* 1996;139:61–90.

3. Weng JR, Tsai CH et al. A potent indole-3-carbinol–derived antitumor agent with pleiotropic effects on multiple signaling pathways in prostate cancer cells. *Cancer Res.* 2007;67:7815–7824.

4. Bonnesen C, Eggleston IM, Hayes JD. Dietary indoles and isothiocyanates that are generated from cruciferous vegetables can both stimulate apoptosis and confer protection against DNA damage in human colon cell lines. *Cancer Res.* 2001;61:6120.

5. Izutani Y, Yogosawa S, Sowa Y, Sakai T. Brassinin induces G1 phase arrest through increase of p21 and p27 by inhibition of the phosphatidylinositol 3-kinase signaling pathway in human colon cancer cells. *Int J Oncol.* 2012;40(3):816–24. doi: 10.3892/ijo.2011.1246. Epub 2011 October 27.

6. Davidson MH, Maki KC. Nutritional and health benefits of inulin and oligofructose. *J Nutr.* 1999;129:1474S–1477S.

7. Moshfegh AJ, Friday JE, Goldman JP, Ahuja JKC. Presence of inulin and oligofructose in the diets of Americans. *J Nutr.* 1999:129(7):1407S–1411S.

8. Cherbut C. Inulin and oligofructose in the dietary fibre concept. *Br J Nutr.* 2002;87:S159–S162.

9. Roberfroid M. Dietary fiber, inulin, and oligofructose: A review comparing their physiological effects. *Crit Rev Food Sci Nutr.* 1993;33(2):103–148.

10. Jellin JM, Gregory PJ et al. *Natural Medicine Comprehensive Database.* Therapeutic Research Faculty. 2013. http://www.naturaldatabase.com. Accessed July 11, 2012.

11. Institute of Medicine. *Dietary Reference Intakes for Vitamin A, Vitamin K, Arsenic, Boron, Chromium, Copper, Iodine, Iron, Manganese, Molybdenum, Nickel, Silicon, Vanadium, and Zinc.* Washington, DC: National Academy Press; 2001; 258.

12. Nutrition. Feinberg School of Medicine. Northwestern University Nutrition Fact Sheet: Iodine. http://nuinfo-proto4.northwestern.edu/nutrition/factsheets/iodine.html. Accessed October 7, 2009.

13. Román GC. Nutritional disorders in tropical neurology. *Handb Clin Neurol.* 2013;114:381–404. doi: 10.1016/B978-0-444-53490-3.00030-3.

14. Whitney E, DeBruyne LK, Pinna K, Rolfes SR. *Nutrition for Health and Health Care,* 4th edn. Belmont, CA: Cengage Learning; 2011.

15. National Institutes of Health. Office of Dietary Supplements. Iron fact sheet. http://ods.od.nih.gov/factsheets/Iron-HealthProfessional/. Accessed April 15, 2015.

16. Procter SB, Campbell CG. Position of the Academy of Nutrition and Dietetics: Nutrition and lifestyle for a healthy pregnancy outcome. *J Acad Nutr Diet.* 2014;114:1099–1103.

17. Jagetia GC, Reddy TK. Alleviation of iron induced oxidative stress by the grape fruit flavanone naringin *in vitro. Chem Biol Interact.* 2011;190:121–128. Epub 2011 February 20.

18. Tillem J, Hardy M. Soy foods and breast cancer risk reduction. *Altern Med Alert.* 1999;2:109–113.

19. Kim SH, Kim CW, Jeon SY, Go RE, Hwang KA, Choi KC. Chemopreventive and chemotherapeutic effects of genistein, a soy isoflavone, upon cancer development and progression in preclinical animal models. *Lab Anim Res.* 2014;30(4):143–150. doi: 10.5625/lar.2014.30.4.143. Epub 2014 December 24.

I

20. U.S. Department of Agriculture. Agricultural Research Service. 2008. USDA Database for the Isoflavone Content of Selected Foods, Release 2.0. Nutrient Data Laboratory Home Page: http://www.ars.usda.gov/nutrientdata/isoflav.

21. Chun OK, Chung SJ, Song WO. Estimated dietary flavonoid intake and major food sources of U.S. adults. *J Nutr.* 2007;137:1244–1252.

22. Messina M, Kucuk O, Lampe JW. An overview of the health effects of isoflavones with an emphasis on prostate cancer risk and prostate-specific antigen levels. *J AOAC Int.* 2006;89(4):1121–1134.

23. Taku K, Umegaki K, Ishimi Y, Watanabe S. Effects of extracted soy isoflavones alone on blood total and LDL cholesterol: Meta-analysis of randomized controlled trials. *Ther Clin Risk Manage.* 2008;4(5):1097–1103.

24. Qin Y, Niu K, Zeng Y, Liu P, Yi P, Zhang T, Zhang QY, Zhu JD, Mi MT. Isoflavones for hypercholesterolaemia in adults. *Cochrane Database Syst Rev.* 2013;6:CD009518. doi: 10.1002/14651858.CD009518.pub2.

25. Taku K, Umegaki K, Sato Y, Taki Y, Endoh K, Watanabe S. Soy isoflavones lower serum total and LDL cholesterol in humans: A meta-analysis of 11 randomized controlled trials. *Am J Clin Nutr.* 2007;85(4):1148–1156.

26. Wang H, Murphy PA. Isoflavone content in commercial soybean foods. *J Agric Food Chem.* 1994;42(8):1666–1673.

27. Messina M, Ho S, Alekel DL. Skeletal benefits of soy isoflavones: A review of the clinical trial and epidemiologic data. *Curr Opin Clin Nutr Metab Care.* 2004;7(6):649–658.

28. Lee YB, Lee HJ, Sohn HS. Soy isoflavones and cognitive function. *J Nutr Biochem.* 2005;16(11):641–649.

29. Lethaby A, Marjoribanks J, Kronenberg F, Roberts H, Eden J, Brown J. Phytoestrogens for menopausal vasomotor symptoms. *Cochrane Database Syst Rev.* 2013;12:CD001395. doi: 10.1002/14651858.CD001395.pub4.

30. Newton KM. Isoflavones hold limited promise for the treatment of menopausal vasomotor symptoms. *Evidence Based Med.* 2014;19(5):178. doi: 10.1136/ebmed-2014-110000. Epub 2014 June 17.

31. Academy of Nutrition and Dietetics Evidence Analysis Library. Is there a dose–response relationship of the soy protein and/or isoflavone effects on cholesterol levels? http://andevidencelibrary.com/conclusion.cfm?conclusion_statement_id=95. Accessed July 29, 2013.

32. US Department of Agriculture. Database for the Isoflavone Content of Selected Foods. http://www.ars.usda.gov/SP2UserFiles/Place/80400525/Data/isoflav/Isoflav_R2.pdf. Accessed August 30, 2015.

33. Doerge DR, Sheehan DM. Goitrogenic and estrogenic activity of soy isoflavones. *Environ Health Perspect.* 2002;110(Suppl 3):349–353.

34. Craig WJ. Phytochemicals: Guardians of our health. *J Am Diet Assoc.* 1997;97(10):S199–S204.

35. Burke YD, Stark J, Roach SL, Sen SE, Crowell PL. Inhibition of pancreatic cancer growth by the dietary isoprenoids farnesol and geraniol. *Lipids.* 1997;32(2):151–156. doi: 10.1007/s11745-997-0019-y.

36. Shapiro TA, Fahey JW, Wade KL, Stephenson KK, Talalay P. Human metabolism and excretion of cancer chemoprotective glucosinolates and isothiocyanates of cruciferous vegetables. *Cancer Epidemiol Biomarkers Prev.* 1998;7:1091–1100.

37. Bhattacharya A, Li Y, Wade KL, Paonessa JD, Fahey JW, Zhang Y. Allyl iso-thiocyanate-rich mustard seed powder inhibits bladder cancer growth and muscle invasion. *Carcinogenesis.* 2010;31(12):2105–2110.
38. Lin CM, Preston JF 3rd, Wei CI. Antibacterial mechanism of allyl isothiocya-nate. *J Food Prot.* 2000;63(6):727–734.
39. Fimognari C, Turrini E, Ferruzzi L, Lenzi M, Hrelia P. Natural iso-thiocyanates: Genotoxic potential versus chemoprevention. *Mutat Res.* 2012;750(2):107–131. Epub 2011 December 10.
40. Miller PE, Snyder DC. Phytochemicals and cancer risk: A review of the epidemiological evidence. *Nutr Clin Pract.* 2012;27(5):599–612. doi: 10.1177/0884533612456043. Epub 2012 August 9.
41. Zhang Y. Allyl isothiocyanate as a cancer chemopreventive phytochemical. *Mol Nutr Food Res.* 2010;54(1):127–135.

I

J

Jasmine rice (Oryza sativa L.)

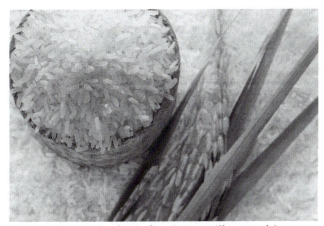

Jasmine rice. (Image from Praisaeng/Shutterstock.)

definition

An Asian variety of long- or medium-grain rice noted for being aromatic and flavorful when cooked owing to the presence of the chemical 2-acetyl-1-pyrrolin.[1,2] Jasmine rice is primarily grown in Thailand and readily commercially available. Nutritionally, jasmine rice, like all rice, is rich in starch, and enriched jasmine rice is a source of thiamin, niacin, iron, and folic acid.[3]

scientific findings

Rice is a high-glycemic index food; people with diabetes may benefit from lower-glycemic index foods such as rice noodles.[4]

bioactive dose

Not known.

safety

Presumed safe when consumed in normal dietary quantities by non-allergic individuals.

Jerusalem artichoke (Helianthus tuberosus)

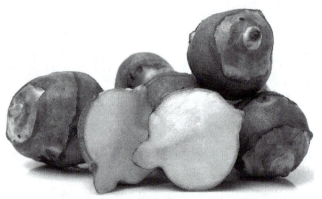

Jerusalem artichoke. (Image from Jiang Hongyan/Shutterstock.)

definition

Specie of sunflower with an edible root, also called a sun root or sun choke. It is neither from Jerusalem nor an artichoke. Its elongated finger-like tubers, which have a crisp texture, are cooked and eaten. Similar to water chestnuts in taste, Jerusalem artichoke tubers resemble potatoes except that the tuber carbohydrate is primarily inulin (and not starch).[5]

scientific findings

Fructans from Jerusalem artichokes reduced insulin response, compared to fructose, an effect attributed to fructans' slowing of GI transit time, in a small (n = 8) trial of healthy subjects.[6]

bioactive dose

Not known.

safety

Presumed safe when consumed in normal dietary quantities by non-allergic individuals.

Jicama (Pachyrhizus erosus)

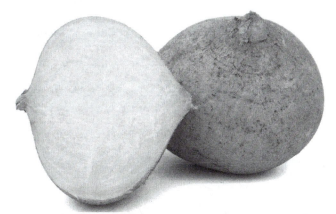

Jicama. (Image from Binh Thanh Bui/Shutterstock.)

definition

Also called "Mexican potato" and "yambean." A sweet, starchy tuber[7] native to Mexico and Central America pronounced "hecama." Jicama can weigh up to 6 lbs, has crunchy flesh, and contains fewer than 25 cal per 1/2 cup. In addition, raw jicama is a good source of vitamin C[8] and contains lignin and phenolic compounds.[9] Jicama tastes like a combination of water chestnut and apple and is used as a substitute for water chestnut in Asian cooking. It is also eaten fresh as thin slices or strips with vegetable dip or lime juice, in salads, and in stir fries.

scientific findings

See also *phenolic compounds.*

bioactive dose

Not known.

safety

Presumed safe when consumed in normal dietary quantities by non-allergic individuals.

Juniper berry (Juniperus communis L.)

definition

Cone of a shrub that appears berry-like, although not a true berry. It contains the phytochemicals limonene, myrcene, and phenolics.[10,11] Juniper berry flavors gin. The juniper berry is commonly used in bath salts for treating rheumatism.[12]

scientific findings

Juniper has *in vitro* antioxidant properties that may help inhibit lipid peroxidation *in vitro*.[11] An experimental study showed juniper berry to be hepatoprotective in rats.[13]

bioactive dose

Not known. A typical oral dose of juniper berry is 1–2 g three times daily, or one cup of the tea three to four times daily. The tea is prepared by steeping 1 teaspoon of the crushed juniper berry, about 2–3 g, in 150 mL boiling water for 10 min and then straining. Juniper should be used up to a maximum of 10 g of the dried berry per day, which should be used no longer than 4 weeks without physician consultation.[12]

safety

Juniper, juniper berry, and juniper extract are likely safe when used orally in amounts commonly found in foods.[12] Juniper berry oil should only be used under medical supervision.[12] *J. communis* extract adversely affected fertility and was abortifacient in studies using albino rats.[14] Juniper should not be used in pregnancy because it can increase uterine tone, interfere with fertility and implantation, and cause abortion.[12] Juniper should not be used during lactation because there is insufficient information to evaluate its safety.[12] Prolonged use of high doses can increase the potential for severe side effects such as convulsions or kidney damage.[12]

References

1. Cordeiro GM, Christopher MJ, Henry RJ, Reinke RF. Identification of microsatellite markers for fragrance in rice by analysis of the rice genome sequence. *Mol Breed.* 2002;9(4):245–250.
2. Bradbury LMT, Fitzgerald TI, Henry RJ, Jin Q, Waters DLE. The gene for fragrance in rice. *Plant Biotechnol J.* 2005;3(1):363–370.
3. Guerrero RTL, Gebhardt SE, Holden J, Kretsch MJ, Todd K, Novotny R, Murphy SP. White rice sold in Hawaii, Guam, and Saipan often lacks nutrient enrichment. *J Am Diet Assoc.* 2009;109(10):1738–1743.

4. Chan HM, Brand-Miller JC, Holt SH, Wilson D, Rozman M, Petocz P. The glycaemic index values of Vietnamese foods. *Eur J Clin Nutr.* 2001;55(12):1076–1083.

5. University of Wisconsin Agricultural Extension Service. Jerusalem artichokes. *Alternative Field Crops Manual.* http://www.hort.purdue.edu/newcrop/afcm/jerusart.html. Accessed January 18, 2012.

6. Rumessen JJ, Bodé S, Hamberg O, Gudmand-Høyer E. Fructans of Jerusalem artichokes: Intestinal transport, absorption, fermentation, and influence on blood glucose, insulin, and C-peptide responses in healthy subjects. *Am J Clin Nutr.* 1990;52:675–681.

7. Mélo EA, Stamford TL, Silva MP, Krieger N, Stamford NP. Functional properties of yam bean (*Pachyrhizus erosus*) starch. *Bioresour Technol.* 2003; 89(1):103–106.

8. Produce for Better Health Foundation. Fruit and Veggies More Matters. Jicama. http://www.fruitsandveggiesmorematters.org/?page_id=1350. Accessed January 2, 2012.

9. Aquino-Bolanos EN, Mercado-Silva E. Effects of polyphenol oxidase and peroxidase activity, phenolics and lignin content on the browning of cut jicama. *Postharvest Biol Technol.* 2004;33(3):275–283.

10. Shabmir F, Ahmadi AL, Mirza M, Korori SAA. Secretory elements of needles and berries of *Juniperus communis* L. ssp. *communis* and its volatile constituents. *Flavour Fragrance J.* 2003;18(5):425–428.

11. Elmastaşa M, Gülçinb I, Beydemirb S, İrfan Küfrevioğlub O, Aboul-Eneinc HY. A study on the *in vitro* antioxidant activity of Juniper (*Juniperus communis* L.) fruit extracts. *Anal. Lett.* 2006;39(1):47–65. doi: 10.1080/00032710500423385.

12. Jellin JM, Gregory PJ et al. Natural Medicine Comprehensive Database. Therapeutic Research Faculty. 2013. http://www.naturaldatabase.com. Accessed July 11, 2012.

13. Jones SM, Zhong Z, Enomoto N, Schemmer P, Thurman RG. Dietary juniper berry oil minimizes hepatic reperfusion injury in the rat. *Hepatology.* 1998;28(4):1042–1050.

14. Final report on the safety assessment of *Juniperus communis* extract, *Juniperus oxycedrus* extract, *Juniperus oxycedrus* tar, *Juniperus phoenicea* extract, and *Juniperus virginiana* extract. *Int J Toxicol.* 2001;20(Suppl 2):41–56.

K

Kaempferol

definition

Common dietary flavonoid found in a wide variety of plant foods such as tea, broccoli, cabbage, kale, beans, endive, leek, tomato, and strawberry.[1]

scientific findings

According to a review of kaempferol, some epidemiological studies have found a positive association between the consumption of foods containing kaempferol and a reduced risk of developing cancer and cardiovascular disease.[1] Although two epidemiologic studies reported little association between dietary intake of kaempferol and lung cancer, a population-based case–control study (n = 558 lung cancer cases and 837 controls) found an inverse association between kaempferol intake and lung cancer among tobacco smokers.[2] Some experimental research has shown kaempferol and some of its glycosides to have a wide range of pharmacological activities, including analgesic, antiallergic, anticancer, antidiabetic, anti-inflammatory, antimicrobial, antiosteoporotic, antioxidant, antiapoptotic, anxiolytic, cardioprotective, estrogenic/antiestrogenic, and neuroprotective.[1,3]

bioactive dose

Not known.

safety

Presumed safe when consumed in normal dietary quantities by non-allergic individuals.

Kale (*Brassica oleracea* var. *acephala*)

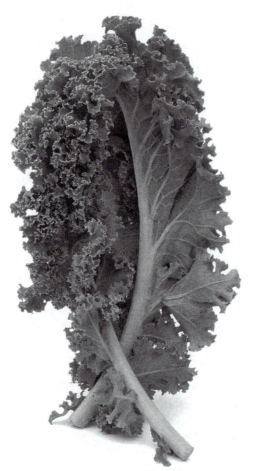

Kale. (Image from Binh Thanh Bui/Shutterstock.)

definition

Dark green leafy Brassica vegetable that is an excellent source of folate, vitamin C, β-carotene, vitamin K, and a good source of magnesium, in addition to supplying lutein, xeaxanthin, and allyl isothiocyanate.[4,5] Kale leaves and stems are chopped, sautéed with or without meat for flavoring, and served as greens or baked into kale chips. Baby kale is more tender than kale and is used as a salad green. The leaves of curly kale (*Brassica oleracea* L. convar. *acephala* var. *sabellica*) were found to contain dozens of different phenolic compounds in a laboratory analysis.[6]

scientific findings

Kale seeds exhibited antioxidant properties *in vitro*.[7]

bioactive dose

Not known.

safety

Presumed safe when consumed in normal dietary quantities by non-allergic individuals. The thiocyanate component of kale may induce hypothyroid effects in some individuals when kale is consumed and the amount may vary by individual.[8]

Key lime (Citrus aurantifolia)

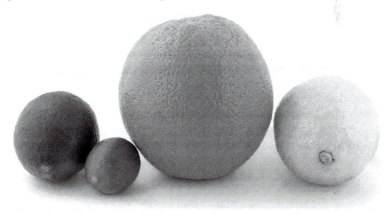

Note the small size of Key lime, second from left in this picture featuring lime and other citrus fruits. (Image from Alexandar Iotzov/Shutterstock.)

definition

Miniature lime named for one of its growing places, the Florida Keys. Adds zesty flavor to marinades, salads, and Key lime pie; also used to make limeade and to flavor and garnish beverages. A good source of vitamin C and flavonoids.[9]

scientific findings

Lime essential oil from lime peel reduced body weight in laboratory animals.[10]

bioactive dose

Not known.

safety

Presumed safe when consumed in normal dietary quantities by nonallergic individuals.[11] Lime juice administered enterally blocked ovulation and compromised fertility in laboratory animals.[12] Lime juice also reduced the effectiveness of warfarin in laboratory animals.[13] Although lime peel is considered to be "likely safe" when used orally in medicinal amounts, lime oil from lime peel contains photosensitizing constituents.[14]

Kiwifruit (Actinidia chinensis)

definition

Also called kiwi. Small green- or gold-fleshed fruit that is eaten fresh and, depending on the variety, is a source of vitamins C and E, phenolics, carotenoids, lutein, and xeaxanthin.[15,16] When its small, edible black seeds are consumed, one small, whole kiwifruit supplies 2 g of fiber.[16]

scientific findings

In experimental research, kiwifruit improved markers of immune function in mice.[17] Kiwifruit polysaccharides increased fibroblast activity in an *in vitro* study, which may have implications for human collagen synthesis.[18] According to a review, kiwi may improve laxation, aid digestion, and promote healthy gut microflora in humans, and, in addition, it has antioxidant and antiplatelet aggregatory properties.[19]

bioactive dose

Not known.

safety

Presumed safe when consumed in normal dietary quantities by non-allergic individuals.

Kumquat (Fortunella sp. Swingle)

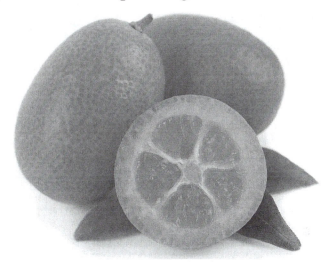

Kumquat. (Image from Volosina/Shutterstock.)

K

definition

Miniature citrus genus orange that is approximately the size and shape of a large olive. Its very thin peel is edible; however, its distinctive green seeds are bitter and are not intended to be eaten. Kumquats are a source of flavones, vitamin C, and the carotenoids α-carotene, β-crytopoxanthin, lutein, and xeaxanthin.[20] Kumquats can be eaten raw and whole or can be used to make marmalade. Canned, peeled kumquats are often served as desserts in Chinese restaurants.

scientific findings

See also *citrus.*

bioactive dose

Not known.

safety

Presumed safe when consumed in normal dietary quantities by non-allergic individuals.

References

1. Calderón-Montaño JM, Burgos-Morón E, Pérez-Guerrero C, López-Lázaro M. A review on the dietary flavonoid kaempferol. *Mini Rev Med Chem.* 2011;11(4):298–344.

2. Cui Y, Morgenstern H, Greenland S, Tashkin DP, Mao JT, Cai L, Cozen W, Mack TM, Lu QY, Zhang ZF. Dietary flavonoid intake and lung cancer— A population-based case–control study. *Cancer.* 2008;112(10):2241–2248. doi: 10.1002/cncr.23398.

3. Xiao J, Sun GB, Sun B, Wu Y, He L, Wang X, Chen RC, Cao L, Ren XY, Sun XB. Kaempferol protects against doxorubicin-induced cardiotoxicity *in vivo* and *in vitro. Toxicology.* 2012;292(1):53–62.

4. US Department of Agriculture. Agricultural Research Service. Nutrient Data Laboratory. Kale, raw. http://www.nal.usda.gov/fnic/foodcomp/cgi-bin/list_nut_edit.pl. Accessed January 4, 2012.

5. Fernandes F, Guedes de Pinho P, Valentão P, Pereira JA, Andrade PB. Volatile constituents throughout *Brassica oleracea* L. var. *acephala* germination. *J Agric Food Chem.* 2009;12;57(15):6795–6802.

6. Olsen H, Aaby K, Borge GIA. Characterization and quantification of flavonoids and hydroxycinnaminic acids in curly kale (*Brassica oleracea* L. convar. *acephala* var. *sabellica*) by HPLC-DAD-ESI-MS. *J Agric Food Chem.* 2009;57(7):2816–2825.

7. Ferreres F, Fernandes F, Sousa C, Valentão P, Pereira JA, Andrade PB. Metabolic and bioactivity insights into *Brassica oleracea* var. *acephala. J Agric Food Chem.* 2009;57(19):8884–8892.

8. Román GC. Autism: Transient in utero hypothyroxinemia related to maternal flavonoid ingestion during pregnancy and to other environmental antithyroid agents. *J Neurol Sci.* 2007;262(1–2):15–26.

9. Martí N, Mena DP, Cánovas JA, Micol V, Saura D. Vitamin C and the role of citrus juices as functional food. *Nat Prod Commun.* 2009;4(5):677–700.

10. Asnaashari S, Delazar A, Habibi B, Vasfi R, Nahar L, Hamedeyazdan S, Sarker SD. Essential oil from *Citrus aurantifolia* prevents ketotifen-induced weight-gain in mice. *Phytother Res.* 2010;24(12):1893–1897.

11. U.S. Government Publishing Office. Food and drugs. Substances Generally Recognized as Safe. http://www.ecfr.gov/cgi-bin/text-idx?rgn=div5&node=21:3.0.1.1.13#se21.3.182_11. Accessed January 21, 2015.

12. Salawu AA, Osinubi AA, Dosumu OO, Kusemiju TO, Noronha CC, Okanlawon AO. Effect of the juice of lime (*Citrus aurantifolia*) on estrous cycle and ovulation of Sprague-Dawley rats. *Endocr Pract.* 2010;16(4):561–565.

13. Adepoju G, Adeyemi T. Evaluation of the effect of lime fruit juice on the anticoagulant effect of warfarin. *J Young Pharm.* 2010;2(3):269–272.

14. Jellin JM, Gregory PJ et al. *Natural Medicine Comprehensive Database.* Therapeutic Research Faculty. 2013. http://www.naturaldatabase.com. Accessed July 11, 2012.

15. Nishiyama I, Fukuda T, Oota T. Genotypic differences in chlorophyll, lutein, and beta-carotene contents in the fruits of actinidia species. *J Agric Food Chem.* 2005;53(16):6403–6407.

16. US Department of Agriculture. Agricultural Research Service. Nutrient Database. Kiwifruit, green, raw. http://www.nal.usda.gov/fnic/foodcomp/cgi-bin/list_nut_edit.pl. Accessed May 12, 2011.

K

17. Hunter DC, Denis M, Parlane NA, Buddle BM, Stevenson LM, Skinner MA. Feeding ZESPRI GOLD Kiwifruit puree to mice enhances serum immunoglobulins specific for ovalbumin and stimulates ovalbumin-specific mesenteric lymph node cell proliferation in response to orally administered ovalbumin. *Nutr Res.* 2008;28(4):251–257.

18. Deters AM, Schröder KR, Hensel A. Kiwi fruit (*Actinidia chinensis* L.) polysaccharides exert stimulating effects on cell proliferation via enhanced growth factor receptors, energy production, and collagen synthesis of human keratinocytes, fibroblasts, and skin equivalents. *J Cell Physiol.* 2005;202(3):717–722.

19. Skinner MA, Loh JM, Hunter DC, Zhang J. Gold kiwifruit (*Actinidia chinensis* 'Hort16A') for immune support. *Proc Nutr Soc.* 2011;70(2):276–280.

20. US Department of Agriculture. Agricultural Research Service. National Nutrient Database. Kumquats, fresh. http://www.nal.usda.gov/fnic/food-comp/cgi-bin/list_nut_edit.pl. Accessed January 4, 2012.

K

L

Lactose

definition

Disaccharide that requires intestinal lactase for its digestion. In lactase deficiency, lactose maldigestion causes bloating, gas, abdominal pain, loose stools, and osmotic diarrhea. Lactose is a common food additive, appearing on label ingredient listings of breads, cereals, breakfast drinks, salad dressings, and cake mixes. Approximately 20% of prescription drug products and 5% of over-the-counter drug products may contain lactose.[1]

scientific findings

Lactose improves the absorption of calcium.[2] Lactose intolerance is a risk factor for low bone density[3] because milk avoidance limits calcium and vitamin D consumption.

bioactive dose

Not known.

safety

Presumed safe when consumed in normal dietary quantities, except by lactose-intolerant individuals who may experience symptoms after consuming even minute amounts of lactose.

Legume

definition

High-protein member of the Fabaceae family (formerly called Leguminosae), including starchy beans, such as black beans, garbanzo beans (also called chickpeas), kidney beans, lentils, pinto beans, and lima beans, but not string beans; and peas, such as black-eyed peas and split peas. Although recommended as a substitute for meat protein, only 7.9% of Americans consume legumes on a daily basis.[4] Eating approximately

1/2 cup of dry beans or peas increases intakes of fiber, protein, folate, zinc, iron, and magnesium without appreciably contributing to fat or saturated fat intake.[4] Legumes contain phytochemicals such as enzyme inhibitors, phytohemagglutinins (lectins), phytoestrogens, oligosaccharides, saponins, and phenolic compounds.[5] White beans can be substituted for other legumes, for example, chili can be made with 1/2 red kidney beans and 1/2 white beans; white beans are used to make minestrone soup.

scientific findings

A review of epidemiological evidence on diet and mortality in older adults found that in general, dietary patterns that demonstrated greater adherence to diets that emphasized whole fruits and vegetables, whole grains, low-fat dairy, lean meats, and legumes and nuts were inversely associated with mortality in adults aged 60 and older.[6] Legumes may help to control blood sugar in people with diabetes[7] due to their soluble fiber content. *In vitro*, white bean extract has been shown to block the carbohydrate-digesting enzyme α-amylase and is therefore being investigated for its potential to reduce carbohydrate absorption.[8] In a 4-week randomized, double-blind, placebo-controlled study (n = 25 healthy subjects), consumption of 1000 mg of white bean extract (equal to approximately 4 cups of legumes) or placebo twice a day before meals in conjunction with a multicomponent weight-loss program, including diet, exercise, and behavioral intervention, significantly reduced the weight and waist size of test subjects.[9] Legumes have a low glycemic index.[10] A high-legume, low-glycemic index diet improved serum leptin levels in insulin-resistant, middle-aged men.[10] A high-legume, high-fiber, low-glycemic index diet, compared to a healthy American diet, each eaten for 4 weeks, improved serum lipid profiles in men in a randomized, controlled crossover feeding study (n = 64 middle-aged men).[11]

bioactive dose

While there is no daily recommendation for legumes *per se*, ChooseMyPlate. gov promotes legume consumption and suggests adults aged 19–50 ingest 5–5.5 oz equivalents (1 oz equivalent = 1/4 cup of cooked beans) daily from all protein sources.[12]

safety

Presumed safe when consumed in normal dietary quantities by non-allergic individuals.

Lemon (Citrus limon)

definition

Popular citrus fruit used to add tang to salads and seafood, to marinate, and to make juice drinks. Its citrate content is the highest among citrus fruits.[13] Lemon juice is an excellent source of vitamin C and is also a source of liminoid, β-cryptoxanthin, lutein, xeaxanthin, coumarins, hesperetin, quercetin, and myricetin.[14,15]

scientific findings

Lemon essential oil from lemon peel, when sprayed as an aerosol, reduced *Staphylococci*, *Streptococci*, and *Sarcina* in the air.[16] Lemonade has been studied in small groups of patients to evaluate its ability to increase urinary citrate levels, a desirable effect in preventing kidney stones. Drinking lemonade compared to taking potassium citrate improved urine volume, a desirable effect, in a small prospective, cross-over design trial (n = 21 subjects at risk for stone formation). Lemonade, however, did not improve urinary citrate or urinary pH while potassium citrate did, and neither treatment improved uric acid level.[17] In a second small trial (n = 12 patients who were either noncompliant with or intolerant of pharmacological citrate therapy), patients supplemented their routine diet with lemonade citrate (made with 4 oz of reconstituted lemon juice) consumed at uniform intervals throughout the day. "Citrate supplementation with lemonade increased urinary citrate levels more than two-fold without changing total urinary volume."[18] In a third trial, 11 men and women, mean age 52.7 years, were treated with lemonade therapy for a mean of 44.4 months. The control group, 11 men and women mean age 54.5 years, were treated with potassium citrate for a mean of 42.5 months. Of the 11 patients on lemonade, 10 demonstrated increased urinary citrate levels, and all potassium citrate therapy subjects demonstrated an increase in urinary citrate. During lemonade therapy, the stone formation rate decreased from 1.00 to 0.13 stones per patient per year. Researchers in this trial concluded that lemonade appears to be a reasonable alternative for patients with hypocitraturia who cannot tolerate first line therapy due to its significant citraturic effect.[13]

bioactive dose

Not known.

safety

Presumed safe when consumed in normal dietary quantities by non-allergic individuals.

Lemongrass (Cymbopogon citratus)

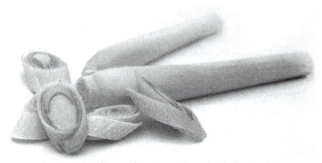

Lemongrass. (Image from tarmizi razali/Shutterstock.)

L

definition

Tropical grass used in cooking that resembles a small hard stalk. Lemongrass is chopped finely and used as a spice in Thai cooking to impart intense lemon flavor. Lemongrass tea has been used in traditional medicine to treat hypertension and diabetes.[19]

scientific findings

Lemongrass essential oil, when sprayed as an aerosol, reduced airborne microorganism contaminants.[16] Laboratory research suggests that anti-inflammatory compounds in lemongrass work by inhibiting the release of pro-inflammatory cytokines.[20] Lemongrass attenuated animal liver damage in an experimental study.[21]

bioactive dose

Not known.

safety

Presumed safe when consumed in normal dietary quantities by non-allergic individuals.

Lettuce (Lactuca sativa)

definition

Salad green available in different varieties, such as Bibb, a tender lettuce that grows in small, loose heads, and lola rosa (also spelled lolla rossa and lolla rosa), a loose-leaf lettuce variety that has a mild taste, green leaves at its base, and ruffled burgundy leaves near the ends.[22] *Lactuca*, the Roman name for lettuce, comes from "lac" (milk) because wild lettuce contains a milky sap. Lettuce was traditionally eaten at the end of the evening meal because it was thought to produce a mild, sedative effect; it may also have been eaten at the beginning of a meal to enhance appetite.[22] Nutritional content varies by variety. Bibb is a source of folate, vitamin A, and vitamin K,[23] and contains the phytochemical xeaxanthin.[24] Lola rosa is a source of vitamin K, potassium, calcium, copper, manganese, fiber, β-carotene, lutein, xeaxanthin, quercetin, and, concentrated in its intense red-pigmented parts, anthocyanins.[25-29]

scientific findings

A lettuce-derived protein elicited antibodies with positive reactivity against human immunodeficiency virus isolates in a laboratory study, as well as systemic and local immune responses when administered to mice.[30]

bioactive dose

Not known.

safety

Presumed safe when consumed in normal dietary quantities by non-allergic individuals.

Licorice (Glycyrrhiza glabra)

definition

Root of the licorice shrub that is processed as a flavoring agent and included in some authentically flavored licorice foods and candies, though most "licorice" candy sold in the United States is actually flavored with anise, not licorice, and therefore is not a source of licorice or active licorice compounds.[31] True licorice extract contains the active ingredients glycyrrhizin and glycyrrhizic acid. The body converts glycyrrhizin to a metabolite compound, glycyrrhetinic acid.[32] Deglycyrrhizinated licorice extracts are also available to make licorice candy. Licorice has a history of use for gastrointestinal symptoms[31] and chronic hepatitis.[33]

scientific findings

There are not enough reliable data to determine whether licorice is effective for any health condition.[34] Glycyrrhizic acid was attributed to improving lipoprotein lipase activity, insulin sensitivity,[35] and dyslipidemia[36] in obese laboratory animals.

bioactive dose

Not known.

safety

Licorice is likely safe when used orally in amounts commonly found in foods.[37] Licorice glycyrrhizin, glycyrrhizic acid, and/or glycyrrhetinic acid may cause increased potassium excretion, sodium and water retention, body weight gain, hypertension, hypokalemia, alkalosis, suppression of the renin–angiotensin–aldosterone system, and muscular paralysis.[33,38,39] Habitual licorice ingestion, which has been defined as "consuming 30 g or more of licorice daily for several weeks" can cause severe adverse events including hypertension, hypokalemia, alkalosis, weakness, paralysis, and occasionally encephalopathy in otherwise healthy people.[37] Additionally, ingestion of antituberculosis agents containing licorice and long-term ingestion of licorice-containing agents for chronic gastritis, chronic hepatitis, or chronic dermatitis were implicated in 59 cases of glycyrrhizin (licorice)-induced hypokalemic myopathy involving quadriplegia, muscle pain, peripheral dysesthesia in the extremities, and numbness.[40] Large amounts of *G. glabra* must be avoided in pregnancy because it may increase the risk of preterm labor.[31,41]

Lignan

definition

Phytoestrogen that is prominent in the Western diet,[42] classes of which include enterolactone and enterodiol.[43] Lignan is found in flaxseed, pumpkin seed, sesame seed, soybean, broccoli, whole grains, beans, peas, and some berries.[43,44] Lignan should not be confused with lignin (a polymer of phenolic compounds that occurs naturally in plants).[45]

scientific findings

Although additional research is required to understand the association between lignan exposure and breast cancer risk, a meta-analysis of 21 epidemiologic studies concluded that "high lignan exposure might be associated with a reduced breast cancer risk in postmenopausal women."[42] GI microorganisms interacting with lignan enterodiol and enterolactone have generated bioactive compounds that retarded experimentally induced cancer.[46]

bioactive dose

Not known.

safety

Presumed safe when consumed in normal dietary quantities by non-allergic individuals.

Liminoid

definition

Prominent group of secondary metabolites, some of which have a bitter flavor,[47] that are found in tangerine, grapefruit, and other *Citrus* genus fruits and their juices. Examples of limonoids include aglycones, such as limonin, and glucosides, such as limonin glucoside.[48,49]

scientific findings

Compounds belonging to this group have exhibited biological activities such as antibacterial, antifungal, antimalarial, anticancer, and antiviral, in laboratory studies.[50]

bioactive dose

Not known.

safety

Presumed safe when consumed in normal dietary quantities by non-allergic individuals.

Limonene

definition

Terpene found in high concentration in orange, lemon, mandarin, lime, and grapefruit oils.[51] Ingested when the zest, or peel of citrus fruits, is consumed; also used as a flavoring agent in fruit juices, soft drinks, baked goods, ice cream, and pudding.[51]

scientific findings

Limonene exhibited chemopreventive activity against rat mammary cancer.[52,53] Preliminary data suggest that limonene has shown some efficacy in the chemoprevention and chemotherapy of human malignancies, according to a review.[52]

safety

Presumed safe when consumed in normal dietary quantities by non-allergic individuals.

L

Lingonberry (*Vaccinium vitis-idaea*)

definition

Relative of a cranberry that is a popular fresh fruit in Scandinavian countries, but is available for sale in the United States as jam. Contains anthocyanins, flavonols, resveratrol, and procyanidin.[54] Lingonberry has been used for its antioxidant properties in traditional medicine.

scientific findings

In laboratory studies, the phenolics in lingonberries were effective free radical scavengers[54] and were antimicrobial against *Staphylococcus aureus*.[55]

bioactive dose

Not known.

safety

Presumed safe when consumed in normal dietary quantities by non-allergic individuals.

Lutein

definition

Xanthophyll carotenoid that commonly occurs with xeaxanthin in foods. Lutein and xeaxanthin are considered to be one of the major categories of carotenoids[56] and are responsible for the yellow color in foods and the macula region of the retina.[57] Dark green vegetables are a source of lutein: there are 44 mg of lutein/cup of cooked kale, 26 mg/cup of cooked spinach, and 3 mg/cup of broccoli.[37]

scientific findings

The macular pigment may protect retinal cells from damage due to light by absorbing blue light. There is also "epidemiological evidence that the amount of macular pigment is inversely associated with the incidence of age-related macular degeneration."[57] A meta-analysis reported that dietary lutein (and xeaxanthin) is not significantly associated with a reduced risk of early age-related macular degeneration, whereas an increase in the intake of these carotenoids may be protective against late age-related macular degeneration.[58] Age-related macular degeneration is an irreversible process that is a major cause of blindness in the elderly.[57] Epidemiology suggests a reduced risk of developing severe cataracts in people consuming higher amounts of lutein in their diet.[37] People consuming 6.9–11.7 mg of lutein per day through diet had the lowest risk of developing age-related macular degeneration and cataracts, according to two large cohort studies (n = 36,644 men; n = 77,466 women).[37] Population research suggests that increasing intake of dietary lutein does not decrease the risk of developing coronary heart disease.[37]

bioactive dose

A dose of 6 mg of food lutein has been used for reducing the risk of cataract and age-related macular degeneration.[37]

safety

Presumed safe when consumed in normal dietary quantities by non-allergic individuals. Dietary lutein intake of 6.9–11.7 mg/day is considered "high intake" and appears to be safe.[37]

Lychee fruit (also spelled litchi, *Litchi chinensis*)

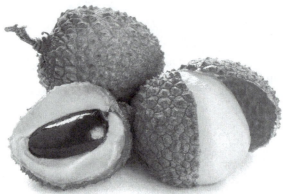

Lychee. (Image from Subbotina Anna/Shutterstock.)

definition

Small, oval-shaped fruit with an inedible skin, whose white or pink-ish white flesh tastes like a grape. Lychee is a source of vitamin C, all B vitamins except B12, calcium, iron, potassium, and polyphenolic compounds.[59,60] Lychee fruit can be eaten fresh or peeled, pitted and canned in syrup.

scientific findings

Polyphenolic compounds from lychee fruits were strong antioxidants in laboratory studies.[60]

bioactive dose

Not known.

safety

Presumed safe when consumed in normal dietary quantities by non-allergic individuals.

Lycopene (Solanum lycopersicum)

definition

Carotenoid antioxidant that imparts pink and red pigments to plant foods such as watermelon, pink grapefruit, guava, and tomatoes. Approximately 85% of the dietary lycopene intake in the United States is from tomatoes.[61]

One cup (240 mL) of tomato juice provides about 23 mg of lycopene. Dietary lycopene intake increases plasma levels of lycopene.[62] Lycopene is found primarily as *trans*-lycopene in food sources; some *trans*-lycopene is converted into *cis*-lycopene due to body metabolism of lycopene.[63]

scientific findings

The Food and Drug Administration found no association between lycopene intake and reduced risk of breast, colorectal, endometrial, gastric, lung, ovarian, prostate, or pancreatic cancer in its 2004 review of lycopene for qualified health claim status.[64] Lycopene may help to alleviate cellular oxidative stress.[65] Observational studies in many countries have shown that the risk for some types of cancer is lower in individuals who have higher levels of lycopene in their blood.[66] Whereas some epidemiological research suggests that a low serum concentration of lycopene is associated with age-related macular degeneration risk,[67] pooled results from nine prospective cohort studies (n = 149,203 people) found that intake of certain carotenoids, including lycopene, had little or no effect on the primary prevention of early age-related macular degeneration.[68] A small clinical trial (n = 55: 34 patients with age-related macular degeneration and 21 control subjects) found that lycopene levels in age-related macular degeneration patients was significantly decreased in serum, in LDL, and in HDL.[67] A review of epidemiological evidence on lycopene and cardiovascular disease in women found that higher serum lycopene levels were associated with reduced risk of cardiovascular disease in some, but not all, studies. In men, it appeared that dietary intake of lycopene was not associated with a reduced risk of cardiovascular disease.[37] Men's consumption of 12 g/day of dietary lycopene and women's consumption of 6.5 mg/day of dietary lycopene was associated with a decreased risk of lung cancer in nonsmoking men and women in an observational study.[37] Epidemiological research shows no association between dietary lycopene intake and the risk of developing colon cancer.[37] A meta-analysis that included 10 clinical trials found no evidence of an association between lycopene intake and the risk for having type 2 diabetes.[62] Circulating lycopene was protective against human papilloma virus progression to cervical neoplasia, according to the findings of a small case–control study in women (n = 32 subjects with incident cervical dysplasia and 113 control subjects with normal cervical cytology), a nonsignificant finding due to small sample size.[69] In a case–control study, a 56% reduction in human papilloma virus persistence risk was observed in women with the highest plasma lycopene concentrations compared with women with the lowest plasma lycopene concentrations.[63] "Lycopene induces responses in human prostate epithelial cells that are antiproliferative, antioxidative, and anti-inflammatory, as well as downregulating targets in the androgen receptor signaling pathway."[70]

It has been suggested that lycopene is negatively associated with the risk of prostate cancer.[71] In a large epidemiological study, a cohort of the Health Professionals Follow-up Study (n = 47,894 subjects initially free of diagnosed cancer), increased dietary lycopene intake from foods was associated with a lower risk of developing prostate cancer: Researchers found that combined lycopene intake from tomatoes, tomato sauce, tomato juice, and pizza, which accounted for 82% of lycopene intake, was inversely associated with the risk of prostate cancer for consumption frequency greater than 10 servings per week versus less than 1.5 servings per week.[72] The Prostate Cancer Prevention Trial (n = 9559 participants) found no association between dietary intake of lycopene and prostate cancer risk.[73] An analysis of The Prostate Cancer Prevention Trial reiterated that findings suggest no association between serum lycopene and prostate cancer risk.[74] Three randomized clinical trials (n = 154 participants) found "no statistical difference in prostate-specific antigen levels between men randomized to receive lycopene and control subjects."[75] There is "insufficient evidence to either support, or refute, the use of lycopene for the prevention of prostate cancer, and no robust evidence from randomized clinical trials to identify the impact of lycopene consumption upon the incidence of prostate cancer, prostate symptoms, prostate specific antigen levels or adverse events."[75]

L

bioactive dose

Not known.

safety

Presumed safe when consumed in normal dietary quantities by non-allergic individuals. Some research suggests that lycopene, in significant quantities as are found in large doses, for example, in dietary supplements but not foods, might worsen established cancers of the prostate.[61]

References

1. Whitney E, Rolfes SR. *Understanding Nutrition*, 11th edn. Belmont, CA: Thomson Higher Education; 2008.
2. Cámara-Martos F, Amaro-López MA. Influence of dietary factors on calcium bioavailability: A brief review. *Biol Trace Elem Res.* 2002;89(1):43–52.
3. Savaiano D. Lactose intolerance: An unnecessary risk for low bone density. *Nestle Nutr Workshop Ser Pediatr Program.* 2011;67:161–171. Epub 2011 February 16.
4. Mitchell DC, Lawrence FR, Hartman TJ, Curran JM. Consumption of dry beans, peas, and lentils could improve diet quality in the US population. *J Am Diet Assoc.* 2009;109(5):909–913. doi: 10.1016/j.jada.2009.02.029.

5. Huang WY, Davidge ST, Wu J. Bioactive natural constituents from food sources-potential use in hypertension prevention and treatment. *Crit Rev Food Sci Nutr.* 2013;53(6):615–630. doi: 10.1080/10408398.2010.550071.

6. Ford DW, Jensen GL, Hartman TJ, Wray L, Smiciklas-Wright H. Association between dietary quality and mortality in older adults: A review of the epidemiological evidence. *J Nutr Gerontol Geriatr.* 2013;32(2):85–105. doi: 10.1080/21551197.2013.779622.

7. No author. Beans may help control blood sugar in people with diabetes. *Harv Health Lett.* 2013;38(3):8.

8. Udani J, Hardy M, Madsen DC. Blocking carbohydrate absorption and weight loss: A clinical trial using phase 2 brand proprietary fractionated white bean extract. *Altern Med Rev.* 2004;9(1):63–69.

9. Udani J, Singh BB. Blocking carbohydrate absorption and weight loss: A clinical trial using a proprietary fractionated white bean extract. *Altern Ther Health Med.* 2007;13(4):32–37.

10. Zhang Z, Lanza E, Ross AC, Albert PS, Colburn NH, Rovine MJ, Bagshaw D, Ulbrecht JS, Hartman TJ. A high-legume low-glycemic index diet reduces fasting plasma leptin in middle-aged insulin-resistant and -sensitive men. *Eur J Clin Nutr.* 2011;65(3):415–418. Epub 2011 January 5.

11. Zhang Z, Lanza E, Kris-Etherton PM, Colburn NH, Bagshaw D, Rovine MJ, Ulbrecht JS et al. A high legume low glycemic index diet improves serum lipid profiles in men. *Lipids.* 2010;45(9):765–775. doi: 10.1007/s11745-010-3463-7. Epub 2010 August 24.

12. US Department of Agriculture. Choose MyPlate.gov. How much food from the protein foods group is needed daily? http://myplate.gov/printpages/MyPlateFoodGroups/ProteinFoods/food-groups.protein-foods-amount.pdf. Accessed July 28, 2013.

13. Kang DE, Sur RL, Haleblian GE, Fitzsimons NJ, Borawski KM, Preminger GM. Long-term lemonade based dietary manipulation in patients with hypocitraturic nephrolithiasis. *J Urol.* 2007;177(4):1358–1362.

14. US Department of Agriculture. Agricultural Research Service. Nutrient Data Laboratory. US Department of Agriculture. Lemon juice, raw. http://ndb.nal.usda.gov/ndb/foods/show/2274?fg=&man=&lfacet=&format=&count=&max=25&offset=&sort=&qlookup=lemon+juice. Accessed January 8, 2012.

15. US Department of Agriculture. Agricultural Research Center. Phytochemical Database. Citrus limon. http://www.pl.barc.usda.gov/usda_rrcp/rrecipe_detail.cfm?code=69685564&id=62&ThisName=sd1. Accessed January 8, 2012.

16. Janssen AM, Scheffer JJC, Svendsen AB. Antimicrobial activities of essential oils. A 1976–1986 literature review on possible applications. *Pharm Weekbl* [*Sci*]. 1987;9:193–197.

17. Koff SG, Paquette EL, Cullen J, Gancarczyk KK, Tucciarone PR, Schenkman NS. Comparison between lemonade and potassium citrate and impact on urine pH and 24-hour urine parameters in patients with kidney stone formation. *Urology.* 2007;69(6):1013–1016.

18. Seltzer MA, Low RK, McDonald M, Shami GS, Stoller ML. Dietary manipulation with lemonade to treat hypocitraturic calcium nephrolithiasis. *J Urol.* 1996;156(3):907–909.

L

19. Campos J, Schmeda-Hirschmann G, Leiva E, Guzmán L, Orrego R, Fernández P, González M et al. Lemon grass (*Cymbopogon citratus* (D.C) Stapf) polyphenols protect human umbilical vein endothelial cell (HUVECs) from oxidative damage induced by high glucose, hydrogen peroxide and oxidised low-density lipoprotein. *Food Chem.* 2014;151:175–181. doi: 10.1016/j. foodchem.2013.11.018. Epub 2013 November 14.

20. Salim E, Kumolosasi E, Jantan I. Inhibitory effect of selected medicinal plants on the release of pro-inflammatory cytokines in lipopolysaccharide-stimulated human peripheral blood mononuclear cells. *J Nat Med.* 2014;68(3):647–653. Epub 2014 May 6.

21. Rahim SM, Taha EM, Al-janabi MS, Al-douri BI, Simon KD, Mazlan AG. Hepatoprotective effect of *Cymbopogon citratus* aqueous extract against hydrogen peroxide-induced liver injury in male rats. *Afr J Tradit Complementary Altern Med.* 2014;11(2):447–451.

22. Yuma County Cooperative Extension. Lolla rosa. http://cals.arizona.edu/ fps/sites/cals.arizona.edu.fps/files/cotw/Lolla_Rosa.pdf. Accessed January 1, 2012.

23. US Department of Agriculture. Agricultural Research Service. National Nutrient Database. Bibb lettuce. http://www.nal.usda.gov/fnic/foodcomp/ cgi-bin/list_nut_edit.pl. Accessed March 23, 2011.

24. Yang Z, Zhang Z, Penniston KL, Binkley N, Tanumihardjo SA. Serum carotenoid concentrations in postmenopausal women from the United States with and without osteoporosis. *Int J Vitam Nutr Res.* 2008;78(3):105–111. doi: 10.1024/0300-9831.78.3.105.

25. Crozier A, Lean MEJ, McDonald MS, Black C. Quantitative analysis of the flavonoid content of commercial tomatoes, onions, lettuce, and celery. *J Agric Food Chem.* 1997;45(3):590–595.

26. Koudela M, Petříková K. Nutrients content and yield in selected cultivars of leaf lettuce (*Lactuca sativa* L. var. crispa). *Hort Sci (Prague).* 2008;35(3):99–106.

27. US Department of Agriculture. Agricultural Research Service. Nutrient Data Lab. Red leaf lettuce. http://www.nal.usda.gov/fnic/foodcomp/cgi-bin/list_nut_edit.pl. Accessed January 8, 2012.

28. Lazic B, Lazic S, Sekulic P. Effect of species and variety on the content of macroelements and micronutrients in lettuce. *Acta Hort.* (*ISHS*) 2002;579:609–612 http://www.actahort.org/books/579/579_107.htm. Accessed July 11, 2010.

29. US Department of Agriculture. Agricultural Research Service. Phytochemical Database. *Lactuca sativa* (Romaine lettuce). http://www. pl.barc.usda.gov/usda_rrcp/rrecipe_detail.cfm?code=69685564&id=55&ThisName=sd1. Accessed January 8, 2012.

30. Govea-Alonso DO, Rubio-Infante N, García-Hernández AL, Varona-Santos JT, Korban SS, Moreno-Fierros L, Rosales-Mendoza S. Immunogenic properties of a lettuce-derived C4(V3)6 multiepitopic HIV protein. *Planta.* 2013;238(4):785–792. Epub 2013 July 30.

31. DerMarderosian A, Beutler J. *Review of Natural Products,* 5th edn. St. Louis, MO: Wolters Kluwer Health; 2008.

32. Werbach MR, Murray MT. *Botanical Influences on Illness,* 2nd ed. Tarzana, CA: Third Line Press, Inc.; 2000.

33. Fujiwara Y, Kikkawa R, Nakata K, Kitamura E, Takama T, Shigeta Y. Hypokalemia and sodium retention in patients with diabetes and chronic hepatitis receiving insulin and glycyrrhizin. *Endocrinol J.* 1983;30(2):243–249.

34. National Institutes of Health. National Center for Complementary and Alternative Medicine. Licorice root. http://nccam.nih.gov/health/licoriceroot/D318_Herbs.pdf. Accessed April 2, 2011.

35. Eu CH, Lim WY, Ton SH, bin Abdul Kadir K. Glycyrrhizic acid improved lipoprotein lipase expression, insulin sensitivity, serum lipid and lipid deposition in high-fat diet-induced obese rats. *Lipids Health Dis.* 2010;29(9):81.

36. Lim WY, Chia YY, Liong SY, Ton SH, Kadir KA, Husain SN. Lipoprotein lipase expression, serum lipid and tissue lipid deposition in orally-administered glycyrrhizic acid-treated rats. *Lipids Health Dis.* 2009;8:31.

37. Jellin JM, Gregory PJ. *Natural Medicine Comprehensive Database.* Therapeutic Research Faculty. 2013. http://www.naturaldatabase.com. Accessed July 11, 2012.

38. Heikens J, Fliers E, Endert E, Ackermans M, van Montfrans G. Liquorice-induced hypertension—A new understanding of an old disease: Case report and brief review. *Neth J Med.* 1995;47:230–234.

39. Cosmetic Ingredient Review Expert Panel. Final report on the safety assessment of glycyrrhetinic acid, potassium glycyrrhetinate, disodium succinoyl glycyrrhetinate, glyceryl glycyrrhetinate, glycyrrhetinyl stearate, stearyl glycyrrhetinate, glycyrrhizic acid, ammonium glycyrrhizate, dipotassium glycyrrhizate, disodium glycyrrhizate, trisodium glycyrrhizate, methyl glycyrrhizate, and potassium glycyrrhizinate. *Int J Toxicol.* 2007;26(2):79–112.

40. Shintani S, Murase H, Tsukagoshi H, Shiigai T. Glycyrrhizin (licorice)-induced hypokalemic myopathy. Report of 2 cases and review of the literature. *Eur Neurol.* 1992;32(1):44–51.

41. National Institutes of Medicine. National Center for Complementary and Alternative Medicine. Licorice root. http://nccam.nih.gov/health/root/. Accessed April 2, 2011.

42. Buck K, Zaineddin AK, Vrieling A, Linseis en J, Chang-Claude J. Meta-analyses of lignans and enterolignans in relation to breast cancer risk. *Am J Clin Nutr.* 2010;92(1):141–153.

43. Birt DF, Shull JD, Yaktine AL. Chemoprevention of cancer. In: Shils ME, Olson JA, Shike M, Ross CA, eds . *Modern Nutrition in Health and Disease*, 9th edn. Baltimore, MD: Williams & Wilkins; 1998.

44. Touré A, Xueming X. Flaxseed lignans: Source, biosynthesis, metabolism, antioxidant activity, bio-active components, and health benefits. *Comp Rev Food Sci F.* 2010;9(3):261–269.

45. Baurhoo B, Ruiz-Feria CA, Zhao X. Purified lignin: Nutritional and health impacts on farm animals—A review. *Anim Feed Sci Technol.* 2008;144(3–4):175–184.

46. Davis CD, Milner JA. Gastrointestinal microflora, food components and colon cancer prevention. *J Nutr Biochem.* 2009;20(10):743–752. Epub 2009 August 27.

47. Manners GD. Citrus limonoids: Analysis, bioactivity, and biomedical prospects. *J Agric Food Chem.* 2007;55(21):8285–8294. Epub 2007 September 25.

48. Fong CH, Hasegawa S, Herman Z, Ou P. Limonoid glucosides in commercial citrus juices. *J Food Sci.* 1989;54:1505–1506. doi: 10.1111/j.1365-2621.1989.tb05146.x.

49. Vikram A, Jayaprakasha GK. Simultaneous determination of citrus limonoid aglycones and glucosides by high performance liquid chromatography. *Anal Chim Acta.* 2007;590(2):180–186. Epub 2007 March 18.

50. Roy A, Saraf S. Limonoids: Overview of significant bioactive triterpenes distributed in plants kingdom. *Biol Pharm Bull.* 2006;29(2):191–201.

51. Sun J. D-limonene: Safety and clinical applications. *Altern Med Rev.* 2007;12(3):259–264.

52. Crowell PL. Monoterpenes in breast cancer chemoprevention. *Breast Cancer Res Treat.* 1997;46(2–3):191–197.

53. Miller JA, Hakim IA, Chew W, Thompson P, Thomson CA, Chow HH. Adipose tissue accumulation of d-limonene with the consumption of a lemonade preparation rich in d-limonene content. *Nutr Cancer.* 2010;62(6):783–788.

54. Zheng W, Wang SY. Oxygen radical absorbing capacity of phenolics in blueberries, cranberries, chokeberries, and lingonberries. *J Agric Food Chem.* 2003;51(2):502–509.

55. Kylli P, Nohynek L, Puupponen-Pimiä R, Westerlund-Wikström B, Leppänen T, Welling J, Moilanen E, Heinonen M. Lingonberry (*Vaccinium vitis-idaea*) and European cranberry (*Vaccinium microcarpon*) proanthocyanidins: Isolation, identification, and bioactivities. *J Agric Food Chem.* 2011;59(7):3373–3384. Epub 2011 March 3.

56. Lee HS, Cho YH, Park J, Shin HR, Sung MK. Dietary intake of phytonutrients in relation to fruit and vegetable consumption in Korea. *J Acad Nutr Diet.* 2013;113(9):1194–1199. doi: 10.1016/j.jand.2013.04.022. Epub 2013 July 3.

57. Krinsky NI, Landrum JT, Bone RA. Biologic mechanisms of the protective role of lutein and xeaxanthin in the eye. *Annu Rev Nutr.* 2003;23:171–201.

58. Ma L, Dou HL, Wu YQ, Huang YM, Xu XR, Zou ZY, Lin XM. Lutein and xeaxanthin intake and the risk of age-related macular degeneration: A systematic review and meta-analysis. *Br J Nutr.* 2012;107(3):350–359.

59. US Department of Agriculture. Agricultural Research Service. Nutrient Data Laboratory. Litchee fruit. http://ndb.nal.usda.gov/ndb/foods/show/2 281?fg=&man=&lfacet=&format=&count=&max=25&offset=&sort=&qlook up=lychee+fruit. Accessed July 7, 2013.

60. Purdue University Center for New Crops and Plant Products. Lychee *Litchi chinensis* sonn. *Nephelium litchi* cambess. http://www.hort.purdue.edu/newcrop/morton/lychee.html. Accessed January 8, 2012.

61. US National Library of Medicine. National Institutes of Health. Medline Plus. Lycopene. http://www.nlm.nih.gov/medlineplus/druginfo/natural/554.html. Accessed March 16, 2011.

62. Valero MA, Vidal A, Burgos R, Calvo FL, Martínez C, Luengo LM, Cuerda C. Meta-analysis on the role of lycopene in type 2 diabetes mellitus. *Nutr Hosp.* 2011;26(6):1236–1241. doi: 10.1590/S0212-16112011000600007.

63. Sedjo RL, Roe DJ, Abrahamsen M, Harris RB, Craft N, Baldwin S, Giuliano AR. Vitamin A, carotenoids, and risk of persistent oncogenic human papillomavirus infection. *Cancer Epidemiol Biomarkers Prev.* 2002;11(9):876–884.

64. Kavanaugh CJ, Trumbo PR, Ellwood KC. The U.S. Food and Drug Administration's evidence-based review for qualified health claims: Tomatoes, lycopene, and cancer. *J Natl Cancer Inst.* 2007;99(14):1074–1085. Epub 2007 July 10.

65. Chen J, Song Y, Zhang L. Effect of lycopene supplementation on oxidative stress: An exploratory systematic review and meta-analysis of randomized controlled trials. *J Med Food.* 2013;16(5):361–374. doi: 10.1089/jmf.2012.2682. Epub 2013 April 30.

L

66. American Cancer Society. Lycopene. http://www.cancer.org/Treatment/ TreatmentsandSideEffects/ComplementaryandAlternativeMedicine/ DietandNutrition/lycopene. Accessed January 29, 2012.

67. Cardinault N, Abalain JH, Sairafi B, Coudray C, Grolier P, Rambeau M, Carré JL, Mazur A, Rock E. Lycopene but not lutein nor xeaxanthin decreases in serum and lipoproteins in age-related macular degeneration patients. *Clin Chim Acta*. 2005;357(1):34–42.

68. Chong EW, Wong TY, Kreis AJ, Simpson JA, Guymer RH. Dietary antioxidants and primary prevention of age-related macular degeneration: Systematic review and meta-analysis. *BMJ*. 2007;335(7623):755. Epub 2007 October 8.

69. Kanetsky PA, Gammon MD, Mandelblatt J, Zhang Z-F, Ramsey E, Dnistrian A, Norkusg EP, Wright Jr. TC. Dietary intake and blood levels of lycopene: Association with cervical dysplasia among non-hispanic, black women. *Nutr Cancer*. 1998;31(1):31–40.

70. Sporn MB, Liby KT. Is lycopene an effective agent for preventing prostate cancer? *Cancer Prev Res (Phila)*. 2013;6(5):384–386. doi: 10.1158/1940-6207. CAPR-13-0026. Epub 2013 March 12.

71. Vance TM, Su J, Fontham ET, Koo SI, Chun OK. Dietary antioxidants and prostate cancer: A review. *Nutr Cancer*. 2013;65(6):793–801. doi: 10.1080/01635581.2013.806672.

72. Giovannucci E, Ascherio A, Rimm EB, Stampfer MJ, Colditz GA, Willett WC. Intake of carotenoids and retinol in relation to risk of prostate cancer. *J Natl Cancer Inst*. 1995;87(23):1767–1776.

73. Kristal AR, Arnold KB, Neuhouser ML, Goodman P, Platz EA, Albanes D, Thompson IM. Diet, supplement use, and prostate cancer risk: Results from the prostate cancer prevention trial. *Am J Epidemiol*. 2010;172(5):566–577. doi: 10.1093/aje/kwq148. Epub 2010 August 6.

74. Giovannucci E. Commentary: Serum lycopene and prostate cancer progression: A re-consideration of findings from the prostate cancer prevention trial. *Cancer Causes Control*. 2011;22(7):1055–1059. doi: 10.1007/s10552-011-9776-x. Epub 2011 May 15.

75. Ilic D, Forbes KM, Hassed C. Lycopene for the prevention of prostate cancer. *Cochrane Database Syst Rev*. 2011;(11):CD008007. doi: 10.1002/14651858. CD008007.pub2.

L

M

Magnesium

definition

Fourth most abundant mineral in the body, magnesium is necessary for reactions in energy metabolism, vitamin D metabolism and/or action, bone cell activity, regulating the electrical activity of the heart, helping to maintain normal muscle and nerve function, immunity, helping to regulate blood sugar levels, and maintaining normal blood pressure.[1-3] Magnesium is a constituent of bone[4] and most body magnesium is found in bone.[3] Magnesium is withdrawn from bone to maintain blood levels when dietary intake of magnesium is inadequate.[5] Good sources of magnesium include dark green vegetables, such as broccoli, and dark green leafy vegetables, such as curly kale. The chlorophyll molecule contains magnesium.[3] Other good sources include whole grains, such as oatmeal and raisin bran (the bran and germ contain magnesium); nuts and peanut butter; legumes; halibut; and cocoa products.[3] The following foods supply approximately 100 mg: 4 slices of whole grain bread, 1 cup of beans, 1/4 cup of nuts, 1/2 cup of cooked spinach, or 3 bananas.[3] Hard, mineral-rich water, known to be a source of certain cardioprotective nutrients, including magnesium, is associated with decreased arterial blood pressure and blood lipids.[6]

Approximately one-half of the U.S. population has magnesium intakes below their RDA,[7] but children aged 4–8 appear to meet their magnesium RDA.[4] Among the groups with lowest intake are African-Americans and older adults in every racial and ethnic group.[2]

scientific findings

Hypomagnesemia occurs due to vomiting, diarrhea, alcohol abuse, protein malnutrition, prolonged nutritionally inadequate intravenous fluid use, poorly controlled diabetes, and use of diuretic medications.[2,8] Magnesium deficiency can initially result in muscle cramps, hypertension, coronary and cerebral vasospasms, loss of appetite, nausea, vomiting, fatigue, and weakness.[2] As magnesium deficiency worsens, numbness, tingling, muscle contractions and cramps, seizures, sudden changes in behaviors, personality changes, abnormal heart rhythms, and coronary spasms can occur.[2] A meta-analysis of 37 published studies investigating the association of magnesium and attention deficit hyperactivity disorder concluded that no well-controlled clinical trial has yet been published to support the efficacy of magnesium for attention deficit hyperactivity disorder treatment.[9] A large cross-sectional study of adult men and women (n = 1120 men and 1384 women aged 18–74) found that dietary magnesium intake was inversely associated with fasting blood glucose levels.[10] Magnesium deficiency can negatively affect insulin sensitivity in type 2 diabetes.[11] Magnesium deficiency leads to loss of bone mass, abnormal bone growth, and skeletal weakness.[12] In experimental research, magnesium deficiency in animal bone cells increased formation of osteoclasts.[12] Magnesium deficiency slows the bone mass accretion in childhood and adolescence, and accelerates bone loss after menopause or in old age.[11] Both magnesium deficiency and high magnesium blood levels have been observed in patients with restless leg syndrome.[11]

bioactive dose

The RDA for magnesium for adult women aged 31–50 is 320 mg and for men aged 31–50 is 420 mg.

safety

When ingested as a naturally occurring substance in foods, magnesium has not been associated with any adverse events (AEs).[2] The UL for magnesium is based upon nonfood sources; total magnesium from supplementary sources should not exceed 350 mg for adults. Excess magnesium from nonfood sources (e.g., dietary supplements or magnesium salts used pharmacologically) is associated with AEs such as diarrhea.[2]

Mango (Mangifera indica)

definition

Juicy, orange-fleshed tropical fruit, eaten fresh or dried, that is a source of potassium, fatty acids, and numerous phytochemicals including polyphenols, terpenoids, steroids, phenolic esters, flavan-3-ols, and mangiferin, a xanthone.[13]

scientific findings

In vitro and *in vivo* models, mango has exerted antioxidant, iron chelator, anti-inflammatory, antinociceptive, antitumor, and immunomodulatory properties.[13–15]

bioactive dose

Not known.

safety

Presumed safe when consumed in normal dietary quantities by non-allergic individuals.

Marjoram, sweet (Origanum majorana)

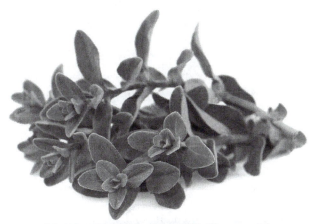

Marjoram. (Image from Scisetti Alfio/Shutterstock.)

M

definition

Mint family herb that contains phenolics and terpenoids.[16] Used fresh or dried to flavor cooked vegetable- or protein-based dishes and pairs well with carrot, mushroom, pea, zucchini, and tomato, chicken, duck, eggs, fish such as halibut and tuna, and lamb chops.[17] It has been historically used for "rhinitis and colds in infants and toddlers, gastritis, stimulating appetite, as a digestive aid, antispasmodic, antiflatulent, and astringent, to promote circulation, healthy sleep, [and to] treat mood swings."[11]

scientific findings

Marjoram essential oils exhibited antimicrobial and antifungal properties in laboratory studies.[18,19]

dioactive dose

Not known.

safety

Presumed safe when consumed in normal dietary quantities by non-allergic individuals.

Melatonin

definition

Also called *N*-acetyl-5-methoxytryptamine.[20] Pineal gland hormone produced by the metabolism of serotonin[20] and a phytochemical that is ubiquitous in the plant kingdom,[21] found in foods such as corn, rice, barley, ginger,[20,22] and other plant foods.

scientific findings

In laboratory studies, melatonin suppressed tumor angiogenesis[23] and has been shown to be a scavenger of hydroxyl radicals.[20]

bioactive dose

Not known.

safety

Presumed safe when consumed in normal dietary quantities by non-allergic individuals.

M

Monounsaturated fatty acid

definition

Dietary triglycerides whose fatty acids predominately contain one double bond. Monounsaturated fatty acid is the major triglyceride found in canola, olive, peanut, and sunflower oils; avocados; and nuts and seeds. The Mediterranean diet is high in monounsaturated fats, in addition to omega-3-fatty acid and plant foods, and it is low in saturated fat, trans fat, and cholesterol.[24,25]

scientific findings

Replacing saturated and trans fats with monounsaturated fats and polyunsaturated fats reduces LDL cholesterol.[26] A meta-analysis and review incorporating 12 studies found that high monounsaturated fat intakes (>12%) were associated with lower body fat mass, total cholesterol, LDL cholesterol, HDL cholesterol, triacylglycerols, systolic and diastolic blood pressures, and C-reactive protein.[27] A Mediterranean diet may reduce the risk of all-cause mortality, cardiovascular disease, type 2 diabetes, obesity, certain cancers, and Alzheimer's disease.[25,28] In a prospective observational study, greater monounsaturated fat intakes were associated with less cognitive decline in women.[29] Monounsaturated fat intake was found to be inversely associated with age-related hearing loss.[30]

bioactive dose

For lowering coronary heart disease risk, the National Cholesterol Education Program recommends consuming up to 20% of total kcals from monounsaturated fat.[8]

safety

Presumed safe when consumed in normal dietary quantities by non-allergic individuals.

Mulberry (Morus rubrum)

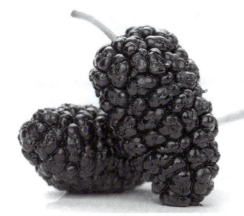

Mulberry. (Image from ravl/Shutterstock.)

M

definition

Blackberry look-alike whose red species, *Morus rubrum,* is cultivated in the United States.[31] Excellent source of vitamin C, good source of manganese and vitamin K,[32] and source of anthocyanin[33] and resveratrol.[34] While black mulberry, *Morus nigra,* native to Iran, has been planted only to a limited extent in America, primarily on the Pacific Coast, red or American mulberry, *Morus rubrum,* grows from Massachusetts to Kansas and down to the Gulf coast.[35]

scientific findings

M. nigra contains numerous phytochemicals including β-sitosterol, which exerted anti-inflammatory effects in a laboratory study.[36] *M. nigra* exhibited neuroprotective and biomembrane-protective, antioxidant effects in a laboratory study.[37]

bioactive dose

Not known.

safety

Presumed safe when consumed in normal dietary quantities by non-allergic individuals.

Mung bean (Phaseolus aureus)

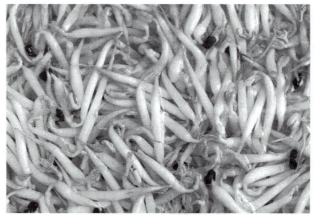

Mung bean sprouts. (Image from Chokchai Suksatavonraphan/Shutterstock.)

definition

Pea-sized, oblong-shaped legume that may be red or green depending on the variety. A source of vitamin K, iron, magnesium, phosphorus, potassium, and phytochemicals, including phenolics, vanillic acid, caffeic acid, chlorogenic acid, coumaric acid, flavonoids, and terpenoids.[38,39] The whole bean is cooked and coupled with rice; for example, mung dal is a bright-yellow soup-like entrée commonly served in Indian restaurants. Mung bean sprouts may be purchased ready-to-eat and can be home-grown from mung bean seeds. They are common in Asian cooking, and are a source of phenolics and flavonoids.

scientific findings

Mung bean sprouts and seed extracts exerted antidiabetic effects in animals with type 2 diabetes,[40] and antioxidant effects in laboratory research.[41] Extracts made from mung bean sprout exerted antitumor effects in laboratory studies.[42]

bioactive dose

Not known.

safety

Presumed safe when consumed in normal dietary quantities as foods by nonallergic individuals.

Mushroom, maitake (Grifola frondosa)

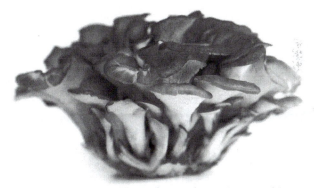

Maitake mushroom. (Image from soulgems/Shutterstock.)

M

definition

Also called hen of the woods. Mild-tasting mushroom whose white stems branch from its base in clustered, grayish brown masses; it has spoon-shaped caps.[43,44] Both caps and stems are edible and are cooked by grilling, roasting, searing, or preparing in ways similar to button mushrooms. Maitake mushroom contains 22 cal per 1 cup and supplies 4 mg of niacin (20% DV), 786 IU of vitamin D (200% DV), 21 µg of folate (5% DV), and small amounts (5 g) of carbohydrate,[45] including the polysaccharides lentinan and D-fraction, which are among the most studied of its bioactive constituents.

scientific findings

Maitake mushroom polysaccharides exerted antitumor and immune activity in laboratory studies.[46–49] Clinical evidence does not support that maitake mushroom is effective in treating or preventing cancer in humans.[50] Maitake mushroom exhibited antidiabetic properties in experimental research and in two cases of patients with type 2 diabetes.[51–53] It is presumed, based upon laboratory findings, that its hypoglycemic effect may be due to insulin sensitization or activation of insulin receptors in insulin-targeted cells.[53] More evidence is needed to evaluate the effectiveness of maitake mushroom in lowering blood sugar. More evidence is needed to evaluate maitake mushroom effectiveness in inducing ovulation in polycystic ovary syndrome, for which it was found to be effective in a 12-week clinical trial (n = 80 patients with polycystic ovary syndrome).[11,54] In *in vitro* and *in vivo* studies, *Grifola frondosa* extracts or compounds demonstrated neuroprotective effects, including reduced beta amyloid-induced neurotoxicity, and exerted anti-neuroinflammatory effects.[55] Maitake mushroom reduced blood pressure and improved dyslipidemia in animal studies.[11,56]

bioactive dose

Not known.

safety

Presumed safe when used in normal dietary quantities by nonallergic individuals. Dried maitake mushroom powder was safely used in doses up to 2.25 g daily for up to 28 weeks and maitake mushroom polysaccharides 1–1.5 g daily was safely used for up to 2 years.[55]

M

Mushroom, oyster (Pleurotus ostreatus)

definition

Fleshy, mild-flavored mushroom tastes like oyster when cooked with butter. It is white-to-brown in color with a small, stub-like stalk, having whitish or yellow-tinged gills.[57] Grows wild and is commercially sold fresh or dried.

scientific findings

Oyster mushroom exhibited anti-inflammatory properties in laboratory studies.[58] Antitumor and immunomodulating factors have been isolated in oyster mushroom.[59]

bioactive dose

Not known.

safety

Presumed safe when consumed in normal dietary quantities by non-allergic individuals. Allergies to mushrooms have been reported.

Mushroom, shiitake *(Lentinus edodes)*

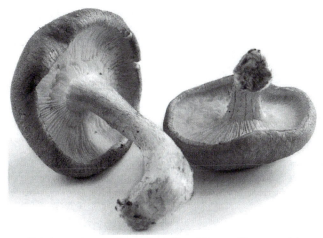

Shiitake mushroom. (Image from Elena Elisseeva/Shutterstock.)

definition

Also spelled *shitake*. Brown and white fungus that has a meat-like texture and is a source of riboflavin, niacin, vitamin B6, phosphorus, and selenium.[60,61] Shiitake are the second most popular edible mushroom marketed globally[44,62] and are used fresh or rehydrated from dried form.

scientific findings

Chemical analysis of shiitake mushrooms have isolated antibiotic, anticarcinogenic, and antiviral compounds.[62] In laboratory studies, shiitake constituents have demonstrated immunomodulatory properties[63]; and lentinan, a polysaccharide flavonoid,[64] was immunomodulatory and demonstrated antitumor effects in an animal model.[65] Shiitake mushrooms decreased hypertension in rats.[66] Shiitake mushroom extract given three times daily for 6 months did not prevent prostate cancer disease progression, as determined by prostate-specific antigen levels, in a clinical trial (n = 62 men with prostate cancer, mean age 73.2 years who had two consecutive elevated prostate specific antigen readings during a 3-month study period) that found shiitake mushroom extract to be "ineffective in the treatment of clinical prostate cancer."[67] Shiitake mushroom alkaloids have exhibited anticarcinogenic properties in laboratory studies.[68]

bioactive dose

Not known.

M

safety

Presumed safe when consumed in normal dietary quantities by non-allergic individuals.

Mustard seed (Brassica alba)

definition

Small round seeds of the mustard plant that has been grown since ancient times. Contains phenolics, isothiocyanate, glucosinsolates, and brassinin.[69] Commercial mustard is made by grinding the seed and vinegar into a paste. Traditionally, mustard powder is used to "brighten and clear the voice" when it is stirred with honey to form balls, and one or two of these honey balls are taken on an empty stomach.[55]

scientific findings

In a laboratory study, mustard exhibited chemoprotective properties, which were attributed to its allyl isothiocyanate content.[70] Flavonoids have been isolated in shoots, roots, and extracts of *Brassica alba*.[71]

M

bioactive dose

Not known.

safety

Presumed safe when consumed in normal dietary quantities by non-allergic individuals.

References

1. Shils ME. Magnesium. In: Shils ME, Olson JA, Shike M, Ross AC (eds.). *Modern Nutrition in Health and Disease*, 9th edn. Baltimore, MD: Williams & Wilkins; 1999:169–192.
2. Institute of Medicine. *Dietary Reference Intakes for Calcium, Phosphorus, Magnesium, Vitamin D and Fluoride*. Washington DC: National Academy Press; 1997.
3. National Institutes of Health. Office of Dietary Supplements. Dietary Supplement Fact Sheet: Magnesium. http://ods.od.nih.gov/factsheets/Magnesium-HealthProfessional/. Accessed May 30, 2011.
4. Abrams SA, Chen Z, Hawthorne KM. Magnesium metabolism in 4 to 8 year old children. *J Bone Miner Res*. 2014;29(1):118–122. Epub 2013 June 20. doi: 10.1002/jbmr.2021. [Epub ahead of print].
5. Hedrick FH, Mikesky AE, Burgoon LA. *Practical Applications in Sports Nutrition*, 3rd edn. Burlington MA: Jones & Bartlett Learning; 2012.

6. Bastos P, Araújo JR, Azevedo I, Martins MJ, Ribeiro L. Effect of a natural mineral-rich water on catechol-O-methyltransferase function. *Magnesium [Epub ahead of print].Res.* 2014;27(3):131–141. doi: 10.1684/mrh.2014.0369.
7. DeBruyne LK, Pinna K. *Nutrition for Health and Health Care,* 5th edn. Belmont, CA: Wadsworth Cengage Learning; 2014.
8. Whitney E, DeBruyne LK, Pinna K, Rolfes SR. *Nutrition for Health & Health Care,* 4th edn. Belmont CA: Wadsworth Cengage; 2007.
9. Ghanizadeh A. A systematic review of magnesium therapy for treating attention deficit hyperactivity disorder. *Arch Iran Med.* 2013;16(7):412–417. doi: 013167/AIM.0010.
10. Mirmiran P, Shab-Bidar S, Hosseini-Esfahani F, Asghari G, Hosseinpour-Niazi S, Azizi F. Magnesium intake and prevalence of metabolic syndrome in adults: Tehran lipid and glucose study. *Public Health Nutr.* 2012;15(4):693–701. [Epub ahead of print.]
11. Jellin JM, Gregory PJ. Natural Medicine Comprehensive Database. Therapeutic Research Faculty. 2013. http://www.naturaldatabase.com. Accessed March 30, 2015.
12. Belluci MM, Schoenmaker T, Rossa-Junior C, Orrico SR, de Vries TJ, Everts V. Magnesium deficiency results in an increased formation of osteoclasts. *J Nutr Biochem.* 2013;24(8):1488–1498. Epub 2013 March 18. doi: 10.1016/j.jnutbio.2012.12.008. [Epub ahead of print.]
13. Rodeiro I, Cancino L, González JE, Morffi J, Garrido G, González RM, Nuñez A, Delgado R. Evaluation of the genotoxic potential of *Mangifera indica* L. extract (Vimang), a new natural product with antioxidant activity. *Food Chem Toxicol.* 2006;44(10):1707–1713. Epub 2006 May 26.
14. Martínez G, Delgado R, Pérez G, Garrido G, Núñez Sellés AJ, León OS. Evaluation of the *in vitro* antioxidant activity of *Mangifera indica* L. extract (Vimang). *Phytother Res.* 2000;14(6):424–427.
15. Garrido G, González D, Lemus Y, García D, Lodeiro L, Quintero G, Delporte C, Núñez-Sellés AJ, Delgado R. *In vivo* and *in vitro* anti-inflammatory activity of *Mangifera indica* L. extract (Vimang). *Pharmacol Res.* 2004;50(2):143–149.
16. US Department of Agriculture. Agricultural Research Service. Beltsville Agricultural Research Center. *Origanum majoram.* http://www.pl.barc.usda.gov/usda_plant/plant_detail.cfm?code=28969643&plant_id=416&ThisName=ps721. Accessed June 4, 2011.
17. Dornenburg A, Page K. *Culinary Artistry.* New York: Van Nostrand Reinhold; 1996.
18. Deans SG, Svoboda KP. The antimicrobial properties of marjoram (*Origanum majorana* L.) Volatile Oil. *Flavour Fragrance J.* 1990;5(3):187–190.
19. Charai M, Faid M, Mosaddak M. Chemical composition and antimicrobial activities of two aromatic plants: *Origanum majorana* L. and *O. compactum* Benth. *J Essent Oil Res.* 1996;8(6): 657–564.
20. Badria FA. Melatonin, serotonin, and tryptamine in some Egyptian food and medicinal plants. *J Med Food.* 2002;5(3):153–157.
21. Kolár J, Macháčková I. Melatonin in higher plants: Occurrence and possible functions. *J Pineal Res.* 2005;39(4):333–341.
22. Tan DX, Manchester LC, Simopoulos AP, Maldonado MD, Flores LJ, Terron MP. Melatonin in edible plants (phytomelatonin): Identification, concentrations, bioavailability and proposed functions. *World Rev Nutr Diet.* 2007;97:211–230.

M

23. Park SY, Jang WJ, Yi EY, Jang JY, Jung Y, Jeong JW, Kim YJ. Melatonin suppresses tumor angiogenesis by inhibiting HIF-1alpha stabilization under hypoxia. *J Pineal Res.* 2010;48(2):178–184.

24. Mayo Clinic the New Mediterranean Diet Pyramid. Nutrition-wise blog. http://www.mayoclinic.com/health/mediterranean-diet-pyramid/ MY00663. Accessed July 15, 2013.

25. Schröder H. Protective mechanisms of the Mediterranean diet in obesity and type 2 diabetes. *J Nutr Biochem.* 2006;18(3):149–160.

26. Academy of Nutrition and Dietetics Evidence Analysis Library. What is the relation between LDL-Cholesterol and replacing dietary saturated fatty acids with MUFAs and PUFAs in patients with disorders of lipid metabolism? http://andevidencelibrary.com/conclusion.cfm?conclusion_statement_id=20. Accessed July 16, 2013. doi: 10.1111/j.1532-5415.2011.03402.x.

27. Schwingshack L, Strasser B, Hoffmann G. Effects of monounsaturated fatty acids on cardiovascular risk factors: A systematic review and meta-analysis. *Ann Nutr Metab.* 2011;59(2–4):176–186. Epub 2011 December 2.

28. Sofi F, Abbate R, Gensini GF, Casini A. Accruing evidence on benefits of adherence to the Mediterranean diet on health: An updated systematic review and meta-analysis. *Am J Clin Nutr.* 2010;92(5):1189–1196. Epub 2010 September 1.

29. Naqvi AZ, Harty B, Mukamal KJ, Stoddard AM, Vitolins M, Dunn JE. Monounsaturated, trans, and saturated fatty acids and cognitive decline in women. *J Am Geriatr Soc.* 2011;59(5):837–843.

30. Gopinath B, Flood VM, Teber E, McMahon CM, Mitchell P. Dietary intake of cholesterol is positively associated and use of cholesterol-lowering medication is negatively associated with prevalent age-related hearing loss. *J Nutr.* 2011;141(7):1355–1361. Epub 2011 May 25.

31. University of Georgia Cooperative Extension. Mulberry. http://mcdowell. ces.ncsu.edu/Mulberry/. Accessed March 30, 2015.

32. Produce for Better Health Foundation. Fruit and Veggies More Matters. Mulberry http://www.fruitsandveggiesmorematters.org/?page_id=16191. Accessed January 15, 2012.

33. Kim HG, Ju MS, Shim JS, Kim MC, Lee SH, Huh Y, Kim SY, Oh MS. Mulberry fruit protects dopaminergic neurons in toxin-induced Parkinson's disease models. *Br J Nutr.* 2010;104(1):8–16. Epub 2010 February 26.

34. Mukherjee S, Dudley JI, Das DK. Dose-dependency of resveratrol in providing health benefits. *Dose Response.* 2010;8(4):478–500.

35. California Rare Fruit Growers.org. Mulberry. http://www.crfg.org/. Accessed May 30, 2011.

36. Padilha MM, Vilela FC, Rocha CQ, Dias MJ, Soncini R, dos Santos MH, Alves-da-Silva G, Giusti-Paiva A. Anti-inflammatory properties of *Morus nigra* leaves. *Phytother Res.* 2010;24(10):1496–1500.

37. Naderi GA, Asgary S, Sarraf-Zadegan N, Oroojy H, Afshin-Nia F. Antioxidant activity of three extracts of *Morus nigra. Phytother Res.* 2004;18(5):365–369.

38. US Department of Agriculture. Agricultural Research Service. Nutrient Data Laboratory. Mung beans, cooked, boiled without salt. http://ndb.nal .usda.gov/ndb/foods/show/4773. Accessed January 16, 2012.

39. US Department of Agriculture. Agricultural Research Service. Medicinal Plant Database. Phaseolus vulgaris/common bean. http://www.pl.barc. usda.gov/usda_plant/plant_detail.cfm?code=69685564&plant_id=398&y1s27=&ThisName=ps721. Accessed January 16, 2012.

M

40. Yao Y, Chen F, Wang M, Wang J, Ren G. Antidiabetic activity of Mung bean extracts in diabetic KK-Ay mice. *J Agric Food Chem.* 2008;56(19):8869–8873. Epub 2008 September 4.

41. Chon SU. Total polyphenols and bioactivity of seeds and sprouts in several legumes. *Curr Pharm Des.* 2013;19(34):6112–6124.

42. Soucek J, Skvor J, Pouckova P, Matousek J, Slavík T, Matousek J. Mung bean sprout (*Phaseolus aureus*) nuclease and its biological and antitumor effects. *Neoplasma.* 2006;53(5):402–409.

43. Lincoff GH. *The Audubon Society Field Guide to North American Mushrooms.* New York: Alfred A. Knopf; 1992:463–464.

44. Czarnecki J. Mushrooms from the wood: The ultimate recyclers. *A Cook's Book of Mushrooms.* New York, NY: Artisan; 1995:129.

45. US Department of Agriculture. National Nutrient Database. Mushroom, maitake. http://ndb.nal.usda.gov/ndb/foods/show/3635?manu=&fgcd= Accessed September 2, 2015.

46. Ren L, Perera C, Hemar Y. Antitumor activity of mushroom polysaccharides: A review. *Food Funct.* 2012;3(11):1118–1130. doi: 10.1039/c2fo10279j.

47. Wasser SP. Medicinal mushrooms as a source of antitumor and immunomodulating polysaccharides. *Appl Microbiol Biotechnol.* 2002;60(3):258–274. Epub 2002 September 10.

48. Suzuki I, Hashimoto K, Oikawa S, Sato K, Osawa M, Yadomae T. Antitumor and immunomodulating activities of a beta-glucan obtained from liquid-cultured *Grifola frondosa. Chem Pharm Bull.* 1989;37(2):410–413.

49. Vetvicka V, Vetvickova J. Immune-enhancing effects of Maitake (*Grifola frondosa*) and Shiitake (*Lentinula edodes*) extracts. *J. Ann Transl Med.* 2014;2(2):14. doi: 10.3978/j.issn.2305-5839.2014.01.05.

50. American Cancer Society. Maitake Mushrooms. http://www.cancer.org/Treatment/TreatmentsandSideEffects/ComplementaryandAlternative Medicine/DietandNutrition/maitake-mushrooms. Accessed January 15, 2012.

51. Lei H, Zhang M, Wang Q, Guo S, Han J, Sun H, Wu W. MT-α-glucan from the fruit body of the maitake medicinal mushroom *Grifola frondosa* (higher Basidiomyetes) shows protective effects for hypoglycemic pancreatic β-cells. *Int J Med Mushrooms.* 2013;15(4):373–381.

52. Ma X, Zhou F, Chen Y, Zhang Y, Hou L, Cao X, Wang C. A polysaccharide from *Grifola frondosa* relieves insulin resistance of HepG2 cell by Akt-GSK-3 pathway. *Glycoconjugate J.* 2014;31(5):355–363. doi: 10.1007/s10719-014-9526-x. Epub 2014 June 8.

53. Konno S, Tortorelis DG, Fullerton SA, Samadi AA, Hettiarachchi J, Tazaki H. A possible hypoglycemic effect of maitake mushroom on type 2 diabetic patients. *Diabetic Med.* 2001;18(12):1010.

54. Chen JT, Tominaga K, Sato Y, Anzai H, Matsuoka R. A possible monotherapy and a combination therapy after failure with first-line clomiphene citrate. Maitake mushroom (*Grifola frondosa*) extract induces ovulation in patients with polycystic ovary syndrome. *Altern Complementary Med.* 2010;16(12):1295–1299. doi: 10.1089/acm.2009.0696. Epub 2010 October 29.

55. Phan CW, David P, Naidu M, Wong KH, Sabaratnam V. Therapeutic potential of culinary-medicinal mushrooms for the management of neurodegenerative diseases: Diversity, metabolite, and mechanism. *Crit Rev Biotechnol.* 2015;35(3):355–368. doi: 10.3109/07388551.2014.887649.

M

56. Sato M, Tokuji Y, Yoneyama S, Fujii-Akiyama K, Kinoshita M, Chiji H, Ohnishi M. Effect of dietary maitake (*Grifola frondosa*) mushrooms on plasma cholesterol and hepatic gene expression in cholesterol-fed mice. *J Oleo Sci.* 2013;62(12):1049–1058.

57. Lincoff GH. *The Audubon Society Field Guide to North American Mushrooms.* New York: Alfred A. Knopf; 1992:793.

58. Jedinak A, Dudhgaonkar S, Wu QL, Simon J, Sliva D. Anti-inflammatory activity of edible oyster mushroom is mediated through the inhibition of NF-kB and AP-1 signaling. *Nutr J.* 2011;10(1):52. [Epub ahead of print.]

59. Sarangi I, Ghosh D, Bhutia SK, Mallick SK, Maiti TK. Anti-tumor and immunomodulating effects of *Pleurotus ostreatus* mycelia-derived proteoglycans. *Int Immunopharmacol.* 2006;6(8):1287–1297.

60. Turlo J, Gutkowska B, Herold F, Dawidowski M, Słowiński T, Zobel A. Relationship between selenium accumulation and mycelial cell composition in *Lentinula edodes* (Berk.) cultures. *J Toxicol Environ Health A.* 2010;73(17–18):1211–1219.

61. Produce for Better Health Foundation. Fruit and Veggies More Matters. Shitake Mushroom. http://www.fruitsandveggiesmorematters.org/shiitake-mushrooms-nutrition-selection-storage. Accessed January 15, 2012.

62. Bisen PS, Baghel RK, Sanodiya BS, Thakur GS, Prasad GB. *Lentinus edodes*: A macrofungus with pharmacological activities. *Curr Med Chem.* 2010;17(22):2419–2430.

63. Okamoto T, Kodoi R, Nonaka Y, Fukuda I, Hashimoto T, Kanazawa K, Mizuno M, Ashida H. Lentinan from shiitake mushroom (*Lentinus edodes*) suppresses expression of cytochrome P450 1A subfamily in the mouse liver. *BioFactors.* 2004;21(1–4):407–409.

64. Wang JL, Bi Z, Zou JW, Gu XM. Combination therapy with lentinan improves outcomes in patients with esophageal carcinoma. *Mol Med Rep.* 2012;5(3):745–748. doi: 10.3892/mmr.2011.718. Epub 2011 December 19.

65. Borchers AT, Stern JS, Hackman RM, Keen CL, Gershwin ME. Mushrooms, tumors, and immunity. *Proc Soc Exp Biol Med.* 1999;221(4):281–293.

66. Kabir Y, Yamaguchi M, Kimura S. Effect of shiitake (*Lentinus edodes*) and maitake (*Grifola frondosa*) mushrooms on blood pressure and plasma lipids of spontaneously hypertensive rats. *J Nutr Sci Vitaminol.* (Tokyo). 1987;33(5):341–346.

67. deVere White RW, Hackman RM, Soares SE, Beckett LA, Sun B. Effects of a mushroom mycelium extract on the treatment of prostate cancer. *Urology.* 2002;60(4):640–644.

68. Rao JR, Millar BC, Moore JE. Antimicrobial properties of shiitake mushrooms (*Lentinula edodes*). *Int J Antimicrob Agents.* 2009;33(6):591–592.

69. U.S. Department of Agriculture. Agricultural Research Service. *Brassica alba*/Mustard seed. http://www.pl.barc.usda.gov/usda_rrcp/rrecipe_detail.cfm?code=69685564&id=149&ThisName=sd1. Accessed January 16, 2012.

70. Bhattacharya A, Li Y, Wade KL, Paonessa JD, Fahey JW, Zhang Y. Allyl isothiocyanate-rich mustard seed powder inhibits bladder cancer growth and muscle invasion. *Carcinogenesis.* 2010;31(12):2105–2110. Epub 2010 October 1.

71. Poncea MA, Scervinob JM, Erra-Balsellsa R, Ocampoc JA, Godeas AM. Flavonoids from shoots, roots and roots exudates of *Brassica alba*. *Phytochemistry.* 2004;65(23):3131–3134.

M

N

Naringin

definition

Bitter principle of grapefruit and flavonoid that is partly responsible, along with a related compound called naringenin, for grapefruit juice enhancing the bioavailability of certain medications.[1]

scientific findings

In laboratory studies, naringin exhibited antioxidant properties, inhibited tumor growth, and suppressed age-related blood pressure increases in hypertensive rats.[2-4]

bioactive dose

Not known.

safety

Presumed safe when consumed in normal dietary quantities by non-allergic individuals.

Nectarine (Prunus persica nectarina)

definition

Relative of the peach that has smooth, shiny skin. Commonly eaten fresh, the orange and white cultivars of nectarine supply fiber, vitamin C, phenolics, and carotenoids.[5]

scientific findings

Phenolic compounds have exerted antioxidant, anti-inflammatory, and antimicrobial effects.[6-8] Carotenoids exhibited antioxidant activity *in vitro*; whereas, direct evidence of *in vivo* antioxidant activity is limited.[9] Epidemiology suggests that diets high in carotenoid-rich fruits and vegetables reduce the risk of oxidation-dependent diseases such as cancer, atherosclerosis, and macular degeneration.[9] Vitamin C is a cofactor in collagen, carnitine, and neurotransmitter synthesis,[10] is necessary for immune function, and increases intestinal absorption of nonheme iron[10] by either reducing iron from the ferrous ionic state to ferric state or by forming a soluble complex with the iron in the alkaline pH of the small intestine.[11]

bioactive dose

Not known.

safety

Presumed safe when consumed in normal dietary quantities by non-allergic individuals.

Niacin

definition

Also called nicotinic acid, nicotinamide, and vitamin B3.[12] B vitamin necessary for energy metabolism. Niacin sources include protein-containing foods such as legumes and meat, enriched and whole grains, and vegetables such as mushrooms, potatoes, and asparagus.[13] Niacin deficiency causes pellagra, which is characterized by dermatitis, diarrhea, dementia, and, if untreated, death.

scientific findings

Niacin deficiency causes neurodegeneration.[14] Eating protein foods prevents niacin deficiency because they supply tryptophan, an amino acid that is converted into niacin. Inadequate iron, riboflavin, or vitamin B6 status decreases the conversion of tryptophan to niacin.[15]

bioactive dose

Niacin intake is measured in "niacin equivalents" to include niacin *per se* and the conversion of the tryptophan to niacin. The RDA for men is 16 niacin equivalents. The RDA for women is 14 niacin equivalents.

safety

The UL is 35 mg/day of niacin equivalents.

Nitrates and nitrites

definition

Compounds that are present naturally in soil, water (nitrates are the most common chemical contaminant in groundwater),[19] all plants, and in meats.[16] Nitrites are naturally occurring compounds associated with the nitrogen cycle in soil and water; concentrations of nitrites in plants and water are usually very low[16]; however, sodium nitrite is added to cured meats and smoked/salted fish in order to prevent botulism, develop cured meat flavor and color, and retard rancidity, off-odors, and off-flavors and its intake parallels consumption of these processed meats. Both are regulated in water and certain foods by the Environmental Protection Agency and the FDA. Nitrates and nitrites are found in many vegetables, such as spinach and beets, and products made from them, such as commercial baby foods,[17] in addition to fruits.[18,19]

scientific findings

Nitrates and nitrites have physiologic roles in vascular and immune function[20] and the dietary intake of nitrates and nitrites from vegetables and fruits may actually contribute to the blood pressure-lowering effects of the Dietary Approaches to Stop Hypertension (DASH) diet.[20] According to a review, "In humans, dietary nitrate and nitrite sources have been demonstrated to lower blood pressure and decrease oxygen consumption during submaximal and maximal aerobic exercise. In animal models, nitrite has been demonstrated to enhance mucosal blood flow and serve antimicrobial functions, protect against heart attack and stroke, and reverse vascular inflammation from a high fat diet."[20] "However, the adverse effects of nitrates and nitrites are perhaps more well-known than their beneficial effects. Ingested nitrate is reduced to nitrite, which binds to hemoglobin to form methemoglobin,"[19] a compound that, at high levels, adversely affects infant health by interfering with the oxygen-carrying capacity of blood.[19] Nitrates and nitrites are also associated with gastrointestinal cancer and blood disorders.[20,21] A case–control study found, by examining subsequent occurrence of colorectal cancer in a cohort (n = 9985 adult men and women) over a period of 24 years, that "N-nitroso compounds can induce colorectal cancer in humans."[22] Production of butyric acid by certain probiotic bacteria neutralizes the activity of dietary carcinogens such as nitrosamines.[23]

bioactive dose

Not applicable.

safety

The World Health Organization established an acceptable daily nitrate intake of 222 mg/day.[24] A hypothetical nitrate intake while following the DASH diet may range from 174 to 1222 mg, which exceeds the World Health Organization's acceptable daily intake of nitrate for a 60-kg adult by 550%.[20]

Noni (Morinda citrifolia)

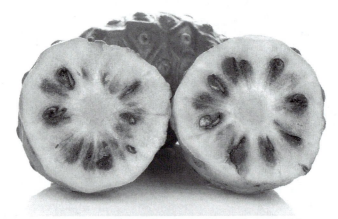

Noni. (Image from Nipaporn Panyacharoen/Shutterstock.)

N

definition

Also called Indian mulberry fruit.[25] A yellow oval-shaped fruit about the size of a potato that when ripe has a yellow, bumpy surface.[26,27] Noni has been used in folk medicine for over 2000 years[28] and also for its immune properties to treat infection.[29] There are anecdotal reports for successful use of noni to treat colds and influenza,[26] but FDA has warned several noni product manufacturers to stop making false claims related to noni product use, including that it treats, cures, or prevents various diseases.[27] Its uniquely purple, sweet juice is used in juice blends. Noni fruit is a good source of vitamins A and C, and is high in potassium.[27]

scientific findings

Noni was shown in laboratory studies to have antioxidant, immune-stimulating, tumor-fighting, anti-inflammatory, and antioxidative properties.[29–31]

bioactive dose

Not known.

safety

Presumed safe when consumed in normal dietary quantities by non-allergic individuals. Noni safety has not been adequately studied.[30] The juice has been linked to liver damage,[25] and its high potassium content contraindicates it for use by people on potassium-restricted diets.[30]

Nori (Porphyra tenera)

definition

Seaweed algae is a source of calcium, iron, iodine, magnesium, zinc, potassium, sodium, and the phytochemicals chlorophyll, β-carotene, and lutein.[32,33] Dried nori is commonly used as a seaweed wrap in making sushi-rice rolls. It is also consumed as a dried vegetable.

scientific findings

Raw nori contains vitamin B12; however, dried nori is not a reliable source of vitamin B12.[34] In a laboratory study, nori was antimutagenic.[35]

N

bioactive dose

Not known.

safety

Presumed safe when consumed in normal dietary quantities by non-allergic individuals.

Nut

definition

High-protein food that is low in saturated fat, high in unsaturated fat, and a rich source of insoluble fiber.[36] At approximately 85 cal per 1/2 oz of mixed nuts, different nuts supply different nutrients and phytochemicals. Typically sold roasted and salted to make trail mixes and nut mixtures, and as nut butters.

scientific findings

Consuming 5 oz of any type of nut per week is associated with a reduced risk of congestive heart failure.[37]

bioactive dose

Not known.

safety

Allergies to nuts have been reported; however, they are presumed safe when consumed in normal dietary quantities by nonallergic individuals.

Nutmeg (Myristica fragrans)

N

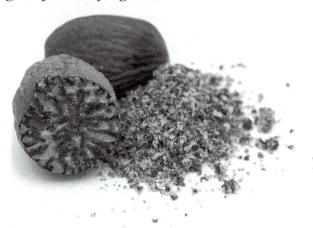

Nutmeg. (Image from Diana Taliun/Shutterstock.)

definition

Ground seed of a tropical evergreen tree fruit. *M. fragrans* contains phenolics, such as myristicin, and terpenoids, such as elemicin.[38] Used to flavor eggnog, pumpkin pie, quiche, and other dishes. It has been used as an antiflatulent effect and for nausea and diarrhea.

scientific findings

In laboratory studies, nutmeg showed antidiabetic properties, possibly due to improvements in insulin sensitivity,[39] insulin secretagogue action, and/or the ability to inhibit intestinal α-glucosidase leading to a slower postprandial glucose response.[40] Myristicin exhibited hepatoprotective effects in experimental research.[41] Elemicin was antimicrobial against the human enteropathogen *Campylobacter jejuni* in a laboratory study.[42]

bioactive dose

Not known. The following doses have been used: for antiflatulent effect, 0.03 mL nutmeg oil; for nausea, gastric upset, or chronic diarrhea, the common dose is 3–5 drops of the essential oil on a sugar lump or in honey; and for diarrhea, 4–6 tablespoons of the powder has been used daily.[43]

safety

Presumed safe when used in normal dietary quantities by nonallergic individuals. Nutmeg significantly inhibited human cytochrome activity in a laboratory study.[44] In traditional medicines, *M. fragrans* may have been used in high doses as a hallucinogenic (over 2 tablespoons of nutmeg consumed at once)[40] and nutmeg seeds are abused because of the psychotropic effects that result after ingesting large doses,[45] which may also induce GI upset. Elemicin was found to be genotoxic in a laboratory study.[46]

References

1. De Castro WV, Mertens-Talcott S, Rubner A, Butterweck V, Derendorf H. Variation of flavonoids and furanocoumarins in grapefruit juices: A potential source of variability in grapefruit juice–drug interaction studies. *J Agric Food Chem*. 2006;54(1):249–255.
2. Jagetia GC, Reddy TK. Alleviation of iron induced oxidative stress by the grapefruit flavanone naringin in vitro. *Chem Biol Interact*. 2011;190(2–3): 121–128. Epub 2011 February 20.
3. Ikemura M, Sasaki Y, Giddings JC, Yamamoto J. Preventive effects of hesperidin, glucosyl hesperidin and naringin on hypertension and cerebral thrombosis in stroke-prone spontaneously hypertensive rats. *Phytother Res*. 2012;26(9):1272–1277. doi: 10.1002/ptr.3724. Epub 2012 January 7.
4. Camargo CA, Gomes-Marcondes MC, Wutzki NC, Aoyama H. Naringin inhibits tumor growth and reduces interleukin-6 and tumor necrosis factor α levels in rats with Walker 256 carcinosarcoma. *Anticancer Res*. 2012;32(1):129–133.
5. Gil MI, Tomás-Barberán FA, Hess-Pierce B, Kader AA. Antioxidant capacities, phenolic compounds, carotenoids, and vitamin C contents of nectarine, peach, and plum cultivars from California. *J Agric Food Chem*. 2002;50(17):4976–4982.
6. Martínez-Valverde I, Periago MJ, Ros G. Nutritional importance of phenolic compounds in the diet. *Arch Latinoam Nutr*. 2000;50(1):5–18.
7. Abidi W, Jiménez S, Moreno MÁ, Gogorcena Y. Evaluation of antioxidant compounds and total sugar content in a nectarine [*Prunus persica* (L.) Batsch] progeny. *Int J Mol Sci*. 2011;12(10):6919–6935. Epub 2011 October 19.

N

8. Crozier A, Jaganath IB, Clifford MN. Dietary phenolics: Chemistry, bioavailability and effects on health. *Nat Prod Rep.* 2009;26(8):1001–1043. Epub 2009 May 13.

9. NIH Office of Dietary Supplements. Dietary Supplement Fact Sheet: Vitamin A and Carotenoids http://ods.od.nih.gov/factsheets/Chromium-HealthProfessional/. Accessed February 8, 2011.

10. Institute of Medicine. *Dietary Reference Intakes for Vitamin C, Vitamin E, Selenium and Carotenoids.* Washington, DC: National Academy Press; 2000.

11. Gropper SS, Smith JL, Groff JL. *Advanced Nutrition and Human Metabolism,* 4th edn. Belmont CA: Wadsworth Cengage Learning; 2005.

12. Institute of Medicine. *Dietary Reference Intakes for Thiamin, Riboflavin, Niacin, Vitamin B6, Folate, Vitamin B12, Pantothenic Acid, Biotin, and Choline.* Washington DC: National Academy Press; 1998.

13. DeBruyne LK, Pinna K. *Nutrition for Health and Health Care,* 5th edn. Belmont, CA: Wadsworth Cengage Learning; 2014.

14. Xu XJ, Jiang GS. Niacin-respondent subset of schizophrenia—A therapeutic review. *Eur Rev Med Pharmacol Sci.* 2015;19(6):988–997.

15. National Institutes of Health. Medline Plus Niacin and Niacinamide. http://www.nlm.nih.gov/medlineplus/druginfo/natural/924.html. Accessed February 12, 2011.

16. Environmental Health Criteria 5. Nitrates, nitrites and N-nitroso compounds. *World Health Organization International Programme on Chemical Safety.* Geneva, Switzerland; 1978. http://www.who.int/ipcs/publications/ehc/ehc_numerical/en/index.html. Accessed July 16, 2013.

17. Phillips WEJ. Naturally occurring nitrate and nitrite in foods in relation to infant methaemoglobinaemia. *Food Cosmet Toxicol.* 1971;9(2):219–228.

18. Dich J, Järvinen R, Knekt P, Penttilä PL. Dietary intakes of nitrate, nitrite and NDMA in the Finnish Mobile Clinic Health Examination Survey. *Food Addit Contam.* 1996;13(5):541–552.

19. Ward MH, deKok TM, Levallois P, Brender P, Gulis G, Nolan BT, VanDerslice J. Workgroup Report: Drinking-water nitrate and health—Recent findings and research needs. *Environ Health Perspect.* 2005;113(11): 1607–1614.

20. Hord NG, Tang Y, Bryan NS. Food sources of nitrates and nitrites: The physiologic context for potential health benefits. *Am J Clin Nutr.* 2009;90(1):1–10. Epub 2009 May 13.

21. Peters JM, Preston-Martin S, London SJ, Bowman JD, Buckley JD, Thomas DC. Processed meats and risk of childhood leukemia (California, USA). *Cancer Causes Control.* 1994;5(2):195–202.

22. Knekt P, Järvinen R, Dich J, Hakulinen T. Risk of colorectal and other gastro-intestinal cancers after exposure to nitrate, nitrite and N-nitroso compounds: A follow-up study. *Int J Cancer.* 1999;80(6):852–856.

23. Kailasapathy K, Chin J. Survival and therapeutic potential of probiotic organisms with reference to *Lactobacillus acidophilus* and *Bifidobacterium* spp. *Immunol Cell Biol.* 2000;78(1):80–88.

24. Michigan State University Today. MSU research supports calls to study health benefits of nitrate, nitrite. http://msutoday.msu.edu/news/2009/msu-research-supports-calls-to-study-health-benefits-of-nitrate-nitrite/. Accessed July 16, 2013.

25. Waldman W, Piotrowicz G, Sein Anand J. Hepatoxic effect of a noni juice consumption—A case report. *Przegl Lek.* 2013;70(8):690–692.
26. Wange M-Y, West BJ, Jarakae Jensen C, Nowicki D, Su C, Palu AK, Anderson G. *Morinda citrifolia* (Noni): A literature review and recent advances in Noni research. *Acta Pharmacol Sin.* 2003;23(12):1127–1141.
27. American Cancer Society. Noni plant. http://www.cancer.org/treatment/ treatmentsandsideeffects/complementaryandalternativemedicine/dietand-nutrition/noni-plant. Accessed April 10, 2015.
28. Zhang X, Li J, Wong DK, Wagner TE, Wei Y. Fermented noni exudate-treated dendritic cells directly stimulate B lymphocyte proliferation and differentiation. *Oncol Rep.* 2009;21(5):1147–1152.
29. Nayak S, Mengi S. Immunostimulant activity of noni (*Morinda citrifolia*) on T and B lymphocytes. *Pharm Biol.* 2010;48(7):724–731. doi: 10.3109/13880200903264434.
30. National Institutes of Health. National Center for Complementary and Alternative Medicine. Herbs at a Glance: Noni. http://nccam.nih.gov/health/noni/. Accessed February 12, 2011.
31. Lin YL, Chang YY, Yang DJ, Tzang BS, Chen YC. Beneficial effects of noni (*Morinda citrifolia* L.) juice on livers of high-fat dietary hamsters. *Food Chem.* 2013;140(1–2):31–38. doi: 10.1016/j.foodchem.2013.02.035. Epub 2013 February 20.
32. Urbano MG, Goñi I. Bioavailability of nutrients in rats fed on edible seaweeds, Nori (*Porphyra tenera*) and Wakame (*Undaria pinnatifida*), as a source of dietary fibre. *Food Chem.* 2002;76(3):281–286.
33. Watanabe F, Takenaka S, Katsura H, Masumder SA, Abe K, Tamura Y, Nakano Y. Dried green and purple lavers (Nori) contain substantial amounts of biologically active vitamin B(12) but less of dietary iodine relative to other edible seaweeds. *J Agric Food Chem.* 1999;47(6):2341–2343.
34. Yamada K, Yamada Y, Fukuda M, Yamada S. Bioavailability of dried asaku-sanori (*Porphyra tenera*) as a source of cobalamin (Vitamin B12). *Int J Vitam Nutr Res.* 1999;69(6):412–418.
35. Higashi-Okaia K, Yanob, Otani S. Identification of antimutagenic substances in an extract of edible red alga, *Porphyra tenera* (Asadusa-nori). *Cancer Lett.* 1996;100(1–2):235–240.
36. Megías-Rangil I, García-Lorda P, Torres-Moreno M, Bulló M, Salas-Salvadó J. Nutrient content and health effects of nuts. *Arch Latinoam Nutr.* 2004;54(2 Suppl 1):83–86.
37. Academy of Nutrition and Dietetics. Evidence Analysis Library. What is the relationship between consuming nuts and the risk of CHD? http://www.adaevidencelibrary.com/conclusion.cfm?conclusion_statement_id=3. Accessed June 4, 2011.
38. De Vincenzi M, De Vincenzi A, Silano M. Constituents of aromatic plants: Elemicin. *Fitoterapia.* 2004;75(6):615–618.
39. Han KL, Choi JS, Lee JY, Song J, Joe MK, Jung MH, Hwang JK. Therapeutic potential of peroxisome proliferators—Activated receptor-alpha/gamma dual agonist with alleviation of endoplasmic reticulum stress for the treatment of diabetes. *Diabetes.* 2008;57(3):737–745.
40. Patil SB, Ghadyale VA, Taklikar SS, Kulkarni CR, Arvindekar AU. Insulin secretagogue, alpha-glucosidase and antioxidant activity of some selected spices in streptozotocin-induced diabetic rats. *Plant Foods Hum Nutr.* 2011;66(1):85–90.

N

41. Morita T, Jinno K, Kawagishi H, Arimoto Y, Suganuma H, Inakuma T, Sugiyama K. Hepatoprotective effect of myristicin from nutmeg (*Myristica fragrans*) on lipopolysaccharide/d-galactosamine-induced liver injury. *J Agric Food Chem*. 2003;51(6):1560–1565.

42. Rossi PG, Bao L, Luciani A, Panighi J, Desjobert JM, Costa J, Casanova J, Bolla JM, Berti L. (E)-Methylisoeugenol and elemicin: Antibacterial components of *Daucus carota* L. essential oil against *Campylobacter jejuni*. *J Agric Food Chem*. 2007;55(18):7332–7336. Epub 2007 August 9.

43. Jellin JM, Gregory PJ et al. *Natural Medicine Comprehensive Database*. Therapeutic Research Faculty. 2013. http://www.naturaldatabase.com. Accessed July 11, 2012.

44. Kimura Y, Ito H, Hatano T. Effects of mace and nutmeg on human cytochrome P450 3A4 and 2C9 activity. *Biol Pharm Bull*. 2010;33(12):1977–1982.

45. Beyer J, Ehlers D, Maurer HH. Abuse of nutmeg (*Myristica fragrans* Houtt.): Studies on the metabolism and the toxicologic detection of its ingredients elemicin, myristicin, and safrole in rat and human urine using gas chromatography/mass spectrometry. *Ther Drug Monit*. 2006;28(4):568–575.

46. Hasheminejad G, Caldwell J. Genotoxicity of the alkenylbenzenes alphaand beta-asarone, myristicin and elimicin as determined by the UDS assay in cultured rat hepatocytes. *Food Chem Toxicol*. 1994;32(3):223–231.

N

O

Oat (Avena sativa)

definition

Versatile whole grain that is commonly used as a hot breakfast cereal, used to make granola, or used in baking. A good source of soluble β-glucan fiber found in the endosperm cell walls of oats.[1] It also supplies the phytochemical avenanthramides.[2]

scientific findings

According to a review, "Intact grains as well as a variety of processed oat and barley foods containing at least 4 g of β-glucan … can significantly reduce postprandial blood glucose."[3] At least 3 g of oat β-glucan consumed daily may reduce plasma total and LDL cholesterol levels by 5%–10% in normocholesterolemic or hypercholesterolemic subjects.[1] Consuming 56–150 g (1/4 cup to 2/3 cup[4]) contains approximately 3.6–10 g of β-glucan.[5]

bioactive dose

A dose of 3–10 g/day of oat β-glucan reduces total cholesterol.[6]

safety

Presumed safe when consumed in normal dietary quantities by nonallergic individuals. Recent research has suggested that only certain strains of oats produce adverse effects in people with celiac disease.[7] Most people with celiac disease can safely eat small amounts of oats, as long as the oats are not contaminated with wheat gluten during processing. People with celiac disease should work closely with their healthcare professional when deciding whether to include oats in their diet.[8]

Okra (Abelmoschus esculentus)

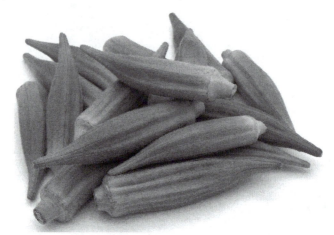

Okra. (Image from Binh Thanh Bui/Shutterstock.)

definition

Green, finger-shaped, antioxidant-rich vegetable,[9] the seeds and skin of which contain flavonols, hydroxycinnamic acid, and quercetin.[10] Mucilaginous fiber in okra imparts a slippery texture and enables its use as a thickening agent in foods. Okra is popular in Southern Creole and Indian cooking, and is eaten fresh, fried, grilled, and in stews.

scientific findings

A. esculentus exhibited antidiabetic and antihyperlipidemic properties in diabetic rats.[11]

bioactive dose

Not known.

safety

Presumed safe when consumed in normal dietary quantities in non-allergic individuals.

Olive (Olea europaea L.)

definition

Marble-sized fruit that has been cultivated in warm climates for more than 7000 years.[12] Olives contain pectin and lipophilic phenolic compounds such as flavonoids. Olive has been used in folk medicine to treat fever and malaria.[12] Usually brined, olives are eaten in salad, sandwiches, and in Mediterranean meals, as a vegetable side dish.

scientific findings

The lipophilic phenolic compounds in olive "are known to possess multiple biological activities such as antioxidant, anticarcinogenic, anti-inflammatory, antimicrobial, antihypertensive, antidyslipidemic, cardio-tonic, laxative, and antiplatelet."[12]

bioactive dose

Not known.

safety

Presumed safe when consumed in normal dietary quantities by non-allergic individuals.

Olive oil (O. europaea)

definition

Monounsaturated oil that is expressed from olives. It is the main fatty component of the Mediterranean diet and a key contributor to the beneficial effects of the Mediterranean diet.[13,14] Extra-virgin olive oil is a source of oleic acid and contains phenolic compounds, including hydroxytyrosol and oleuropein, which provide its characteristic flavor and high stability.[15] Olive oil is now popularly used in place of butter on breads and is used to manufacture numerous products including salad dressings, mayonnaise, and bread spreads.

scientific findings

Olive oil phenolics are powerful antioxidants, both *in vitro* and *in vivo*.[15] An oleic-acid-rich diet in a small study (n = 11 type 2 diabetic subjects) reduced insulin resistance and restored endothelium-dependent vasodilatation, "suggesting an explanation for the anti-atherogenic benefits of a Mediterranean-type diet."[16] There is limited but not conclusive evidence that suggests that consumers may reduce their risk of coronary heart disease if they consume monounsaturated fat from olive oil and olive oil-containing foods in place of foods high in saturated fat, while at the same time not increasing the total number of calories consumed daily. [17]

Olive oil normalized systolic pressure in hypertensive elderly, in a small clinical trial (n = 31 elderly patients with hypertension and n = 31 normotensive elderly patients) in which subjects consumed diets enriched in sunflower oil for 4 weeks, followed by a 4-week washout period, and then a diet enriched with virgin olive oil for 4 weeks.[18]

bioactive dose

Eating about 2 tablespoons (23 g) of olive oil daily may reduce the risk of coronary heart disease when olive oil replaces a similar amount of saturated fat and does not increase total number of calories eaten in a day.[17]

safety

Presumed safe when consumed in normal dietary quantities by non-allergic individuals.

Omega-3 fatty acid

definition

Long-chain polyunsaturated fatty acid family that includes linolenic acid (also called α-linolenic and linolenic acid), EPA, docosapentaenoic acid (DPA), and DHA. The first double bond in the fatty acid chain occurs on the third carbon atom from the end of the fatty acid chain. Linolenic acid must be consumed in the diet—the body cannot make it. Given linolenic acid, the body can make EPA and DHA.[19] Sources of linolenic acid include canola, soybean, and flaxseed oil; nuts such as walnuts; and vegetables such as soybeans. Sources of EPA and DHA include fish. Omega-3 fatty acids perform various physiologic functions, including the relaxation and contraction of muscles, blood clotting, digestion, fertility, cell division, growth, and the movement of calcium and other substances in and out of cells[20] and that have anti-inflammatory properties.[21] Omega-3 fatty acids increase bleeding time and decrease platelet aggregation, blood viscosity, and fibrinogen, thereby decreasing the potential for thrombus formation.[5]

scientific findings

Omega-3 fatty acids reduce serum lipids and lipoproteins, impair platelet aggregation, increase cell membrane fluidity, and lower blood pressure in humans.[22] Omega-3 fatty acids reduce serum triglycerides among type II diabetics.[23] Fish consumption and various cardiovascular disease outcomes in 39 observational and clinical trials of at least 1 year in duration were reviewed, and it was concluded that "consumption of omega-3 fatty acids from fish … reduces all-cause mortality and various cardiovascular disease outcomes."[24] Omega-3 fatty acids appear to have no effect upon most of the clinical outcomes in rheumatoid arthritis, although tender joint count may be reduced.[23] Data are insufficient to draw conclusions about omega-3 fatty acid intake and insulin resistance in type II diabetics, inflammatory bowel disease, renal disease, systemic lupus erythematosus, bone density, or fractures, or the requirement for anti-inflammatory or immunosuppressive drugs.[23] Strong evidence from meta-analyses suggests that omega-3-fatty acids improve bipolar depressive symptoms.[25]

bioactive dose

The AI for linolenic acid is 1.6 g/day for men and 1.1 g/day for women aged 19–50. Scientists generally agree that people should consume fewer omega-6 fatty acids and more omega-3 fatty acids; however, the ideal ratio of omega-6s to omega-3s has not been determined. "For primary prevention of coronary heart disease, approximately 1.2–2 g per day from dietary sources seems to be associated with the greatest benefit; for secondary prevention of coronary heart disease, approximately 1.6 g per day as part of a Mediterranean diet appears to be beneficial."[5] Fatty acid dosing is often determined based on percentage of daily calories. Some researchers suggest that linolenic acid should make up roughly 1% of daily calories. This comes to approximately 2 g based on a 2000 kcal diet.

safety

Presumed safe when consumed in normal dietary quantities by non-allergic individuals.

Omega-6 fatty acid

definition

Long-chain polyunsaturated fatty acid family that includes linoleic acid. Linoleic acid is necessary for growth, and a dietary intake of 1%–2% of total calories as linoleic acid is sufficient to prevent EFA deficiency. Linoleic acid is the precursor of arachadonic acid, which in turn serves as a substrate for prostaglandin synthesis.[26] Sources of linoleic acid include soybean, safflower, sunflower or corn oils, nuts, and seeds.

scientific findings

Consumption of omega-6 fatty acids in place of saturated fats and trans fats is associated with a decreased risk of coronary heart disease[27]; however, a meta-analysis showed that "current evidence does not clearly support cardiovascular guidelines that encourage high consumption of polyunsaturated fatty acids and low consumption of total saturated fats."[28]

U.S. dietary intake of omega-6 PUFA has been estimated to be 6%–8% of total energy intake.[29] A high ratio of dietary n-6 to n-3 PUFAs is being investigated for possible pro-inflammatory physiological effects.[30]

bioactive dose

The AI for linoleic acid is 17 g/day for men aged 19–50 and 12 g/day for women aged 19–50.

safety

Presumed safe when consumed in normal dietary quantities by non-allergic individuals.

Onion (Allium cepa)

definition

Popular bulb vegetable is a source of mineral sulfur and provides flavonoids, anthocyanins (that imparts a red or purple color to certain varieties), and flavonols such as quercetin, which is responsible for the yellow and brown skins of many other varieties.[31] Commonly used in fresh or cooked forms to add a pungent flavoring to all types of cuisines. Onion is used to treat cardiovascular disease in traditional medicine.[32]

scientific findings

Onion exhibited the following properties in experimental studies: antiplatelet aggregatory, hypocholesterolemic, hypolipidemic, antihypertensive, antidiabetic, and antihyperhomocysteinemic effects, antimicrobial, antioxidant, anticarcinogenic, antimutagenic, antiasthmatic, immunomodulatory, and prebiotic effects,[33–35] but clinical trials examining these effects have not been performed. A case–control study (n = 760 patients with a first episode of nonfatal acute myocardial infarction; n = 682 controls) found that a diet rich in onions may have a favorable effect on the risk of acute myocardial infarction.[35] The Netherlands Cohort Study, a large-scale prospective cohort study on diet and cancer (n = 120,852 men and women, aged 55–69 years) did not find an association between the consumption of onions and leeks and the incidence of male and female colon and rectum carcinoma, female breast cancer risk, or risk of lung carcinoma.[36]

bioactive dose

Not known. A typical dose of onion is 50 g of fresh onion per day (approximately 4–5 tablespoons), but 50 g fresh onion juice and 20 g dried onion has also been used.[5]

safety

Presumed safe when consumed in normal dietary quantities by non-allergic individuals.

Orange, sweet (Citrus sinensis)

definition

More commonly known as the navel orange, this popular citrus fruit and its juice are excellent sources of vitamin C, good sources of folate and potassium, and contain numerous phytochemicals, including pectin and flavonoids.[37]

scientific findings

O

Consuming commercial *C. sinensis* juice decreased blood pressure in a single-blind randomized crossover study (n = 22 healthy subjects 18–59 years old) in which subjects were randomly divided into two groups of 11, each consuming 500 mL/day of commercial orange juice twice a day for 4 weeks with breakfast and dinner, followed by a 2-week washout period, followed by natural orange juice for another 4 weeks dosed according to the same schedule. Commercial orange juice significantly reduced diastolic and systolic blood pressure, but natural orange juice did not have significant effects on either diastolic or systolic blood pressure, an effect that was attributed to the higher flavonoid, pectin, and essential oils content of commercial compared to natural orange juice.[37] Consuming 750 mL, but not of 250 or 500 mL, of orange juice daily, for 4 weeks, increased HDL cholesterol by 21% and decreased the LDL–HDL cholesterol ratio by 16% in hypercholesterolemic patients (n = 16 healthy men and 9 healthy women with elevated plasma total and LDL cholesterol and normal plasma triglycerides), while it also raised triglycerides by 30%.[38]

bioactive dose

Not known.

safety

Presumed safe when consumed in normal dietary quantities by non-allergic individuals.

Oregano (Origanum vulgare)

definition

Culinary herb often used as an ingredient in soups, casseroles, sauces, stews, stuffing, and Italian dishes. Oregano has an earthy, oily, aromatic flavor, and contains numerous phytochemicals including phenolics, caffeic acid, and rosmarinic acid.[39]

scientific findings

In laboratory studies, oregano exhibited antifungal[40] and antioxidant[41] properties. Taking 200 mg of the emulsified oil of oregano orally three times daily for 6 weeks eradicated parasites in the stool of infected patients.[5]

bioactive dose

Not known.

safety

Presumed safe when consumed in normal dietary quantities by non-allergic individuals. Oregano is thought to have abortifacient and emmenagogue effects and should therefore not be used by pregnant women.[5]

References

1. Othman RA, Moghadasian MH, Jones PJ. Cholesterol-lowering effects of oat β-glucan. *Nutr Rev.* 2011;69(6):299–309. doi: 10.1111/j.1753-4887.2011.00401.x.
2. US Department of Agriculture. Agricultural Research Service. Medicinal Foods Database. *Avena sativa* (oats). http://www.pl.barc.usda.gov/usda_rrcp/rrecipe_query_result.cfm?code=69685564&ThisName=grain. Accessed January 17, 2012.
3. Tosh SM. Review of human studies investigating the post-prandial blood-glucose lowering ability of oat and barley food products. *Eur J Clin Nutr.* 2013;67(4):310–317. doi: 10.1038/ejcn.2013.25. Epub 2013 February 20.

4. US Department of Agriculture. Agricultural Research Service. Nutrient Data Lab. Cereals, oats. http://ndb.nal.usda.gov/ndb/foods/show/1890?man=&lfacet=&count=&max=35&qlookup=cooked+oats&offset=&sort=&format=Abridged&reportfmt=other&rptfrm=&ndbno=&nutrient1=&nutrient2=&nutrient3=&subset=&totCount=&measureby=&_action_show=Apply+Changes&Qv=1&Q3794=0.66&Q3795=1&Q3796=0.75. Accessed September 6, 2015.

5. Jellin JM, Gregory PJ. *Natural Medicine Comprehensive Database*. Therapeutic Research Faculty. 2013. http://www.naturaldatabase.com. Accessed July 11, 2012.

6. Charlton KE, Tapsell LC, Batterham MJ, O'Shea J, Thorne R, Beck E, Tosh SM. Effect of 6 weeks' consumption of β-glucan-rich oat products on cholesterol levels in mildly hypercholesterolaemic overweight adults. *Br J Nutr*. 2012;107(7):1037–1047. Epub 2011 August 3.

7. Richman E. The safety of oats in the dietary treatment of coeliac disease. *Proc Nutr Soc*. 2012;71(4):534–537. doi: 10.1017/S0029665112000791. Epub 2012 August 29.

8. US Department of Health and Human Services. National Institute of Diabetes and Digestive and Kidney Diseases. http://www.niddk.nih.gov/health-information/health-topics/digestive-diseases/celiac-disease/Pages/facts.aspx#examples. Accessed April 10, 2015.

9. Carlsen MH, Halvorsen BL, Holte K, Bøhn SK, Dragland S, Sampson L, Willey C et al. The total antioxidant content of more than 3100 foods, beverages, spices, herbs and supplements used worldwide. *Nutr J*. 2010;9(3):2–11.

10. Arapitsas P. Identification and quantification of polyphenolic compounds from okra seeds and skins. *Food Chem*. 2008;110(4);1041–1045.

11. Sabitha V, Ramachandran S, Naveen KR, Panneerselvam K. Antidiabetic and antihyperlipidemic potential of *Abelmoschus esculentus* (L.) Moench. in streptozotocin-induced diabetic rats. *J Pharm Bioallied Sci*. 2011;3(3):397–402.

12. Ghanbari R, Anwar F, Alkharfy KM, Gilani AH, Saari N. Valuable nutrients and functional bioactives in different parts of olive (*Olea europaea* L.)—A review. *Int J Mol Sci*. 2012;13(3):3291–3340. doi: 10.3390/ijms13033291. Epub 2012 March 12.

13. Cardeno A, Sanchez-Hidalgo M, de la Lastra AC. An up-date of olive oil phenols in inflammation and cancer: Molecular mechanisms and clinical implications. *Curr Med Chem*. 2013;20(37):4758–4776. Epub 2013 June 25.

14. Badimon L, Vilahur G, Padro T. Nutraceuticals and atherosclerosis: Human trials. *Cardiovasc Ther*. 2010;28(4):202–215.

15. Visiolia F, Gallia C. Biological properties of olive oil phytochemicals. *Crit Rev Food Sci Nutr*. 2002;42(3):209–221.

16. Ryan M, McInerney D, Owens D, Collins P, Johnson A, Tomkin GH. Diabetes and the Mediterranean diet: A beneficial effect of oleic acid on insulin sensitivity, adipocyte glucose transport and endothelium-dependent vasoreactivity. *QJM*. 2000;93(2):85–91.

17. US Food and Drug Administration. FDA Allows Qualified Health Claim to Decrease Risk of Coronary Heart Disease. http://www.fda.gov/newsevents/newsroom/pressannouncements/2004/ucm108368.htm. Accessed July 17, 2013.

18. Perona JS, Cañizares J, Montero E, Sánchez-Domínguez JM, Catalá A, Ruiz-Gutiérrez V. Virgin olive oil reduces blood pressure in hypertensive elderly subjects. *Clin Nutr*. 2004;23(5):1113–1121.

O

19. DeBruyne LK, Pinna K. *Nutrition for Health and Health Care*, 5th edn. Belmont, CA: Wadsworth Cengage Learning; 2014.

20. National Institutes of Health. National Center for Complementary and Alternative Medicine. Omega-3-Fatty Acids. http://nccam.nih.gov/health/omega3/introduction.htm. Accessed January 18, 2012.

21. Simopoulos AP. Omega-3 fatty acids in inflammation and autoimmune disease. *J Am Coll Nutr*. 2002;21(6):495–505.

22. Malasanos TH, Stacpoole, PW. Biological effects of ω-3 fatty acids in diabetes mellitus. *Diabetes Care*. 1991;14(12):1160–1179.

23. MacLean CH, Mojica WA, Morton SC, Pencharz J, Hasenfeld Garland R, Tu W, Newberry SJ et al. Effects of omega-3 fatty acids on lipids and glycemic control in type II diabetes and the metabolic syndrome and on inflammatory bowel disease, rheumatoid arthritis, renal disease, systemic lupus erythematosus, and osteoporosis. Evidence Report/Technology Assessment. No. 89 (Prepared by Southern California/RAND Evidence-based Practice Center, under Contract No. 290-02-0003). AHRQ Publication No. 04-E012-2. Rockville, MD: Agency for Healthcare Research and Quality; March 2004.

24. Wang C, Chung M, Lichtenstein A, Balk E, Kupelnick B, DeVine D, Lawrence A, Lau J. *Effects of Omega-3 Fatty Acids on Cardiovascular Disease*. Rockville, MD: Agency for Healthcare Research and Quality (US); 2004 March. (Evidence Reports/Technology Assessments, No. 94.) Available from: http://www.ncbi.nlm.nih.gov/books/NBK37223.

25. Sarris J, Mischoulon D, Schweitzer I. Omega-3 for bipolar disorder: Meta-analyses of use in mania and bipolar depression. *J Clin Psychiatry*. 2012;73(1):81–86. doi: 10.4088/JCP.10r06710. Epub 2011 August 9.

26. Goodnight Jr. SH, Harris WS, Connor WE, Illingworth DR. Polyunsaturated fatty acids, hyperlipidemia, and thrombosis. *Arteriosclerosis*. 1982(2);2:87–113.

27. The American Heart Association. Frequently Asked Questions About "Better" Fats. http://www.heart.org/HEARTORG/GettingHealthy/NutritionCenter/Frequently-Asked-Questions-About-Better-Fats_UCM_305985_Article.jsp. Accessed July 22, 2013.

28. Chowdhury R, Warnakula S, Phil M, Kunutsor S, Crowe F, Ward HA, Johnson L et al. Association of dietary, circulating, and supplement fatty acids with coronary risk: A systematic review and meta-analysis. *Ann Intern Med*. 2014;160(6):398–406. doi:10.7326/M13-1788.

29. Muhlhausler BS, Ailhaud GP. Omega-6 polyunsaturated fatty acids and the early origins of obesity. *Curr Opin Endocrinol Diabetes Obes*. 2013;20(1):56–61. doi: 10.1097/MED.0b013e32835c1ba7.

30. Kelly OJ, Gilman JC, Kim Y, Ilich JZ. Long-chain polyunsaturated fatty acids may mutually benefit both obesity and osteoporosis. *Nutr Res*. 2013;33(7):521–533. doi: 10.1016/j.nutres.2013.04.012. Epub 2013 June 10.

31. Griffiths G, Trueman L, Crowther T, Thomas B, Smith B. Onions—A global benefit to health. *Phytother Res*. 2002;16(7):603–615.

32. Sengupta A, Ghosh S, Bhattacharjee S. Allium vegetables in cancer prevention: An overview. *Asian Pac J Cancer Prev*. 2004;5(3):237–245.

33. Augusti KT. Therapeutic values of onion (*Allium cepa* L.) and garlic (*Allium sativum* L.). *Indian J Exp Biol*. 1996;34(7):634–640.

34. Osmont KS, Arnt CR, Goldman IL. Temporal aspects of onion-induced antiplatelet activity. *Plant Foods Hum Nutr*. 2003;58(1):27–40.

35. Galeone C, Tavani A, Pelucchi C, Negri E, La Vecchia C. Allium vegetable intake and risk of acute myocardial infarction in Italy. *Eur J Nutr.* 2009;48(2):120–123.
36. Dorant E, van den Brandt PA, Goldbohm RA. A prospective cohort study on the relationship between onion and leek consumption, garlic supplement use and the risk of colorectal carcinoma in The Netherlands. *Carcinogenesis.* 1996;17(3):477–484.
37. Asgary S, Keshvari M. Effects of *Citrus sinensis* juice on blood pressure. *ARYA Atheroscler.* 2013;9(1):98–101.
38. Kurowska EM, Spence JD, Jordan J, Wetmore S, Freeman DJ, Piché LA, Serratore P. HDL-cholesterol-raising effect of orange juice in subjects with hypercholesterolemia. *Am J Clin Nutr.* 2000;72(5):1095–1100.
39. USDA Agricultural Research Service. Herbs. *Origanum vulgare.* http://www.pl.barc.usda.gov/usda_plant/plant_home.cfm. Accessed June 4, 2011.
40. Adam K, Sivropoulou A, Kokkini S, Lanaras T, Arsenakis M. Antifungal activities of *Origanum vulgare* subsp. hirtum, *mentha spicata, lavandula angustifolia,* and *salvia fruticosa* essential oils against human pathogenic fungi. *J Agric Food Chem.* 1998;46(5):1739–1745.
41. Cervato G, Carabelli M, Gervasio S, Cittera A, Cazzola RA, Cestaro B. Antioxidant properties of oregano (*Origanum vulgare*) leaf extracts. *J Food Biochem.* 2000;24(6):453–465.

O

P

Palm

definition

Vegetable harvested from the coconut (*Cocos nucifera*) palm tree.[1] Hearts of palm are sold canned in salt water and are eaten as a salad vegetable. It is high in sodium, but is also a good source of fiber, folate, vitamin C, and iron, and contains less than 1 g of fat, being equal parts saturated and polyunsaturated. Palm oil has been a major source of cooking oil in Asia and Africa.[2] Palm oil, a saturated, tropical oil, is a source of vitamin E.

scientific findings

One cup of canned hearts of palm contains 4.5 g of nonheme iron whose absorption is increased by its vitamin C content (11.5 mg/19% DV).[1] Palm oil does not raise serum cholesterol levels according to a one review; however, The American Heart Association considers palm and other tropical oils to be atherogenic, saturated fats, and advises limiting them for heart health.[2]

bioactive dose

Not known.

safety

Presumed safe when consumed in normal dietary quantities by non-allergic individuals.

Pantothenic acid

definition

B-vitamin that is found in all food groups, hence its name, "pantos," the Greek word referring to "everywhere." Rich sources include peanut butter, liver, kidney, peanuts, almonds, wheat bran, cheese, and lobster.[3] Although refining, cooking, canning, and freezing decrease the pantothenic acid content of foods,[3] dietary intake from eating the average Western diet has been estimated to meet the RDA.[4]

scientific findings

Pantothenic acid is a required coenzyme in fatty acid metabolism.[4] Pantothenic acid deficiency is uncommon but has been observed in patients who receive no pantothenic acid in their diet or who were given a pantothenic acid antagonist.[4] Signs and symptoms of pantothenic acid deficiency include irritability, restlessness, fatigue, apathy, malaise, sleep disturbances, nausea, vomiting, abdominal cramps, numbness, paresthesias, muscle cramps, a staggering gait, hypoglycemia, and an increased sensitivity to insulin.[4]

bioactive dose

The AI is 5 mg/day for adults aged 19–50 years.

safety

No UL has been established for pantothenic acid.

Papaya (Carica papaya L.)

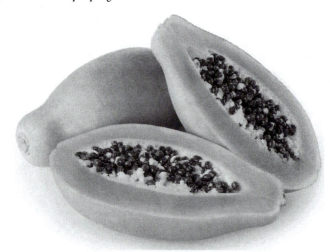

Papaya. (Image from Abramova Elena/Shutterstock.)

definition

Also known as paw-paw (also spelled pawpaw).[5,6] Large, oblong fruit with yellow-green skin that is approximately the size of a football. Papaya is eaten raw in fruit salads and sold as a canned fruit or used to make nectar. Papaya is sweet and has the texture of cantaloupe. One cup of papaya is an excellent source of vitamin C (83 mg, 138% DV), folate (54 µg, 13% DV), and vitamin A (1378 IU, 27% DV) and a good source of fiber (2.5 g, 10% DV) and potassium (264 mg; 7% DV).[7] Papaya is used in folk medicine for contraception,[8] though no scientific evidence supports this use.

scientific findings

Papaya suppressed inflammatory cytokines in the cells of human subjects (n = 12).[9]

bioactive dose

Not known.

safety

Presumed safe when consumed in normal dietary quantities by non-allergic individuals.

P

Paprika (Capsicum annuum)

definition

Dried ground pods of the sweet red or chili pepper that adds earthy or spicy flavor and reddish-brown color to foods such as chili and barbeque sauce. Contains flavonoids and carotenoids, including β-carotene, lutein, and xeaxanthin.[10,11]

scientific findings

Paprika contains antioxidants and has demonstrated free-radical-scavenging ability in laboratory research.[12]

bioactive dose

Not known.

safety

Presumed safe when consumed in normal dietary quantities by non-allergic individuals. Paprika may contain allergens.[13]

Parsley (Petroselinum crispum)

definition

Green culinary herb member of the Apiaceous Apiaceae family, which also includes carrots, parsnips, and celery. The flat-leaf variety is more favored for its flavor, whereas the curly variety is typically used as a garnish or as a main component of tabouleh, the Middle Eastern salad. Parsley is an excellent source of vitamin C and contains phytochemical constituents, including flavones.[14] It has been used in traditional medicine to stimulate menstruation.[15]

scientific findings

Flavones in parsley possess anti-inflammatory properties *in vitro* and in animal models.[14] Parsley and other apiaceous vegetables inhibited anticarcinogenic activity in laboratory research.[16]

bioactive dose

Not known.

safety

Presumed safe when consumed in normal dietary quantities by non-allergic individuals. Adverse effects have been reported from consuming excessive amounts of parsley due to the apiole constituent; for example, 200 g of parsley (about the amount in 3.25 cups of parsley) have been associated with blood dyscrasias, kidney toxicity, and liver toxicities.[15] Components in parsley, including psoralen, bergapten, and xanthotoxin, can cause photosensitization (sensitivity to light).[17]

Passion fruit (Passiflora edulis)

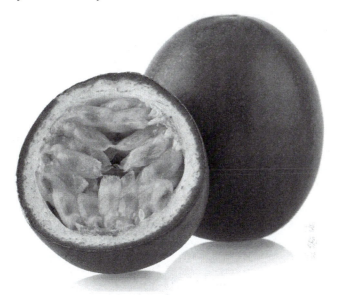

Passion fruit. (Image from Viktar Malyshchyts/Shutterstock.)

definition

Also spelled passionfruit; also called granadilla. Small, purple-skinned fruit that is cut into halves to access its chewy, seed-filled sacs. Eaten fresh and used to make tropical juice blends. A source of terpenoids, flavonoids, and fiber.[18] Passion fruit is used as a folk medicine for its sedative and antihypertensive effects and for treating anxiety and nervousness.[19]

scientific findings

In experimental research, *Passiflora edulis* pulp extract reduced total cholesterol in rats and increased their high-density lipoprotein.[20] In a laboratory study, aqueous extracts of *P. edulis* exhibited an anxiolytic-like activity.[18] Another laboratory study found that a triterpenoid constituent of *P. edulis* Sims possessed antidepressant-like activity in animals.[19]

bioactive dose

Not known.

P

safety

Presumed safe when consumed in normal dietary quantities by non-allergic individuals.

Peach (Prunus persica)

definition

Rosaceae family fruit, which also includes apples, nectarines, plums, pears, and strawberries. Peaches are a source of vitamin C and phytochemicals such as chlorogenic acid, phenolics, anthocyanins, and flavonoids.[21,22] When consumed whole, with the skin intact, peaches are a good source of fiber, with one large peach providing 2.6 g (10% DV) of fiber.[23] Peaches are also commonly consumed canned, dried, as fruit juice, and as nectar.

scientific findings

Raw and canned peaches inhibited LDL oxidation *in vitro*.[24] A prospective case study (n = 75,929 women aged 38–63 years at baseline) examined the associations of specific fruits and vegetables with risk of estrogen receptor-negative breast cancer. Dietary data were collected seven times during a 24-year period. Consuming at least two servings of peaches/nectarines per week was associated with a lower risk of estrogen receptor-negative breast cancer among postmenopausal women compared with nonusers.[25] Chlorogenic acid protected cells from oxidative damage in a laboratory study.[26]

bioactive dose

Not known.

safety

Presumed safe when consumed in normal dietary quantities by non-allergic individuals. A European study showed that the iron, copper, lead, zinc, and tin contents of canned peaches increased over a 2-year period.[27]

Peanut (Arachis hypogaea)

definition

High-protein, high-monounsaturated fat legume that supplies vitamin E; it is also a source of phytochemicals, such as resveratrol.[28] Peanuts are consumed roasted, made into peanut butter, and used in making peanut candy, often paired with chocolate, and other confections. Also used in Thai cooking in noodle-based dishes and on salads.

scientific findings

There is moderate evidence that peanut and other nut consumption improved serum lipid levels.[28] At least five servings (28 g [1 oz] of nuts; or 16 g [1 tablespoon] of peanut butter) was significantly associated with a lower risk of cardiovascular disease (including lower total and LDL cholesterol and apolipoprotein-B-100 concentrations, no effect on HDL cholesterol, and no effect on inflammatory markers) in women with type 2 diabetes in an epidemiological study (n = 54,656 women with type 2 diabetes).[29]

bioactive dose

Not known.

safety

Presumed safe when consumed in normal dietary quantities by non-allergic individuals, peanuts are among the most common foods to cause allergic reactions in children, adolescents, and adults.[30]

Pear (Pyrus communis)

P

definition

White-fleshed fruit that supplies approximately 5–6 g of fiber per medium pear,[31] making it an excellent source of fiber, and flavonoids, such as flavon-3-ols.[32] In addition to many varieties of pear that are consumed fresh, pears are sold canned, dehydrated, dried, and are used to make fruit juice drinks.

scientific findings

In rodents, *Pyrus communis* exerted strong antioxidant activity and protective effects against ethanol- or hydrochloric acid-induced gastric ulcers.[33] Flavonols exert cardioprotective and anticarcinogenic properties *in vitro* and *in vivo*.[34]

bioactive dose

Not known.

safety

Presumed safe when consumed in normal dietary quantities by non-allergic individuals.

Pectin

definition

Fermentable, water-soluble fiber found in grains, legumes, fruits, and vegetables. In foods such as okra, it imparts a unique, gel-like texture that is useful for thickening soups and stews. Pectin in cooked fruit gelatinizes to solidify jams and jellies; oat bran pectin is the viscous material in cooked oatmeal.

scientific findings

Pectin slows the transit of food through the upper GI tract[35] and stimulates epithelial growth within the colon, and thus has been used to manage diarrhea.[36] Pectin significantly reduced diarrhea in a small, double-blind clinical trial (n = 62 boys aged 5–12 months with persistent diarrhea [≥ 14 days]) that randomly assigned subjects to receive a rice-based diet (n = 21); a rice-based diet with 250 g/L of cooked green banana (n = 22); or a rice-based diet with 4 g/kg of pectin (n = 19) for 7 days. Diarrhea significantly improved in the pectin-supplemented and banana groups compared to the rice-only group.[37] Possible mechanisms for pectin to maintain normal stool consistency include that fiber is fermented by anaerobic colonic flora (which constitute the bulk of fecal matter); a lack of dietary fiber may suppress normal colonic metabolism, thereby impairing stool formation/promoting diarrhea; and/or that pectin stimulates epithelial growth in the colon to reduce diarrhea.[38] Pectin, like other soluble fibers, binds bile acids and cholesterol in the small intestine, thereby helping to reduce serum cholesterol.[39]

bioactive dose

The recommended dose used to decrease total cholesterol and triglyceride levels is 15–20 g of pectin daily.[36] For persistent diarrhea in children, 4 g/kg of body weight per day of pectin fiber has been used.[15]

safety

Presumed safe when consumed in normal dietary quantities by non-allergic individuals.

Pepper, sweet bell (Capsicum anuum L.)

definition

Popular salad vegetable that is a good source of vitamins A, C, and E, and provides polyphenols.[40] There are many different cultivars, including green, yellow, orange, and purple bell peppers.

scientific findings

Epidemiology suggests that polyphenols exert cardioprotective effects and laboratory studies suggest that polyphenols exert antioxidant, vasodilatory, anti-inflammatory, antifibrotic, antiapoptotic, and metabolic effects.[41]

bioactive dose

Not known.

safety

Presumed safe when consumed by nonallergic individuals in normal dietary quantities.

Pepper, chili (Capsicum frutescens, Capsicum annuum)

definition

Also spelled chile pepper. Fruit[42] containing pungent compounds, such as capsaicin, that produces a burning sensation upon contact with the skin. *Capsicum annuum* is dried and ground and used to make cayenne pepper. Jalapeño peppers, also called jalapeño chilies, is a variety of *Capsicum frutescens*, that is an excellent source of vitamin C.[43] Different cultivars of chili pepper contain different phytochemicals by color, for example, red habanero peppers contain β-carotene; green serrano and jalapeño peppers contain capsanthin, yellow habanero and Scotch Bonnet peppers contain lutein, and α- and β-carotene, and orange habanero contain antheraxanthin, capsanthin, and xeaxanthin.[44] Native Americans rubbed their gums with pepper pods to relieve toothache.[45] Chili pepper is used as an herbal medicine to treat microbial infection.[46]

scientific findings

Extracts from fresh *C. frutrescens* exhibited antimicrobial effects against *Bacillus cereus*, *Bacillus subtilis*, *Clostridium sporogenes*, *Clostridium tetani*, and *Streptococcus pyogenes* in a laboratory study.[46]

bioactive dose

Not known.

safety

Presumed safe when consumed in normal dietary quantities by non-allergic individuals. Chili pepper consumption may induce liver carcinoma in the rat.[47] Dermatitis can sometimes occur in breast-fed infants when mothers ingest foods heavily spiced with capsicum peppers.[15]

Peppermint (Mentha × piperita)

definition

A cross between water mint (also spelled watermint) and spearmint that contains a menthol constituent[48] thought to be responsible for its sweet fragrance and cooling sensation. When its leaves are finely shredded, it is used as a culinary herb to flavor meat dishes and vegetable or fruit salads. It is also used fresh or dried to make teas, candies, and chewing gum. Peppermint oil is widely used as a spasmolytic agent in irritable bowel syndrome (IBS).[49]

scientific findings

Peppermint oil is antispasmotic due to its calcium channel blocking activity of intestinal smooth muscle.[48] Menthol reduces intestinal motility in animal studies.[49] Peppermint oil improved the symptoms of IBS in clinical trials, and is "likely effective" for IBS.[15,50] In one small randomized, crossover-design clinical trial (n = 26 healthy volunteers) intragastric pressure and motility were improved in healthy volunteers after oral administration of peppermint oil compared to placebo.[49] A prospective, double-blind, placebo-controlled study (n = 74) randomized IBS patients to receive either peppermint oil or placebo three times daily for six weeks, finding that "at six weeks of therapy, abdominal pain … markedly improved … in [the] peppermint oil group compared with … [the] placebo group and the difference was statistically highly significant."[48] A third study showed "significant improvement in pain after three weeks treatment with peppermint oil compared to placebo, but after six weeks, there were no differences between treatment and placebo groups."[15]

bioactive dose

Not known. For irritable bowel syndrome (IBS), the usual medicinal dose is "1–2 capsules three times daily of enteric coated peppermint oil. Each capsule provides approximately 0.2 mL of peppermint oil or 180–225 mg peppermint oil."

safety

Presumed safe when consumed in normal dietary quantities by non-allergic individuals. Peppermint may aggravate heartburn, presumably by its direct effects upon sensory neurons.[50]

Persimmon (Diospyros kaki)

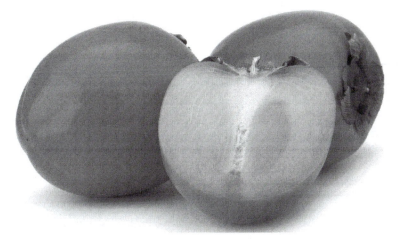

Persimmon. (Image from EM Arts/Shutterstock.)

P

definition

Strong-flavored fruit whose phytochemical content is responsible for its characteristic mouthfeel and aftertaste. It resembles a small orange tomato in appearance (color, firmness, and the calyx or stem at the top center of the fruit), and it is typically most palatable when ripe. Unripe persimmon is strongly astringent. Persimmon is a source of dietary fiber and polyphenols.[51]

scientific findings

Tannin in persimmon bound bile acids *in vitro*.[52] Both fresh and dried persimmon possess high contents of bioactive compounds and have a high antioxidant potential and free-radical scavenging capacity.[51]

bioactive dose

Not known.

safety

Presumed safe when consumed in normal dietary quantities by non-allergic individuals. Consumption of persimmons, particularly unpeeled persimmons, has been associated with the development of bezoars (a concretion formed in the alimentary canal from plant fibers); a case report of 15 patients cautioned that patients who have undergone ulcer surgery should avoid unpeeled persimmons.[53]

Phenolic compounds

definition

Phytochemicals, such as phenolic lipids and phenolic acids, that include chlorogenic acid, hesperidin, kaempferol, luteolin, myricetin, naringenin, p-coumaric acid, rosmarinic acid, and quercetin. Phenolic compounds found in herbs include rosmarinic acid in thyme, rosemary, and oregano. Phenolic compounds are also found in coffee beans and coffee, fruits (apples, blueberries, cherries, grapes, oranges, prunes, pears, and strawberries), oats, potatoes, soybeans, and wine.[54]

scientific findings

Phenolic compounds have exerted antioxidant, anti-inflammatory, and antimicrobial effects in laboratory studies.[55–58] Epidemiological studies suggest that the consumption of fruits and vegetables is associated with a reduced incidence of cardiovascular disease, diabetes, cancer, and stroke. The disease-protective effects are due, in part, to phenolic compounds.[57]

P

bioactive dose

Not known.

safety

Presumed safe when consumed in normal dietary quantities by non-allergic individuals.

Phloretin

definition

Flavonoid found in plant foods such as apples and citrus fruits.[59]

scientific findings

Shown to exert antioxidant properties *in vitro*.[60] Phloretin exerted a chemoprotective activity against the carcinogen aflatoxin B in a laboratory study.[61]

bioactive dose

Not known.

safety

Presumed safe when consumed in normal dietary quantities by non-allergic individuals.

Phosphorus

definition

Mineral that is involved in energy transfer during energy metabolism, is a component of hydroxyapatite crystal of bone, is part of cellular phospholipid membranes, and is involved in numerous body-wide functions, such as maintaining normal pH.[62] Found in abundance in high-protein foods, such as meat, fish, poultry, eggs, and milk. Phosphate salts are also common food additives; for example, as the acidulant phosphoric acid in some soda beverage products.[62] Phosphorus is actually so ubiquitous in foods that nearly total starvation is required to produce a phosphorus deficiency, and phosphorus intake from the average American diet is typically higher than the RDA.[62]

scientific findings

Phosphorus deficiency resulting in hypophosphatemia causes cellular dysfunction, symptoms of which include anorexia, anemia, muscle weakness, bone pain, rickets, osteomalacia, general debility, increased susceptibility to infection, paresthesias, ataxia, confusion, and even death.[62]

bioactive dose

The RDA for adults is 700 mg/day.

safety

The UL for adults is 4 g/day.

Phytate (Phytic acid)

definition

Primary storage compound of phosphorus in seeds.[63] It binds to calcium, iron, potassium, magnesium, manganese, and zinc in the gut and renders them inabsorbable.[63,64] Phytates are found in legumes, seeds, and the husks of whole grains.

scientific findings

Phytic acid is an antioxidant.[65]

bioactive dose

Not known.

safety

Presumed safe when consumed in normal dietary quantities by non-allergic individuals. Diets that provide >40 g of fiber per day may contain phytate levels that adversely impact the absorption of minerals.[54]

Phytoestrogen

definition

P

Phenolic compound that can exert estrogenic and antiestrogenic properties.[66] When circulating estrogen level is low, phytoestrogens are thought to become estrogenic; when circulating estrogen level is high, phytoestrogens are thought to become antiestrogenic.[67] Sources of phytoestrogens include whole grains, fruits, vegetables, such as alfalfa, anise, pumpkin seeds, and soy products such as soybeans, soy flour, soymilk, tofu, and textured vegetable protein made from soybeans, with soy foods being the richest food sources.[54,66,68]

scientific findings

A meta-analysis found that phytoestrogens appear to reduce the frequency of hot flashes (hot flushes) in perimenopausal or postmenopausal women experiencing menopausal symptoms, though authors stated the data were inconclusive.[67] Another meta-analysis found that "No conclusive evidence shows that phytoestrogen supplements effectively reduce the frequency or severity of hot flashes and night sweats in perimenopausal or postmenopausal women."[69] A meta-analysis of observational studies showed higher phytoestrogen intake from foods (dietary supplements were excluded) was associated with a reduced ovarian cancer risk.[70]

bioactive dose

Not known.

safety

Presumed safe when consumed in normal dietary quantities by non-allergic individuals. Estrogenic adverse effects may occur as a result of consuming phytoestrogens. Estrogen-like effects seem to be infrequent and increase with long-term therapy.[71]

Pineapple (Anasas comosus)

definition

Yellow, fibrous-fleshed, juicy tropical fruit of the Bromeliacea family. It is consumed fresh, canned, and as juice. An excellent source of vitamin C, pineapple supplies vitamin A, and all B vitamins except vitamin B12.[72] Pineapple is a natural source of the plant protease bromelain that is used orally as an anti-inflammatory agent.[73] Pineapple is a source of papain, a proteolytic enzyme.

scientific findings

P

In an animal study, pineapple juice significantly decreased plasma triglycerides and delayed gastric emptying.[74] *In vitro* and *in vivo* studies demonstrate that bromelain exhibits various fibrinolytic, antiedematous, antithrombotic, and anti-inflammatory activities,[75] but that there is insufficient evidence to rate its effectiveness for anti-inflammation or other uses in humans.[76] Bromelain also contains chemicals that interfere with the growth of tumor cells and slow blood clotting.[76] Bromelain and papain enhance bioflavonoid absorption.[77]

bioactive dose

Not known.

safety

Presumed safe when consumed in normal dietary quantities by non-allergic individuals.

Pistachio (Pistacia vera)

definition

Small tree nut eaten raw or roasted that is a source of protein, monounsaturated fatty acid, vitamin E, and the antioxidant lutein. Antioxidant
levels are higher in raw pistachios than in roasted pistachios and in natural shells versus in chemically bleached shells.[78]

scientific findings

As part of an antiatherogenic diet, pistachios may contribute to a reduction in serum oxidized-LDL.[79] A meta-analysis of 21 randomized, controlled trials, conducted to evaluate the effect of nut consumption on
blood pressure in adult populations aged ≥18 years, found that total nut
consumption lowered systolic blood pressure in participants without type
2 diabetes, and that pistachios had the strongest impact on reducing systolic and diastolic blood pressure compared to other types of nuts.[80]

bioactive dose

Not known.

safety

Presumed safe when consumed in normal dietary quantities by non-
allergic individuals. Allergies to pistachio nuts have been reported. A case
report of exercise-induced anaphylaxis to pistachio consumed 1/2 h prior
to exercise has been reported.[81]

Plantain (Musa × paradisiaca)

definition

Starchy, green-skinned, banana-like fruit whose skin turns yellow when
ripe. It supplies 65 g of carbohydrate per 1 cup; in addition, it is an excellent source of vitamin A (2227 IU; 45% DV), magnesium (76 mg of magnesium, 19% DV), and potassium (857 mg; 24% DV), and a good source of
vitamin E (2.79 mg of vitamin E, 9% DV)[82] in addition to providing fiber
and flavonoids. Ripe plantains are typically cooked by slicing and frying,
but are not eaten raw.

scientific findings

In a clinical trial (n = 80 hospitalized children ranging in age from 1 to
28 months, who had experienced > or = 14 days of persistent diarrhea),

the experimental group (n = 40) was given a cooked green plantain-based diet; a control group was given a yogurt-based diet. The average duration of diarrhea in the plantain-based diet group was 18 h shorter (significantly different than the yogurt group).[83] Leucocyanidin, a flavonoid having antiulcer properties, has been identified in plantain.[84] A laboratory study found that plantain soluble fiber prevented *Escherichia coli* translocation in intestinal cells, which may have implications in preventing Crohn's disease symtoms.[85]

bioactive dose

Not known.

safety

Presumed safe when consumed in normal dietary quantities by non-allergic individuals.

Plum (Prunus domestica)

definition

Stone fruit that has been cultivated since ancient times. Its different cultivars (including red, purple, yellow, and green varieties) vary in size and nutrient and phytochemical composition. Commonly eaten fresh, dried (as dried plums or prunes), canned, and as part of processed foods, such as baby food. An average, 2"-diameter fresh plum supplies approximately 7.5 g of carbohydrate and 1 g of fiber, in addition to vitamin C, vitamin E, β-carotene, and phytochemicals such as phenolics, quercetin, myrecitin, and kaempferol.[86–88] An analysis of yellow plums found conventional plums to be higher in quercetin than organic plums, but organic plums to be higher in myrecitin and kaempferol than conventional plums.[88] Dried plums/prunes and prune juice are traditionally consumed to relieve constipation. A 100-g serving (10 dried plums or 3/4 cups) of dried plums provides approximately 6.1 g of dietary fiber, 2–3 mg of boron, and 745 mg of potassium,[89,90] making them a good source of fiber and an excellent source of potassium.

scientific findings

Eating 100 g (approximately 3/4 cup) of dried plum for 3 months significantly reduced serum levels of C-reactive protein in a small clinical trial (n = 160 postmenopausal women).[91] Dried plums and prune juice are high in sorbitol (14.7 g and 6.1 g/100 g, respectively), which is a laxative,[89] but soluble and insoluble fiber also promote laxation, the former by retaining water in stool, the latter by providing bulk. Sorbitol is an effective osmotic laxative.[92] In an 8-week, single-blind, randomized crossover study (n = 40 constipated subjects, mean age 38), dried plums (50 g twice a day providing 6 g fiber/day) were found to be more effective than psyllium (11 g twice a day providing 6 g fiber/day) for the treatment of mild to moderate constipation.[93] A laboratory analysis found that phenolic compounds in prunes, pitted prunes, and prune juice inhibited LDL oxidation *in vitro*.[94] Eating dried prunes may improve bone mineral density possibly due to their high boron concentration.[89]

bioactive dose

Not known.

safety

Presumed safe when consumed in normal dietary quantities by non-allergic individuals. A sudden increase in the amount of fiber eaten can cause gastrointestinal distress. Adding high-fiber foods to the diet gradually with sufficient amounts of water is recommended.

Polyunsaturated fatty acids

definition

Oils that include omega-3-fatty acids (n-3) in plants and fish, and omega-6 fatty acids (n-6) in plants. Polyunsaturated fatty acids (PUFAs) are long-chained fatty acids that contain more than one double bond and are liquid at room temperature.

scientific findings

PUFAs are necessary for brain function and must be consumed in the diet to prevent deficiency of essential fatty acids. Essential fatty acid deficiency is characterized by growth, skin, and other abnormalities. Clinical studies suggest that children with attention deficit hyperactivity disorder have lower plasma levels of essential fatty acids.[15] Dietary n-6 PUFAs are associated with improved blood lipids related to cardiovascular disease, in particular when PUFAs replace saturated fatty acids (SFA) and/or trans fatty acids.[95] Energy replacement of SFA with PUFA decreases total cholesterol, LDL cholesterol, and triglycerides, as well as numerous markers of inflammation.[95] PUFA intake significantly decreases risk of cardiovascular disease and has also been shown to decrease the risk of type 2 diabetes.[95] Meta-analyses of randomized, clinical trials found no beneficial effects of LCPUFA supplementation on the physical, visual, and neurodevelopmental outcomes of infants born at term.[96]

bioactive dose

There is no RDA for PUFA *per se.* Omega-3 fatty acid (also called linolenic acid) and omega-6 fatty acid (linoleic acid) each have specific RDAs—see *omega-3 and omega-6 fatty acid.* A dietary intake of 1%–2% of total calories as linoleic acid is sufficient to prevent EFA deficiency; whereas 2%–4% is needed to reverse EFA deficiency.[97]

safety

Presumed safe when consumed in normal dietary quantities by non-allergic individuals.

Pomegranate (Punica granatum)

definition

Orange-sized fruit that has red, leathery skin and contains sacs filled with hundreds of edible seeds encased in juicy red pulp. Pomegranate is high in vitamin C and fiber as well as phytochemicals, including ellagic acid, ellagitannins, punicic acid, anthocyanidins, anthocyanins, estrogenic flavonols, and flavonoids.[98] In traditional medicine, *Punica granatum* has been used as an antiatherogenic, antidiarrheal, and as a treatment for parasitic and microbial infections, ulcers, apthae (mouth inflammations), hemorrhage, and respiratory complications.[98]

scientific findings

Pomegranate constituents, such as ellagic acid, exerted antioxidant properties in experimental research.[98] Drinking pomegranate juice does not seem to relieve symptoms or improve breathing in individuals with chronic obstructive pulmonary disease.[15] There is insufficient evidence to evaluate its use in treating other health conditions for which it has been studied or used, including hyperlipidemia; hypertension, atherosclerosis, gum disease, prostate cancer, coronary stenosis, intestinal worm infestation, obesity, fungal mouth infection, diarrhea, dysentery, sore throat, hemorrhoids, or menopausal symptoms.[15]

bioactive dose

Not known.

safety

Presumed safe when consumed in normal dietary quantities by non-allergic individuals.

Potassium

definition

Main intracellular mineral required for the maintenance of pH balance, blood pressure, and general cellular function.[99] Sources of potassium include fresh foods of all kinds, especially fresh fruits (apricots, dates, bananas), fresh vegetables, soybeans, and dairy products. The average American diet does not meet daily potassium recommendations.[99]

scientific findings

Potassium deficiency affects neural transmission, muscle contraction, blood pressure, and vascular tone.[99] Dietary potassium has significantly lowered blood pressure in both hypertensive and nonhypertensive patients in observational studies, clinical trials, and several meta-analyses.[100] Epidemiologic studies and randomized controlled trials have shown an inverse relationship between fruit and vegetable intake and blood pressure. "The antihypertensive effect of potassium ... appears to occur through several mechanisms that include regulation of vascular sensitivity to catecholamines, promotion of natriuresis, limiting plasma renin activity, and improving endothelial function."[101] Consuming potassium from dietary sources seems to decrease the risk of stroke.[15]

bioactive dose

The AI for adults is 4700 mg/day. Foods that provide at least 350 mg of potassium per serving and that are low in sodium, saturated fat, and cholesterol might help reduce the risk of developing high blood pressure.[15]

safety

Presumed safe when consumed in normal dietary quantities by non-allergic individuals.

Potato, sweet (Ipomoea batatas)

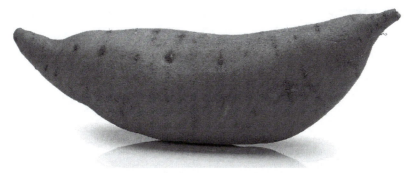

Sweet potato. (Image from Jiang Hongyan/Shitterstock.)

definition

Orange- or yellow-fleshed root vegetable, commonly prepared by steaming, baking, boiling, or frying. One cup of baked sweet potato with its skin is an excellent source of potassium, supplying 950 mg of potassium (30% DV), and, if the skin is consumed, it is a good source of fiber[102]; also a source of phenolics and flavonoids.[103] One baked sweet potato provides over 8800 IU of vitamin A (176% DV) and 141 calories, is rich in complex carbohydrates including fiber, is an excellent source of vitamin C, and is a good source of iron and fiber.[104]

scientific findings

Constituents in sweet potato exerted antioxidant, antiradical, and antiproliferative effects in laboratory studies.[103] In one study, antioxidant activity was directly related to the total amount of phenolics and flavonoids in sweet potato.[103] Eating potassium-rich foods as part of an overall healthy diet helps maintain normal blood pressure.[105]

P

bioactive dose

Not known.

safety

Presumed safe when consumed in normal dietary quantities by non-allergic individuals.

Potato, white (Solanum tuberosum)

definition

Tuber vegetable rich in carbohydrate, resistant starch, vitamin C, potassium, and, when its skin is consumed, fiber. It is commonly eaten boiled, fried, baked, and roasted and is the most important food crop worldwide after rice and wheat.[106] Some of the phytochemicals in white potatoes include glycoalkaloids (which can exert beneficial or harmful effects), aglycones, and phenolic compounds.[107,108]

scientific findings

There is no evidence that the popular white potato protects against cancer.[109] Potassium and dietary fiber have been designated as food components to consume in greater quantity by the 2010 Dietary Guidelines for Americans—potato has them both.[110] The glycoalkaloids in potato inhibited growth of human colon and liver cancer cells.[111] In laboratory studies, solanine, a glycoalkaloid, was found to possess anticarcinogenic and anti-prostate-cancer effects,[112,113] but solanine should not be consumed (see safety section below). Potato peel contains phenolics that exert antioxidant effects.[114]

bioactive dose

Not known.

P

safety

Presumed safe when consumed in normal dietary quantities by non-allergic individuals after cooking and after removing the green layer under the skin and the sprouts (small white shoots that grow out of the eye of the potato) to remove solanine. Solanine is a gastrointestinal and neurological toxin.[115]

Prebiotic

definition

Nondigestible dietary constituent that selectively stimulates the growth and/or activity of beneficial microorganisms in the large intestine. Inulin and fructan (from chicory root), galactooligosaccharides (from lactose), and pyrodextrins (from potato and maize starch) are examples of prebiotic compounds.[116]

scientific findings

Prebiotics beneficially modify gut microbial balance.[115] Some evidence suggests that [prebiotics] may relieve constipation by increasing fecal mass, but more evidence is needed to rate [prebiotics] for this use.[15]

bioactive dose

Not known. For prebiotic effect (to increase fecal bifidobacteria), the typical dose is 4 to 10 grams per day.[15]

safety

Presumed safe when consumed in normal dietary quantities by non-allergic individuals. Overconsumption of prebiotics could cause intestinal discomfort.[117]

Prickly pear (Opuntia sp.)

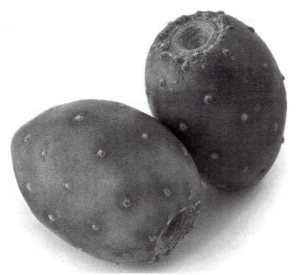

Prickly pear. (Image from Glenn Price/Shutterstock.)

definition

Edible type of cactus eaten fresh without the skin that may be red, purple, yellow, white, or other colors depending upon the cultivar. The flesh is the texture of a common pear, but less juicy. The seeds are large, hard, and difficult to separate from the flesh.[118] Prickly pear contains vitamin C, fiber, flavonoids, and carotenoids.[119] In Mexico, the prickly pear cultivar *Opuntia streptacantha* is traditionally used in the treatment of diabetes mellitus.[120]

scientific findings

Prickly pear contains betalain that exhibited antioxidant properties in a laboratory study.[118] Prickly pear pectin decreased plasma LDL in guinea pigs fed a hypercholesterolemic diet.[121] According to a review, there is some preliminary clinical evidence that a single dose of the specific species of prickly pear cactus called *O. streptacantha* can decrease blood glucose levels by 17%–46% in patients with type 2 diabetes, but it is not known whether extended daily use can consistently lower blood glucose levels and decrease HbA1C levels.[15] *O. streptacantha* juice was confirmed by maltose tolerance test to be an antihyperglycemic agent.[119]

bioactive dose

Not known.

safety

Presumed safe when consumed in normal dietary quantities by non-allergic individuals.

Probiotics

definition

Live microorganisms (in most cases, bacteria) that are similar to beneficial microorganisms found in the human gut.[122] When consumed in adequate amounts they may confer a health benefit to the host.[122,123] For example, *Bifidobacteria* may help to "balance disturbed intestinal microflora and related dysfunction of the human gastrointestinal tract."[124] Some probiotic foods date back to ancient times, such as fermented foods and cultured milk products.[122] *Lactobacillus* in Greek yogurts labeled "fermented with lactobacillus," *Saccharomyces* in beer, and *Bifidobacteria* in kimchi (fermented, spicy Korean cabbage), sourdough bread, kefir, and miso[15] are common examples of foods that contain probiotics. Probiotics are used to: treat diarrhea from rotavirus and diarrhea generally, prevent and treat female genitourinary tract infections, treat IBS, shorten *Clostridium difficile* intestinal infections, prevent and treat pouchitis following surgical removal of the colon, and prevent and manage atopic dermatitis (eczema) in children.[124]

scientific findings

The mechanisms of action of probiotic bacteria include that they produce butyric acid that neutralizes the activity of dietary carcinogens; attach to enterocytes thus inhibiting the binding of enteric pathogens; and promote the growth of beneficial microorganisms in the gastrointestinal tract.[123] In clinical trials examining the benefit of probiotics, findings were that the beneficial effect was usually low [and] ... a strong placebo effect often occurs[15]; moreover, researchers concluded, "the human body can respond differently to the different species and strains of probiotics."[125] There is limited experimental evidence that certain bifidobacteria may protect the host from carcinogenic activity of intestinal flora,[15] but there is no evidence to support or refute the relationship between a patient's intake of probiotics and reduction of cancer symptoms.[126] There is limited evidence supporting some uses of probiotics. Much more scientific knowledge is needed about probiotics, including about their safety and appropriate use.[122]

bioactive dose

Not known.

safety

A probiotic review reported that there is a general lack of adverse event found in probiotic intervention studies, and that "the current literature is not well equipped to answer questions on the safety of probiotic interventions with confidence."[122] *Bifidobacteria* sourced from food are considered to have low pathogenic potential, and are an "extremely rare" cause of infection in humans; and the lack of pathogenicity appears to extend across all age groups and to immunocompromised individuals[123]; however, "there is insufficient reliable information available to evaluate their safe use in pregnancy or lactation."[124]

Protease inhibitors

definition

Proteins in plants that are thought to respond to the attack of insects and pathogenic microorganisms,[127] but that may also impart health benefits to the host when consumed. Found in soy products, broccoli, sprouts, potatoes, and legumes.[54]

scientific findings

Protease inhibitors suppressed enzyme production in cancer, slowed tumor growth, inhibited hormone binding, and inhibited malignant changes in cells in an experimental study.[127]

bioactive dose

Not known.

safety

Presumed safe when consumed in normal dietary quantities by non-allergic individuals.

Protein

definition

Macronutrient whose constituent amino acids are preferentially used to manufacture protein compounds, but which can also be metabolized as a source of energy. All food groups except fruit and oils provide appreciable amounts of protein. Dairy products provide 8 g of protein per 8 oz of milk; protein foods provide 7 g of protein per 1/4 cup of legumes or tofu, 1 egg, 1/2 oz nuts or seeds, 1 tablespoon of peanut butter, or 1 oz of lean cooked meat, poultry, or fish. Grains provide 3 g of protein per 1 slice of bread or 1 cup of cereal. Cooked vegetables provide 2 g of protein per 1 cup of cooked vegetables or 2 cups of raw, leafy salad vegetables. Average healthy Americans exceed their protein RDA.

scientific findings

Protein consumption has minimal influence on glycemic response and insulin requirement.[128] Patients who are malnourished or who are in active disease states generally have higher protein requirements than healthy people.[129] Protein malnutrition is associated with the loss of lean body mass.[128] Protein undernutrition was associated with an increased risk of cataract in a population-based study (n = 2584 subject aged 60–95 years).[130]

bioactive dose

The RDA for protein for healthy adults aged 19–50 years is 0.8 g/kg/day.

safety

No UL for protein has been established.

Psyllium (Plantago ovate)

definition

Seed husk of the herb *Plantago ovate*. Psyllium seed husk is made into cereals and is a chief ingredient in bulk laxatives. Psyllium seed husk contains soluble fiber.

scientific findings

Psyllium is an effective laxative and stool softener[131] that may be effective in relieving the symptoms of IBS, including diarrhea; reducing high blood glucose levels in individuals with type 1 and 2 diabetes (but not in individuals who do not have diabetes); reducing cholesterol in individuals with diabetes who also have high cholesterol; reducing high systolic blood pressure; and managing ulcerative colitis, dysentery, and hemorrhoids.[131] Small clinical trials have shown psyllium fiber to be associated with lower mean daily glucose concentrations, lower postmeal glucose concentrations, fewer hypoglycemic events, lower hemoglobin A1C levels, and lower insulin concentrations in people with diabetes mellitus.[132] Psyllium seems to reduce total and LDL cholesterol, and the LDL-to-HDL ratio.[15]

bioactive dose

Not known.

P

safety

Presumed safe when consumed in normal dietary quantities by non-allergic individuals. Not consuming enough fluid when taking psyllium could lead to choking or obstruction of the esophagus or bowel.[131] Since fiber can speed GI tract transit time and thus limit absorption, psyllium should not be taken within 2 h of many orally administered medications.[133]

Pummelo (Citrus grandis)

definition

Largest citrus family member, weighing two to three pounds on average, resembling an oversized grapefruit but with thicker, loose-fitting skin. Its segments are white- or red-fleshed. Pummelos are excellent sources of vitamin C[134] and a source of flavonoids.

scientific findings

Fresh red pummelo juice is an excellent source of antioxidant compounds that in a laboratory study scavenged superoxide anion free radicals and hydrogen peroxide radicals.[134]

bioactive dose

Not known.

safety

Presumed safe when consumed in normal dietary quantities by non-allergic individuals.

Pumpkin (Cucurbita pepo)

definition

Squash family vegetable that is notably rich in carotenoids and therefore an excellent source of vitamin A (7050 IU per 1/2 cup = 140% DV).[135] Common in baked products, such as muffins and pie.

scientific findings

A review examining natural treatments for benign prostatic hypertrophy found no convincing evidence to support the use of *Curcubita pepo* alone for its treatment.[136] In experimental research, pumpkin exhibited moderate antioxidant activity and moderate to high α-glucosidase and angiotensin-converting enzyme inhibitory activities[137] *in vitro*, which may have implications for the management of hyperglycemia and hypertension. Pumpkin consumption was inversely associated with the development of lung cancer in a case–control study comparing the dietary patterns of subjects with incident lung cancer (n = 371) to controls (n = 496); neither cases nor controls had a neoplasic history.[138]

bioactive dose

Not known.

safety

Presumed safe when consumed in normal dietary quantities by non-allergic individuals.

Pumpkin seed

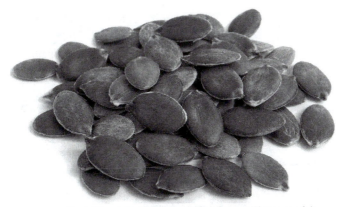

Pumpkin seeds. (Image from Olga Popova/Shutterstock.)

definition

Edible seed of pumpkin (*C. pepo*) when roasted. Pumpkin seeds are a good source of calcium, potassium, magnesium, iron, zinc, and B-vitamins,[139] and contain phosphorus.[140] Pumpkin seeds are also a good source of the γ-tocopherol form of vitamin E[141] and provide selenium.[139]

scientific findings

In a small study (n = 20 boys aged 2–7 years), pumpkin seed treatment as compared with treatment with orthophosphate (the control compound) reduced calcium oxalate bladder stone formation.[139]

bioactive dose

Not known.

safety

Presumed safe when consumed in normal dietary quantities by non-allergic individuals.

References

1. Hayne J, McLaughlin J. Edible palms and their uses. University of Florida Extension. Institute of Food and Agricultural Sciences. Fact Sheet MDCE-00-50-1. November 2000. http://miami-dade.ifas.ufl.edu/old/programs/urbanhort/publications/PDF/EdiblePalms.pdf. Accessed January 3, 2012.

2. Odia OJ, Ofori S, Maduka O. Palm oil and the heart: A review. *World J Cardiol.* 2015;7(3):144–149. doi: 10.4330/wjc.v7.i3.144. Published online 2015 March 26.

3. Kelly GS. Pantothenic acid. Monograph. *Altern Med Rev.* 2011;16(3):263–274.

4. Institute of Medicine. *Dietary Reference Intakes for Thiamin, Riboflavin, Niacin, Vitamin B6, Folate, Vitamin B12, Pantothenic Acid, Biotin and Choline.* Washington DC: National Academy Press; 1998.

5. Office of the Gene Technology Regulator. *Carica papaya* L. in Australia. The Biology and Ecology of Papaya. April 2003. http://www.ogtr.gov.au/internet/ogtr/publishing.nsf/Content/papaya-3/$FILE/papaya.pdf. Accessed July 20, 2013.

6. McKee RA, Adams S, Matthews JA, Smith CJ, Smith H. Molecular cloning of two cysteine proteinases from paw-paw (*Carica papaya*). *Biochem J.* 1986;237(1):105–110.

7. US Department of Agriculture. Agricultural Research Service. Papaya, raw. http://ndb.nal.usda.gov/ndb/foods/show/2350?fgcd=&manu=&lfacet=&format=&count=&max=35&offset=&sort=&qlookup=papaya. Accessed January 19, 2012.

8. Iyer D, Sharma BK, Patil UK. Effect of ether- and water-soluble fractions of *Carica papaya* ethanol extract in experimentally induced hyperlipidemia in rats. *Pharm Biol.* 2011;49(12):1306–1310.

9. Abdullah M, Chai PS, Loh CY, Chong MY, Quay HW, Vidyadaran S, Seman Z, Kandiah M, Seow HF. *Carica papaya* increases regulatory T cells and reduces IFN-γ(+) CD4(+) T cells in healthy human subjects. *Mol Nutr Food Res.* 2011;55(5):803–806.

10. Materska M, Perucka I. Antioxidant activity of the main phenolic compounds isolated from hot pepper fruit (*Capsicum annuum* L.). *J Agric Food Chem.* 2005;5(5):1750–1756.

11. Matsufuji H, Nakamura H, Chino M, Takeda M. Antioxidant activity of capsanthin and the fatty acid esters in paprika (*Capsicum annuum*). *J Agric Food Chem.* 1998;46(9):3468–3472.

12. Park J, Kim S, Moon B. Changes in carotenoids, ascorbic acids, and quality characteristics by the pickling of paprika (*Capsicum annuum* L.) cultivated in Korea. *J Food Sci.* 2011;76(7):C1075–C1080. doi: 10.1111/j.1750-3841.2011.02297.x. Epub 2011 August 5.

13. Leitner A, Jensen-Jarolim E, Grimm R, Wüthrich B, Ebner H, Scheiner O, Kraft D, Ebner C. Allergens in pepper and paprika. Immunologic investigation of the celery-birch-mugwort-spice syndrome. *Allergy.* 1998;53(1):36–41.

14. Hostetler GL, Riedl KM, Schwartz SJ. Endogenous enzymes, heat, and pH affect flavone profiles in parsley (*Petroselinum crispum* var. *neapolitanum*) and celery (*Apium graveolens*) during juice processing. *J Agric Food Chem.* 2012;60(1):202–208. Epub 2011 December 30.

15. Jellin JM, Gregory PJ. Natural Medicine Comprehensive Database. Therapeutic Research Faculty. 2013. http://www.naturaldatabase.com. Accessed July 11, 2012.

16. Peterson S, Lampe JW, Bammler TK, Gross-Steinmeyer K, Eaton DL. Apiaceous vegetable constituents inhibit human cytochrome P-450 1A2 (hCYP1A2) activity and hCYP1A2-mediated mutagenicity of aflatoxin B1. *Food Chem Toxicol.* 2006;44(9):1474–1484. Epub 2006 April 27.

P

17. Beier RC. Natural pesticides and bioactive components in foods. *Rev Environ Contam Toxicol*. 1990;113:47–137.

18. Coleta M, Batista MT, Campos MG, Carvalho R, Cotrim MD, Lima TC, Cunha AP. Neuropharmacological evaluation of the putative anxiolytic effects of *Passiflora edulis* Sims, its sub-fractions and flavonoid constituents. *Phytother Res*. 2006;20(12):1067–1073.

19. Wang C, Xu FQ, Shang JH, Xiao H, Fan WW, Dong FW, Hu JM, Zhou J. Cycloartane triterpenoid saponins from water soluble of *Passiflora edulis* Sims and their antidepressant-like effects. *J Ethnopharmacol*. 2013;148(3):812–817. doi: 10.1016/j.jep.2013.05.010. Epub 2013 May 20.

20. de Souza Mda S, Barbalho SM, Damasceno DC, Rudge MV, de Campos KE, Madi AC, Coelho BR, Oliveira RC, de Melo RC, Donda VC. Effects of *Passiflora edulis* (yellow passion) on serum lipids and oxidative stress status of wistar rats. *J Med Food*. 2012;15(1):78–82. Epub 2011 August 30.

21. Cantín CM, Moreno MA, Gogorcena Y. Evaluation of the antioxidant capacity, phenolic compounds, and vitamin C content of different peach and nectarine (*Prunus persica* [L.] Batsch) breeding progenies. *J Agric Food Chem*. 2009;57(11):4586–4592.

22. Oliveira A, Gomes MH, Alexandre EM, Almeida DP, Pintado M. Impact of pH on the phytochemical profile of pasteurized peach purée during storage. *J Agric Food Chem*. 2014;62(50):12075–12081. doi: 10.1021/jf503913t. Epub 2014 December 4.

23. US Department of Agriculture. Agricultural Research Service. Nutrient Data Laboratory. Peach, raw. http://ndb.nal.usda.gov/ndb/foods/show/23 27?fg=&man=&lfacet=&format=&count=&max=25&offset=&sort=&qlooku p=peach. Accessed July 20, 2013.

24. Yahia EM. The contribution of fruit and vegetable consumption to human health. In: de la Rosa LA, Alvarez-Parrilla E, Gonz´alez-Aguilar GA. *Fruit and Vegetable Phytochemicals. Chemistry, Nutritional Value, and Stability*. Ames, IA: Wiley Blackwell; 26–27.

25. Fung TT, Shiuve SE, Willett WC, Hankinson SE, Hu FB, Holmes MD. Intake of specific fruits and vegetables in relation to risk of estrogen receptor-negative breast cancer among postmenopausal women. *Breast Cancer Res Treat*. 2013;138(3):925–930. doi: 10.1007/s10549-013-2484-3. Epub 2013 March 27.

26. Hoelzl C, Knasmüller S, Wagner KH, Elbling L, Huber W, Kager N, Ferk F et al. Instant coffee with high chlorogenic acid levels protects humans against oxidative damage of macromolecules. *Mol Nutr Food Res*. 2010;54(12):1722–1733.

27. Arvanitoyannis I. The effect of storage of canned juices on content of the metals Fe, Cu, Zn, Pb, Sn, Al, Cd, Sb and Ni. *Nahrung*. 1990;34(2):141–145.

28. American Academy of Nutrition and Dietetics Evidence Analysis Library. What are the health effects related to consumption of nuts? http://andevidencelibrary.com/conclusion.cfm?conclusion_statement_id=251523&highli ght=peanuts&home=1. Accessed July 22, 2013.

29. Li TY, Brennan AM, Wedick NM, Mantzoros C, Rifai N, Hu FB. Regular consumption of nuts is associated with a lower risk of cardiovascular disease in women with type 2 diabetes. *J Nutr*. 2009;139(7):1333–1338. doi: 10.3945/jn.108.103622. Epub 2009 May 6.

30. Perry TT, Pesek RD. Clinical manifestations of food allergy. *Pediatr Ann*. 2013;42(6):96–101. doi: 10.3928/00904481-20130522-09.

P

31. US Department of Agriculture. Agricultural Research Service. Nutrient Data Laboratory. Pears, raw. http://ndb.nal.usda.gov/ndb/foods/show/234 2?fg=&man=&lfacet=&format=&count=&max=25&offset=&sort=&qlookup =pears. Accessed July 20, 2013.

32. Knaze V, Zamora-Ros R, Luján-Barroso L, Romieu I, Scalbert A, Slimani N, Riboli E et al. Intake estimation of total and individual flavan-3-ols, proanthocyanidins and theaflavins, their food sources and determinants in the European Prospective Investigation into Cancer and Nutrition (EPIC) study. *Br J Nutr.* 2012;108(6):1095–1108.

33. Hamauzua Y, Foresta F, Hiramatsub K, Sugimotob M. Effect of pear (*Pyrus communis* L.) procyanidins on gastric lesions induced by HCl/ethanol in rats. *Food Chem.* 2007;100(1):255–263.

34. Kahlon TS, Smith GE. *In vitro* binding of bile acids by bananas, peaches, pineapple, grapes, pears, apricots and nectarines. *Chemistry* 2007;101(3):1046–1051.

35. Whitney ER, DeBruyne LK, Pinna K, Rolfes, SR. *Nutrition for Health and Healthcare*, 4th edn. Belmont CA: Cengage Learning; 2011.

36. Der Marderosian A, Beutler J. *The Review of Natural Products*. St. Louis, MO: Wolters Kluwer Health; 2005:978.

37. Rabbani GH, Teka T, Saha SK, Zaman B, Majid N, Khatun M, Wahed MA, Fuchs GJ. Green banana and pectin improve small intestinal permeability and reduce fluid loss in Bangladeshi children with persistent diarrhea. *Dig Dis Sci.* 2004;49(3):475–484.

38. Schultz AA, Ashby-Hughes B, Taylor R, Gillis DE, Wilkins M. Effects of pectin on diarrhea in critically ill tube-fed patients receiving antibiotics. *Am J Crit Care.* 2000;9(6):403–411.

39. Whitney E, DeBruyne LK, Pinna K, Rolfes SR. *Nutrition for Health and Health Care*, 5th edn. Belmont CA: Cengage Learning; 2011.

40. Marín A, Ferreres F, Tomás-Barberán FA, Gil MI. Characterization and quantitation of antioxidant constituents of sweet pepper (*Capsicum annuum* L.). *J Agric Food Chem.* 2004;52(12):3861–3869.

41. Lecour S, Lamont KT. Natural polyphenols and cardioprotection. *Mini Rev Med Chem.* 2011;11(14):1191–1199. Epub 2011 October 28.

42. Yarnes SC, Ashrafi H, Reyes-Chin-Wo S, Hill TA, Stoffel KM, Van Deynze A. Identification of QTLs for capsaicinoids, fruit quality, and plant architecture-related traits in an interspecific *Capsicum* RIL population. *Genome.* 2013;56(1):61–74. doi: 10.1139/gen-2012-0083. Epub 2013 January 1.

43. Horrocks A. Jalapeno Peppers. Utah University Cooperative Extension. 2011. http://extension.usu.edu/files/publications/publication/FN_Food$ense_ 2011-12pr.pdf. Accessed March 11, 2015.

44. Giuffrida D, Dugo P, Torre G, Bignardi C, Cavazza A, Corradini C, Dugo G. Characterization of 12 *Capsicum* varieties by evaluation of their carotenoid profile and pungency determination. *Food Chem.* 2013;140(4):794–802. doi: 10.1016/j.foodchem.2012.09.060. Epub 2012 September 28.

45. Szallasi A, Blumberg PM. Vanilloid (capsaicin) receptors and mechanisms. *Pharmacol Rev.* 1999;51(2):159–212.

46. Cichewicz RH, Thorpe PA. The antimicrobial properties of chile peppers (*Capsicum* species) and their uses in Mayan medicine. *J Ethnopharmacol.* 1996;52(2):61–70.

47. Arpad Szallasi A, Blumber PM. Vanilloid (capsaicin) receptors and mechanisms. *Pharmacol Rev.*1999;51(2):159–212.

P

48. Alam MS, Roy PK, Miah AR, Mollick SH, Khan MR, Mahmud MC, Khatun S. Efficacy of peppermint oil in diarrhea predominant IBS—A double blind randomized placebo-controlled study. *Mymensingh Med J.* 2013;22(1):27–30.

49. Papathanasopoulos A, Rotondo A, Janssen P, Boesmans W, Farre R, Vanden Berghe P, Tack J. Effect of acute peppermint oil administration on gastric sensorimotor function and nutrient tolerance in health. *Neurogastroenterol Motil.* 2013;25(4):e263–271. doi: 10.1111/nmo.12102. Epub 2013 March 12.

50. National Institutes of Health. National Center for Complementary and Alternative Medicine. Herbs at a Glance. Peppermint. http://nccam.nih .gov/health/peppermintoil. Accessed March 17, 2011.

51. Jung ST, Park YS, Zachwieja Z, Folta M, Barton H, Piotrowicz J, Katrich E, Trakhtenberg S, Gorinstein S. Some essential phytochemicals and the antioxidant potential in fresh and dried persimmon. *Int J Food Sci Nutr.* 2005;56(2):105–113.

52. Takekawa K, Matsumoto K. Water-insoluble condensed tannins content of young persimmon fruits-derived crude fibre relates to its bile acid-binding ability. *Nat Prod Res.* 2012;26(23):2255–2258. Epub 2012 January 18.

53. Benharroch D, Krugliak P, Porath Avi, Zurgil E, Niv Y. Pathogenetic aspects of persimmon bezoars: A case-control retrospective study. *J Clin Gastroent.* 1993;17(2):149–152.

54. Whitney ER, Rolfes SR. *Understanding Nutrition,* 12th edn. Belmont CA: Wadsworth Cengage; 2011.

55. Martínez-Valverde I, Periago MJ, Ros G. Nutritional importance of phenolic compounds in the diet. *Arch Latinoam Nutr.* 2000;50(1):5–18.

56. Abidi W, Jiménez S, Moreno MÁ, Gogorcena Y. Evaluation of antioxidant compounds and total sugar content in a nectarine (*Prunus persica* [L.] Batsch) progeny. *Int J Mol Sci.* 2011;12(10):6919–6935. Epub 2011 October 19.

57. Crozier A, Jaganath IB, Clifford MN. Dietary phenolics: Chemistry, bioavailability and effects on health. *Nat Prod Rep.* 2009;26(8):1001–1043. Epub 2009 May 13.

58. Shaheen UY. *p*-Coumaric acid ester with potential antioxidant activity from the genus *Salvia. Free Radicals Antioxid.* 2011;1(1):23–27.

59. Roowi S, Crozier A. Flavonoids in tropical citrus species. *J Agric Food Chem.* 2011;59(22):12217–12225. Epub 2011 October 19.

60. San Miguel SM, Opperman LA, Allen EP, Zielinski J, Svoboda KK. Antioxidants counteract nicotine and promote migration via RacGTP in oral fibroblast cells. *J Periodontol.* 2010;81(11):1675–1690.

61. Gao SS, Chen XY, Zhu RZ, Choi BM, Kim SJ, Kim BR. Dual effects of phloretin on aflatoxin B(1) metabolism: Activation and detoxification of aflatoxin B(1). *Biofactors.* 2012;38(1):34–43. doi: 10.1002/biof.190. Epub 2012 January 18.

62. Institute of Medicine. *Dietary Reference Intakes for Calcium, Phosphorus, Magnesium, Vitamin D and Fluoride.* National Academy Press: Washington DC; 1997.

63. Bohn L, Meyer AS, Rasmussen SK. Zhejiang J. Phytate: Impact on environment and human nutrition. A challenge for molecular breeding. *J Zhejiang Univ SC-B.* 2008;9(3):165–191.

64. Cheryan M. Phytic acid interactions in food systems. *Crit Rev Food Sci Nutr.* 1980;13(4):297–335.

P

65. Khatiwada J, Verghese M, Davis S, Williams LL. Green tea, phytic acid, and inositol in combination reduced the incidence of azoxymethane-induced colon tumors in Fisher 344 male rats. *J Med Food.* 2011;14(11):1313–1320. Epub 2011 April 18.

66. Bidlack WR, Wang W. Designing functional foods. In: Shils ME, Olson JA, Shike M, Ross CA. *Modern Nutrition in Health and Disease,* 8th edn. Baltimore, MD: Williams and Wilkins; 1994.

67. Chen MN, Lin CC, Liu CF. Efficacy of phytoestrogens for menopausal symptoms: A meta-analysis and systematic review. *Climacteric.* 2015;18(2):260–269. Epub 2014 December 1.

68. Richter D, Abarzua S, Chrobak M, Vrekoussis T, Weissenbacher T, Kuhn C, Schulze S et al. Effects of phytoestrogen extracts isolated from pumpkin seeds on estradiol production and ER/PR expression in breast cancer and trophoblast tumor cells. *Nutr Cancer.* 2013;65(5):739–745. doi: 10.1080/01635581.2013.797000.

69. Lethaby A, Marjoribanks J, Kronenberg F, Roberts H, Eden J, Brown J. Phytoestrogens for menopausal vasomotor symptoms. *Cochrane Database Syst Rev.* 2013;12:CD001395. doi: 10.1002/14651858.CD001395.pub4.

70. Qu XL, Fang Y, Zhang M, Zhang YZ. Phytoestrogen intake and risk of ovarian cancer: A meta-analysis of 10 observational studies. *Asian Pac J Cancer Prev.* 2014;15(21):9085–9091.

71. Girardi A, Piccinni C, Raschi E, Koci A, Vitamia B, Poluzzi El, De Ponti F. Use of phytoestrogens and effects perceived by postmenopausal women: Result of a questionnaire-based survey. *BMC Complement Altern Med.* 2014;14:262. doi: 10.1186/1472-6882-14-262.

72. US Department of Agriculture. Agricultural Research Service. Nutrient Data Laboratory. Pineapple, raw all varieties. http://ndb.nal.usda.gov/ndb/foods/show/2385?man=&lfacet=&count=&max=35&qlookup=pineapple&offset=&sort=&format=Abridged&reportfmt=other&rptfrm=&ndbno=&nutrient1=&nutrient2=&nutrient3=&subset=&totCount=&measureby=&_action_show=Apply + Changes&Qv=1&Q4520=0.5&Q4521=1&Q4522=1&Q4523=1&Q4524=1. Accessed July 21, 2013.

73. Errasti ME, Caffini NO, Pelzer LE, Rotelli AE. Anti-inflammatory activity of *Bromelia hieronymi*: Comparison with bromelain. *Planta Med.* 2013;79(3–4): 207–213. doi: 10.1055/s-0032-1328201. Epub 2013 January 30.

74. Daher CF, Abou-Khalil J, Baroody GM. Effect of acute and chronic grapefruit, orange, and pineapple juice intake on blood lipid profile in normolipidemic rat. *Med Sci Monit.* 2005;11(12):BR465–BR472. Epub 2005 November 24.

75. Pavan R, Jain S, Shraddha, KA. Properties and therapeutic application of bromelain: A review. *Biotechnol Res Int.* 2012;2012:976203. doi: 10.1155/2012/976203. Epub 2012 December 10.

76. National Institutes of Health Medline Plus. Bromelain. http://www.nlm.nih.gov/medlineplus/druginfo/natural/895.html. Accessed July 21, 2013.

77. Shoskes DA, Zeitlin SI, Shahed A, Rajfer J. Quercetin in men with category III chronic prostatitis: A preliminary prospective, double-blind, placebo-controlled trial. *Urol.* 1999;54(6):960–963.

78. Seeram NP, Zhang Y, Henning SM, Lee R, Niu Y, Lin G, Heber D. Pistachio skin phenolics are destroyed by bleaching resulting in reduced antioxidative capacities. *J Agric Food Chem.* 2006;54(19):7036–7040.

79. Kay CD, Gebauer SK, West SG, Kris-Etherton PM. Pistachios increase serum antioxidants and lower serum oxidized-LDL in hypercholesterolemic adults. *J Nutr.* 2010;140(6):1093–1098.

80. Mohammadifard N, Salehi-Abarghouei A, Salas-Salvadó J, Guasch-Ferré M, Humphries K, Sarrafzadegan N. The effect of tree nut, peanut, and soy nut consumption on blood pressure: A systematic review and meta-analysis of randomized controlled clinical trials. *Am J Clin Nutr.* 2015 March 25. pii: ajcn091595. [Epub ahead of print].

81. Porcel S, Sánchez AB, Rodríguez E, Fletes C, Alvarado M, Jiménez S, Hernández J. Food-dependent exercise-induced anaphylaxis to pistachio. *J Investig Allergol Clin Immunol.* 2006;16(1):71–73.

82. US Department of Agriculture. Agricultural Research Service. Nutrient Database. Plaintains, yellow, fried Latino restaurant. http://ndb.nal.usda .gov/ndb/foods/show/2458?fg=&man=&lfacet=&format=&count=&max=2 5&offset=&sort=&qlookup=plantain. Accessed June 16, 2013.

83. Jiménez-Escrig A, Rincón M, Pulido R, Saura-Calixto F. Guava fruit (*Psidium guajava* L.) as a new source of antioxidant dietary fiber. *J Agric Food Chem.* 2001;49(11):5489–5493.

84. Lewis DA, Fields WN, Shaw GP. A natural flavonoid present in unripe plantain banana pulp (*Musa sapientum* L. var. *paradisiaca*) protects the gastric mucosa from aspirin-induced erosions. *J Ethnopharmacol.* 1999;65(3): 283–288.

85. Roberts CL, Keita AV, Duncan SH, O'Kennedy N, Söderholm JD, Rhodes JM, Campbell BJ. Translocation of Crohn's disease *Escherichia coli* across M-cells: Contrasting effects of soluble plant fibres and emulsifiers. *Gut.* 2010;59(10):1331–1339. doi: 10.1136/gut.2009.195370. Epub 2010 September 2.

86. USDA Agricultural Research Service. Phytochemical Database. *Prunus domestica.* http://www.pl.barc.usda.gov/usda. Accessed June 11, 2011.

87. US Department of Agriculture. Agricultural Research Service. National Nutrient Database. Plum, raw. http://ndb.nal.usda.gov/ndb/foods/show/2 398?fgcd=&manu=&lfacet=&format=&count=&max=35&offset=&sort=&ql ookup=plum. Accessed March 17, 2015.

88. Lombardi-Boccia G, Lucarini M, Lanzi S, Altero Aguzzi A, Cappelloni M. Nutrients and antioxidant molecules in yellow plums (*Prunus domestica* L.) from conventional and organic productions: A comparative study. *J Agric Food Chem.* 2004;52(1):90–99.

89. Stacewicz-Sapuntzakis M, Bowen PE, Hussain EA, Damayanti-Wood BI, Farnsworth NI. Chemical composition and potential health effects of prunes: A functional food? *Crit Rev Food Sci Nutr.* 2001;41(1):251–286.

90. US Department of Agriculture. Agricultural Research Service. National Nutrient Database. Prune. http://ndb.nal.usda.gov/ndb/foods/show/2407? man=&lfacet=&count=&max=35&qlookup=prune&offset=&sort=&format= Abridged&reportfmt=other&rptfrm=&ndbno=&nutrient1=&nutrient2=&n utrient3=&subset=&totCount=&measureby=&_action_show=Apply + Cha nges&Qv=1&Q4564=0.60. Accessed March 17, 2015.

91. Chai SC, Hooshmand S, Saadat RL, Payton ME, Brummel-Smith K, Arjmandi BH. Daily apple versus dried plum: Impact on cardiovascular disease risk factors in postmenopausal women. *J Acad Nutr Diet.* 2012;112(8):1158–1168. doi: 10.1016/j.jand.2012.05.005.

92. National Library of Medicine. PubMed Health. Sorbitol (by mouth). http://www.ncbi.nlm.nih.gov/pubmedhealth/PMHT0012194/?report=details. Accessed April 11, 2015.

93. Attaluri A, Donahoe R, Valestin J, Brown K, Rao SSC. Randomised clinical trial: Dried plums (prunes) vs. psyllium for constipation. SS. *Aliment Pharmacol Ther.* 2011;33(7):822–828. doi: 10.1111/j.1365-2036.2011.04594.x. Epub 2011 February 15.

94. Donovan J, Meyer AS, Waterhouse AL. Phenolic composition and antioxidant activity of prunes and prune juice (*Prunus domestica*). *J Agric Food Chem.* 1998;46(4):1247–1252. doi: 10.1021/jf970831x.

95. Academy of Nutrition and Dietetics Evidence Analysis Library. What is the effect of dietary intake of n-6 polyunsaturated fatty acids (PUFA) on increased risk of cardiovascular disease and type 2 diabetes, including intermediate markers such as lipid and lipoprotein levels and inflammation? http://andevidencelibrary.com/conclusion.cfm?conclusion_statement_id=251538&highlight=pufas&home=1. Accessed July 22, 2013.

96. Simmer K, Patole SK, Rao SC. Long-chain polyunsaturated fatty acid supplementation in infants born at term. *Cochrane Database Syst Rev.* 2008;(1):CD000376. doi: 10.1002/14651858.CD000376.pub2.

97. Goodnight Jr. SH, Harris WS, Connor WE, Illingworth DR. Polyunsaturated fatty acids, hyperlipidemia, and thrombosis. *Arteriosclerosis.* 1982(2);2:87–113.

98. Viladomiu M, Hontecillas R, Lu P, Bassaganya-Riera J. Preventive and prophylactic mechanisms of action of pomegranate bioactive constituents. *Evid Based Complement Alternat Med.* 2013;2013:789764. doi: 10.1155/2013/789764. Epub 2013 April 30.

99. Institute of Medicine. *Dietary References for Water, Potassium, Sodium, Chloride and Sulfate.* Washington DC: National Academy Press; 2005.

100. Houston MC. The importance of potassium in managing hypertension. *Curr Hypertens Rep.* 2011;13(4):309–317. doi: 10.1007/s11906-011-0197-8.

101. Kanbay M, Bayram Y, Solak Y, Sanders PW. Dietary potassium: A key mediator of the cardiovascular response to dietary sodium chloride. *J Am Soc Hypertens.* 2013;7(5):395–400. doi: 10.1016/j.jash.2013.04.009. Epub 2013 June 1.

102. US Department of Agriculture. Agricultural Research Service. Nutrient Data Laboratory. Sweet potato, cooked, candied, home prepared. http://ndb.nal.usda.gov/ndb/foods/show/3285?fg=&man=&lfacet=&format=&count=&max=25&offset=&sort=fd_s&qlookup=sweet + potato. Accessed July 29, 2013.

103. Huang D-J, Lin C-D, Chen H-J, Lin Y-H. Antioxidant and antiproliferative activities of sweet potato constituents. *Bot Bull Acad Sin.* 2004;45:179–186.

104. Texas Agrilife A&M Extension. What is the difference between a sweet potato and a yam? http://aggie-horticulture.tamu.edu/archives/parsons/vegetables/sweetpotato.html. Accessed March 25, 2015.

105. US Department of Agriculture. ChooseMyPlate.gov. Why is it important to eat vegetables? http://myplate.gov/food-groups/vegetables-why.html. Accessed August 1, 2013.

106. Camire ME, Kubow S, Donnelly DJ. Potatoes and human health. *Crit Rev Food Sci Nutr.* 2009;49(10):823–840. doi: 10.1080/10408390903041996.

107. Milner SE, Brunton NP, Jones PW, O'Brien NM, Collins SG, Maguire AR. Bioactivities of glycoalkaloids and their aglycones from *Solanum* species. *J Agric Food Chem.* 2011;59(8):3454–3484. Epub 2011 March 14.

108. Friedman M. Potato glycoalkaloids and metabolites: Roles in the plant and in the diet. *J Agric Food Chem.* 2006;54(23):8655–8681.
109. National Cancer Institute. Fruit and vegetable consumption. http://progressreport.cancer.gov/prevention/fruit_vegetable. Accessed April 8, 2015.
110. King JC, Slavin JL. White potatoes, human health, and dietary guidance. *Adv Nutr.* 2014;4(3):393S–401S. doi: 10.3945/an.112.003525.
111. Lee KR, Kozukue N, Han JS, Park JH, Chang EY, Baek EJ, Chang JS, Friedman M. Glycoalkaloids and metabolites inhibit the growth of human colon (HT29) and liver (HepG2) cancer cells. *J Agric Food Chem.* 2004;52(10):2832–2839.
112. Lu MK, Shih YW, Chang Chien TT, Fang LH, Huang HC, Chen PS. α-Solanine inhibits human melanoma cell migration and invasion by reducing matrix metalloproteinase-2/9 activities. *Biol Pharm Bull.* 2010;33(10):1685–1691.
113. Zhang J, Shi GW. Inhibitory effect of solanine on prostate cancer cell line PC-3 *in vitro. Zhonghua Nan Ke Xue.* 2011;17(3):284–287.
114. Kähkönen MP, Hopia AI, Vuorela HJ, Rauha J-P, Pihlaja K, Kujala TS, Heinonen M. Antioxidant activity of plant extract containing phenolic compounds. *J Agric Food Chem.* 1999;47(10):3954–3962.
115. University of Alaska Fairbanks Cooperative Extension Service. Green potatoes causes and concerns. http://www.uaf.edu/files/ces/publications-db/catalog/anr/FGV-00337.pdf. Accessed April 15, 2015.
116. MacFarlane S, MacFarlane GT, Cummings JH. Prebiotics in the gastrointestinal tract. *Aliment Pharm Ther.* 2066;24:701–714. doi: 10.1111/j.1365-2036.2006.03042.x.
117. Ooi L-G, Liong M-T. Cholesterol-lowering effects of probiotics and prebiotics: A review of *in vivo* and *in vitro* findings. *Int J Mol Sci.* 2010;11:2499–2522. doi:10.3390/ijms11062499.
118. Butera B, Tesoriere L, Di Gaudio F, Bongiorno A, Allegra M, Pintaudi AM, Kohen RM, Livrea MA. Antioxidant activities of Sicilian prickly pear (*Opuntia ficus indica*) fruit extracts and reducing properties of its betalains: Betanin and indicaxanthin. *J Agric Food Chem.* 2002;50(23):6895–6901.
119. Kuti JO. Antioxidant compounds from four *Opuntia* cactus pear fruit varieties. *Food Chem.* 2004;85(4):527–533.
120. Becerra-Jiménez J, Andrade-Cetto A. Effect of *Opuntia streptacantha* Lem. on alpha-glucosidase activity. *J Ethnopharmacol.* 2012;139(2):493–496. doi: 10.1016/j.jep.2011.11.039. Epub 2011 December 1.
121. Fernandez ML, Un ECK, Trejo A, McNamara DJ. Prickly pear (*Opuntia* sp.) Pectin alters hepatic cholesterol metabolism without affecting cholesterol absorption in guinea pigs fed a hypercholesterolemic diet. *J Nutr.* 1994;124:817–824.
122. National Institutes of Health. National Center for Complementary and Alternative Medicine. NCCAM Overview of Probiotics. http://nccam.nih.gov/health/probiotics/. Accessed January 22, 2012.
123. Safety of Probiotics Used to Reduce Risk and Prevent or Treat Disease, Structured Abstract. Agency for Healthcare Research and Quality, Rockville, MD. http://www.ahrq.gov/clinic/tp/probiotictp.htm. Accessed June 6, 2011.
124. Kailasapathy K, Chin J. Survival and therapeutic potential of probiotic organisms with reference to *Lactobacillus acidophilus* and *Bifidobacterium* spp. *Immunol Cell Biol.* 2000;78:80–88. doi:10.1046/j.1440-1711.2000.00886.x.
125. Hakansson A, Molin G. Gut microbiota and inflammation. *Nutrients.* 2011;3(6):637–682. Epub 2011 June 3.
126. Academy of Nutrition and Dietetics Evidence Analysis Library. Is there a relationship between a patient's intake of probiotics to reduce symptoms

P

and the reduction of symptoms associated with cancer in all cancer patients? http://andevidencelibrary.com/evidence.dfm?evidence_summary_id=250466. http://www.andeal.org/topic.cfm?cat=1591&conclusion_statement_id=250243&highlight=probiotics&home=1. Accessed 7 April, 2015.

127. De Leo F, Volpicella M, Licciulli Liuni S, Gallerani R, Ceci LR. PLANT-PIs: A database for plant protease inhibitors and their genes. *Nucleic Acids Res.* 2002;30(1):347–348.

128. Academy of Nutrition and Dietetics. What is the relationship between protein intake and metabolic outcomes in persons with type 1 and type 2 diabetes? http://andevidencelibrary.com/conclusion.cfm?conclusion_statement_id=250525. Accessed July 20, 2013.

129. Academy of Nutrition and Dietetics. What evidence suggests that the protein requirements of patients with various cancer types undergoing chemotherapy are different than the RDA? http://andevidencelibrary.com/conclusion.cfm?conclusion_statement_id=250525. Accessed July 20, 2013.

130. Delcourt C, Dupuy AM, Carriere I, Lacroux A, Cristol JP. Pathologies Oculaires Liées à l'Age Study Group. Albumin and transthyretin as risk factors for cataract: The POLA study. *Arch Ophthalmol.* 2005;123(2):225–232.

131. National Institutes of Health. Medline Plus. Blond Psyllium. http://www.nlm.nih.gov/medlineplus/druginfo/natural/866.html. Accessed June 6, 2011.

132. Hall M, Flinkman T. Do fiber and psyllium fiber improve diabetic metabolism? *Consult Pharm.* 2012;27(7):513–516. doi: 10.4140/TCP.n.2012.513.

133. Harkness R, Bratman S. *Mosby's Handbook of Drug-Herb and Drug-Supplement Interactions.* Mosby: St. Louis, MO; 2003.

134. Tsai H-L, Chang SKC, Chang S-J. Antioxidant content and free radical scavenging ability of fresh red pummelo (*Citrus grandis* [L.] Osbeck) juice and freeze-dried products. *J Agric Food Chem.* 2007;55(8):2867–2872. doi: 10.1021/jf0633847.

135. US Department of Agriculture. National Nutrient Database. Pumpkin, cooked. http://ndb.nal.usda.gov/ndb/foods/show/3177?fgcd=&manu=&lfacet=&format=&count=&max=35&offset=&sort=&qlookup=cooked+pumpkin. Accessed January 17, 2015.

136. Wilt TJ, Ishani A, Rutks I, MacDonald R. Phytotherapy for benign prostatic hyperplasia. *Public Health Nutr.* 2000;3(4A):459–472.

137. Kwon YI, Apostolidis E, Kim YC, Shetty K. Health benefits of traditional corn, beans, and pumpkin: *In vitro* studies for hyperglycemia and hypertension management. *J Med Food.* 2007;10(2):266–275.

138. Tarrazo-Antelo AM, Ruano-Ravina A, Abal Arca J, Barros-Dios JM. Fruit and vegetable consumption and lung cancer risk: A case-control study in Galicia, Spain. *Nutr Cancer.* 2014;66(6):1030–1037. doi: 10.1080/01635581.2014.936951. Epub 2014 August 1.

139. Stibilj V, Kreft I, Smrkolj P, Osvald J. Enhanced selenium content in buckwheat (*Fagopyrum esculentum* Moench) and pumpkin (*Cucurbita pepo* L.) seeds by foliar fertilization. *Eur Food Res Technol.* 2004;219:142–144.

140. Suphakarn VS, Yarnnon C, Ngunboonsri P. The effect of pumpkin seeds on oxalcrystalluria and urinary compositions of children in hyperendemic area. *Am J Clin Nutr.* 1987;45(1):115–121.

141. Murkovic M, Hillebrand A, Winkler J, Pfannhauser W. Variability of vitamin E content in pumpkin seeds (*Cucurbita pepo* L). *Z Lebensm Unters F A.* 1996;202(4):275–278.

P

Q

Quercetin

definition

Major flavonoid in the U.S. diet consumed in daily amounts estimated to be 4 or 5 µg[1] through plant foods, especially white fruits and vegetables, such as apples, pears, and onions, but diversely in plant foods of all colors ranging from lolla rosa lettuce and plums to tea, red wine to quinoa.

scientific findings

In experimental research, quercetin reduced inflammation.[2] Quercetin appears to have anti-inflammatory and antioxidant properties.[2] It has been shown, in experimental research, to modify eicosanoid biosynthesis; protect LDL from oxidation; prevent platelet aggregation; relax cardiovascular smooth muscle, which may have antihypertensive and antiarrhythmic effects; and to exert antiviral and carcinostatic properties.[3] Quercetin provided relief of pelvic pain in men with prostatitis (n = 30) taking quercetin 500 mg twice daily for 1 month in a randomized, controlled, clinical trial compared to men taking placebo. In an additional, open-label arm of the study, 17 more prostatitis subjects had significant symptom relief due to quercetin.[4] Epidemiologic studies have reported that frequent consumption of quercetin-rich foods is inversely associated with lung cancer incidence.[1] A case–control study (n = 558 lung cancer cases; n = 837 controls) found that lung cancer was inversely associated with the consumption of quercetin.[1] In a case–control study of 582 patients with incident lung cancer and 582 age-, sex-, and ethnicity-matched control subjects, a statistically significant inverse association was found between lung cancer risk and eating foods containing quercetin.[1]

bioactive dose

Not known.

safety

Presumed safe when consumed in normal dietary quantities by non-allergic individuals.

Quince (Cydonia oblonga)

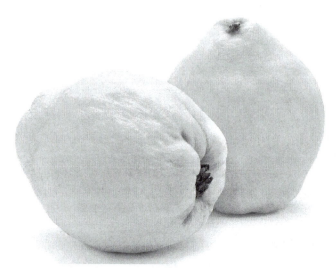

Quince. (Image from Elena Elisseeva/Shutterstock.)

definition

Fruit closely related to apples and pears that is not edible in raw form due to its hard texture and acidic flavor,[5] therefore, it is frequently consumed, with added sweeteners, as jam.[6] Quince jelly and jam are common in Greek cuisine.

Q

scientific findings

Quince pulp, peel, and jam exhibited antioxidant activity in a laboratory study.[6] *C. oblonga* Miller fruit (pulp, peel, and seed) exhibited antiproliferative properties against human kidney and colon cancer cells in a laboratory study.[7]

bioactive dose

Not known.

safety

Presumed safe when consumed in normal dietary quantities by non-allergic individuals.

Quinoa (Chenopodium quinoa)

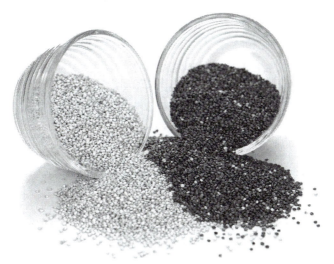

White and red quinoa grain. (Image from cristi180884/Shutterstock.)

definition

Whole grain that is cooked similarly to rice by using one part grain to two parts water and eaten as a side dish. Quinoa is a good source of fiber, zinc, potassium, phosphorus, and supplies omega-6 fatty acid, vitamin E, polyphenols, phytosterols, and flavonoids.[8,9] Though quinoa, compared to other grains, is higher in protein, it lacks the essential amino acids threonine, lysine, and phenylalanine[10] hence, it is not a complete protein, as has been claimed, because it does not contain all essential amino acids.

Q

scientific findings

Quinoa seeds fed to rats reduced serum total cholesterol, glucose, LDL, and triglycerides.[11]

bioactive dose

Not known.

safety

Presumed safe when used in normal dietary quantities by nonallergic individuals.

References

1. Cui Y, Morgenstern H, Greenland S, Tashkin DP, Mao JT, Cai L, Cozen W, Mack TM, Lu QY, Zhang ZF. Dietary flavonoid intake and lung cancer— A population-based case–control study. *Cancer.* 2008;112(10):2241–2248. doi: 10.1002/cncr.23398.
2. Knab AM, Shanely A, Henson D, Jin F, Heinz SA, Austin MD, Neiman DC. Influence of quercetin supplementation on disease risk factors in community-dwelling adults. *J Am Diet Assoc.* 2011;111(4):542–549.
3. Formica JV, Regelson W. Review of the biology of quercetin and related bio-flavonoids. *Food Chem Toxicol.* 1995;33(12):1061–1080.
4. Shoskes DA, Zeitlin SI, Shahed A, Rajfer J. Quercetin in men with category III chronic prostatitis: A preliminary prospective, double-blind, placebo-controlled trial. *Urology.* 1999;54(6):960–963.
5. Purdue University. Quince. http://www.hort.purdue.edu/newcrop/Crops/ Quince.html. Accessed January 27, 2012.
6. Silva BM, Andrade PB, Goncalves AC, Seabra RM, Oliveira MB, Ferreira MA. Influence of jam processing upon the contents of phenolics, organic acids and free amino acids in quince fruit (*Cydonia oblonga* Miller). *Eur Food Res Technol.* 2004;218:385–389.
7. Carvalho M, Silva BM, Silva R, Valento P, Andrade PB, Bastos ML. First report on *Cydonia oblonga* Miller anticancer potential: Differential antiproliferative effect against human kidney and colon cancer cells. *J Agric Food Chem.* 2010;58(6):3366–3370.
8. Abugoch James LE. Quinoa (*Chenopodium quinoa* Willd): Composition, chemistry, nutritional, and functional properties. *Adv Food Nutr Res.* 2009;58:1–31. doi: 10.1016/S1043-4526(09)58001-1.
9. US Department of Agriculture. Agricultural Research Service. National Nutrient Database. Quinoa, cooked. http://ndb.nal.usda.gov/ndb/foods/ show/6539?fgcd=&manu=&lfacet=&format=&count=&max=35&offset= &sort=&qlookup=quinoa. Accessed April 12, 2015.
10. Ruales J, Nair BM. Nutritional quality of the protein in quinoa (*Chenopodium quinoa*, Willd) seeds. *Plant Foods Hum Nutr.* 1992;42(1):1–11.
11. Paśko P, Zagrodzki P, Bartoń H, Chłopicka J, Gorinstein S. Effect of quinoa seeds (*Chenopodium quinoa*) in diet on some biochemical parameters and essential elements in blood of high fructose-fed rats. *Plant Foods Hum Nutr.* 2010;65(4):333–338.

Q

R

Radicchio (Cichorium intybus)

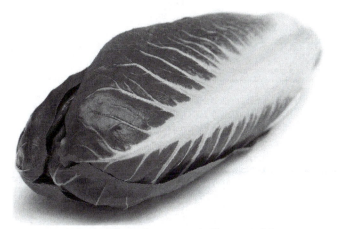

Radicchio. (Image from marmo81/Shutterstock.)

definition

Hardy, variegated, magenta-colored variety of chicory that has a bitter taste and contains phenolics.[1] Used fresh as a salad vegetable, usually mixed with other lettuces to mellow its strong flavor.

R

scientific findings

In a laboratory study, *C. intybus* exhibited antioxidant properties.[2]

bioactive dose

Not known.

safety

Presumed safe when consumed in normal dietary quantities by non-allergic individuals.

Radish (Raphanus sativus)

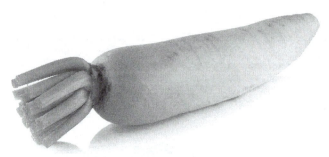

Radish. (Image from amphaiwan/Shutterstock.)

definition

Typically a small, round, white-fleshed vegetable with thin, edible red or white skin that has a sharp, burning flavor. The daikon (above) is a large, conical white variety of radish that is eaten fresh; for example, it may be peeled and grated to be served with sushi or pickled and fermented in Asian cooking. Radish sprouts are a source of glucosinolates and antioxidants.[3] Radishes are so low in calories that they are considered a calorie-free food or so-called "free food" for liberal inclusion in weight management and calorie-controlled diets, and they are also a source of vitamin C.[4] Although there is not sufficient scientific evidence to support the use of radish for any health condition, "a typical dosage is 0.5 tablespoon of pressed radish root juice several times daily up to 50–100 mL per day" has been used orally for peptic disorders; bile duct dyskinesia; loss of appetite; inflammation of the mouth and pharynx; prevention of infection, inflammation or excessive mucus of the respiratory tract; bronchitis; fever; colds; and cough, according to a review of historical use of radish.[5]

scientific findings

See *Brassica vegetables*.

bioactive dose

Not known.

safety

Presumed safe when consumed in normal dietary quantities by non-allergic individuals. Consuming large amounts may lead to gastrointestinal irritation.[5]

Raisin (Vitis vinifera)

definition

Dried grape that is a popular snack food, ingredient in cereal, trail mix, and raisin bread, and that is used in baking and in making confections. Raisins are an excellent source of potassium (100 g of raisins, which is equal to approximately 2/3 cup, supplies 332 cal and 898 mg of potassium),[6] and compared to grapes, contain more fructans, but fewer phenolic compounds,[1] procyanidins, and flavan-3-ols,[7] which are lost during processing. Raisins are a source of both soluble and insoluble fiber.[8]

scientific findings

A small clinical trial found that eating 120 g of sun-dried raisins beneficially modulated the composition of fecal bile acids and short-chain fatty acids in healthy subjects (n = 13).[9] In another small clinical trial (n = 13), 84 g of sun-dried raisins caused beneficial changes in measures of colon health (e.g., intestinal transit time, fecal weight, and fecal bile acid composition).[10]

bioactive dose

Not known.

safety

Presumed safe when consumed in normal dietary quantities by nonallergic individuals.

Raspberry, red (Rubus idaeus)

definition

High vitamin C berry that provides 4 g of fiber per 1/2 cup serving[11] and phytochemicals, including phenolics and anthocyanins,[12] and caffeic acid (not to be confused with caffeine—the two substances are unrelated).[13] (Note to reader: Anthocyanins are a type of phenolic compound, but the study author treats the two as separate entitites.) Eaten raw, frozen, as juice, and in prepared foods, such as desserts and baby food.

scientific findings

Red raspberry muffins exerted measurable antioxidant capacity attributed to raspberry phenolics and anthocyanins.[12] *In vivo* and *in vitro* studies have demonstrated that red raspberry phenolics and ellagitanins form compounds beneficial to colonic cells.[14] In laboratory studies, caffeic acid exhibited antioxidant, immunomodulatory, and anti-inflammatory properties.[15,16] In an experimental model, caffeic acid protected human skin from photo-oxidative damage.[17]

bioactive dose

Not known.

safety

Presumed safe when consumed in normal dietary quantities by non-allergic individuals.

Resveratrol

definition

Polyphenol linked to the "French Paradox" phenomenon, referring to the antiatherogenicity of the typical French diet, known to be high in fat, presumably offset in part due to the inclusion of red wine. Red wine is the major dietary source of resveratrol,[18] but it is also found in grapes, peanuts, and other foods, with white wine having a low content.[19,20]

scientific findings

Resveratrol inhibited LDL oxidation and platelet aggregation, and exerted anti-inflammatory and antiproliferative effects in laboratory research.[20–22] In a 4-week randomized clinical trial (n = 19), resveratrol improved insulin sensitivity in patients with type 2 diabetes: subjects were randomly assigned into a resveratrol group who received resveratrol (a 5-mg dose twice a day) and a control group receiving placebo. After the fourth week, in the resveratrol group, insulin resistance was significantly reduced.[23]

bioactive dose

Not known.

safety

Presumed safe when consumed in normal dietary quantities by non-allergic individuals.

Rhubarb (Rheum officinale)

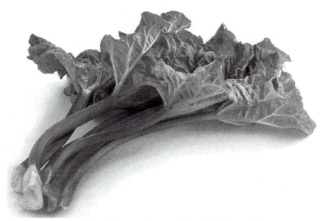

Rhubarb. (Image from photogal/Shutterstock.)

definition

Vegetable consisting of edible stalks, also called petioles, meaning the portion from the stem to the leaf. Rhubarb leaves are not consumed. Rhubarb is tart and must be sweetened heavily before making it into pie, jam, jelly, and sauces. Rhubarb is an excellent source of vitamin K, and though it contains 344 cups of calcium, its calcium is poorly absorbed.[24,25] It is also a source of the phytochemical anthraquinone.[26] Rhubarb's dried root has been used to treat constipation and diarrhea.

scientific findings

Anthraquinone exhibited antiviral properties in laboratory studies.[27,28]

R

bioactive dose

Not known.

safety

Rhubarb leaves are poisonous[29]; however, rhubarb stalks, petioles, and products made from these plant parts are presumed safe when consumed in normal dietary quantities by nonallergic individuals. Several reports of anthroquinones' mutagenicity or other generic or carcinogenenic effects have been reported.[30]

Riboflavin

definition

Also referred to as vitamin B2. Water soluble vitamin that functions as a coenzyme in redox reactions.[31] The best sources of riboflavin include milk and enriched grain products. The average person in the United States meets daily riboflavin requirements.[31]

scientific findings

Deficiency symptoms of riboflavin, characterized by low riboflavin levels in the blood (ariboflavinosis) include sore throat, edema of the pharyngeal and oral mucosa, angular stomatitis, magenta tongue, and impaired metabolism of vitamin B6.[31] Higher intake of riboflavin was associated with reduction in the progression of age-related lens opacification, according to the findings of a sample of Nurses' Health Study participants (n = 408 women aged 52–74 years at baseline). In this study, lens density was assessed at baseline and at the end of 5 years and correlated with subjects' usual dietary intake and use of dietary supplements, which were assessed prior to baseline.[32]

bioactive dose

Not known.

safety

Presumed safe when consumed in normal dietary quantities by non-allergic individuals.

R

Rosemary (Rosmarinus officinalis)

definition

Culinary herb that has a pine-like flavor used fresh or dried to season meat, poultry, pasta, sauces, stuffing, potatoes, peas, and lima beans. Contains rosmarinic acid, which has been described as "one of the most important and well known natural antioxidant compounds."[33]

scientific findings

In experimental studies, rosemary exhibited anti-inflammatory, antispasmodic, analgesic, antirheumatic, carminative, cholagogue, diuretic, expectorant, antiepileptic, and neuroprotective properties.[33–35]

bioactive dose

Not known.

safety

Presumed safe when consumed in normal dietary quantities by non-allergic individuals.

Rutabaga (Brassica napobrassica)

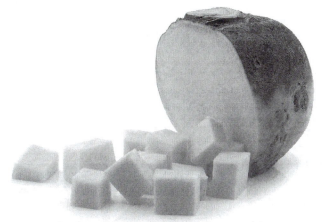

Rutabaga. (Image from 17494494/Shutterstock.)

definition

Yellow-fleshed root vegetable that has a cabbage-like flavor. Its name means "round root." A good source of vitamin C and potassium; also contains glucosinolates.[36,37] Rutabaga is peeled, cooked by boiling, and mashed, possibly with potatoes and carrots, or added to soups, stews, or soufflés.

scientific findings

See *Brassica oleracea.*

bioactive dose

Not known.

safety

Presumed safe when consumed in normal dietary quantities by non-allergic individuals. High levels of goitrogens have been found in rutabaga.[38] Cooking, especially by boiling, destroys goitrogens.

References

1. Innocenti M, Gallori S, Giaccherini C, Ieri F, Vincieri FF Mulinacci N. Evaluation of the phenolic content in the aerial parts of different varieties of *Cichorium intybus* L. *J Agric Food Chem.* 2005;53(16):6497–6502.

2. Sultana S, Perwaiz S, Iqbal M, Athar M. Crude extracts of hepatoprotective plants, *Solanum nigrum* and *Cichorium intybus* inhibit free radical-mediated DNA damage. *J Ethnopharmacol.* 1995;45(3):189–192.

3. Zhou C, Zhu Y, Luo Y. Effects of sulfur fertilization on the accumulation of health-promoting phytochemicals in radish sprouts. *J Agric Food Chem.* 2013;61(31):7552–7559. Epub 2013 July 25.

4. Produce for Better Health Foundation. Daikon radish. http://www.fruit-sandveggiesmorematters.org/daikon-radish. Accessed March 13, 2015.

5. Jellin JM, Gregory PJ et al. Natural Medicine Comprehensive Database. Therapeutic Research Faculty. 2013. http://www.naturaldatabase.com. Accessed July 11, 2012.

6. US Department of Agriculture. Agricultural Research Service. Nutrient Data Laboratory. Raisins, seedless. http://ndb.nal.usda.gov/ndb/foods/sho w/2387?fg=&man=&lfacet=&format=&count=&max=25&offset=&sort=&ql ookup=raisin. Accessed July 27, 2013.

7. Karadeniz F, Durst RW, Wrolstad RE. Polyphenolic composition of raisins. *J Agric Food Chem.* 2000;48(11):5343–5350.

8. Bell SJ. A review of dietary fiber and health: Focus on raisins. *J Med Food.* 2011;14(9):877–883. doi: 10.1089/jmf.2010.0215. Epub 2011 April 10.

9. Spiller GA, Story JA, Furumoto EJ, Chezem JC, Spiller M. Effect of tartaric acid and dietary fibre from sun-dried raisins on colonic function and on bile acid and volatile fatty acid excretion in healthy adults. *Br J Nutr.* 2003;90(4):803–807.

10. Spiller GA, Story JA, Lodics TA, Pollack M, Monyan S, Butterfield G, Spiller M. Effect of sun-dried raisins on bile acid excretion, intestinal transit time, and fecal weight: A dose–response study. *J Med Food.* 2003;6(2):87–91.

11. US Department of Agriculture. Agricultural Research Service. Nutrient Data Laboratory. Raspberry, raw. http://ndb.nal.usda.gov/ndb/foods/show/2475?qlookup=raspberry%2C+raw&fg=&format=&man=&lfacet=&max=25 &new=1. Accessed January 26, 2012.

12. Rosales-Soto MU, Powers JR, Alldredge JR. Effect of mixing time, freeze-drying and baking on phenolics, anthocyanins and antioxidant capacity of raspberry juice during processing of muffins. *J Sci Food Agric.* 2012;92(7):1511–1518. Epub 2012 January 6.

13. Lloyd AJ, Favé G, Beckmann M, Lin W, Tailliart K, Xie L, Mathers JC, Draper J. Use of mass spectrometry fingerprinting to identify urinary metabolites after consumption of specific foods. *Am J Clin Nutr.* 2011;94(4):981–991. Epub 2011 August 24.

14. González-Barrio R, Edwards CA, Crozier A. Colonic catabolism of ellagitannins, ellagic acid, and raspberry anthocyanins: *In vivo* and *in vitro* studies. *Drug Metab Dispos.* 2011;39(9):1680–1688. Epub 2011 May 27.

15. Olthof MR, Hollman PC, Katan MB. Chlorogenic acid and caffeic acid are absorbed in humans. *J Nutr.* 2001;131(1):66–71.

R

16. Natarajan K, Singh S, Burke TR, Grunberger D, Aggarwal BB. Caffeic acid phenethyl ester is a potent and specific inhibitor of activation of nuclear transcription factor NF-kappa B. *Proc Natl Acad Sci USA.* 1996;93(17):9090–9095.

17. Saija A, Tomaino A, Lo Cascio R, Trombetta D, Proteggente A, De Pasquale A, Uccella N, Bonina F. Ferulic and caffeic acids as potential protective agents against photooxidative skin damage. *J Sci Food Agric.* 1999;79(3):476–480.

18. Sun P, Liang JL, Kang LZ, Huang XY, Huang JJ, Ye ZW, Guo LQ, Lin JF. Increased resveratrol production in wines using engineered wine strains *Saccharomyces cerevisiae* EC1118 and relaxed antibiotic or auxotrophic selection. *Biotechnol Prog.* 2015;31(3):650–655. doi: 10.1002/btpr.2057. Epub 2015 February 14.

19. Burns J, Yokota T, Ashihara H, Lean MEJ, Crozier A. Plant foods and herbal sources of resveratrol. *J Agric Food Chem.* 2002;50(11):3337–3340.

20. Frémont L. Biological effects of resveratrol. *Life Sci.* 2000;66(8):663–673.

21. Ramprasath VR, Jones PJ. Anti-atherogenic effects of resveratrol. *Eur J Clin Nutr.* 2010;64(7):660–668. Epub 2010 May 19.

22. Catalog B, Batgirl S, Toga Y, Over NK. Resveratrol: French paradox revisited. *Front Pharmacol.* 2012;17(3):141.

23. Brawny P, Molnar GA et al. Resveratrol improves insulin sensitivity, reduces oxidative stress and activates the Akt pathway in type 2 diabetic patients. *Br J Nutr.* 2011;9:1–7.

24. US Department of Agriculture. Agricultural Research Service. Nutrient Data Laboratory. Rhubarb, frozen, cooked with sugar. http://ndb.nal.usda.gov/ndb/foods/show/2395. Accessed July 27, 2013.

25. Whitney ER, Rolfes SR. *Understanding Nutrition*, 12th edn. Belmont, CA: Cengage; 2011.

26. Yang F, Zhang T, Tian G, Cao H, Liu Q, Ito Y. Preparative isolation and purification of hydroxyanthraquinones from *Rheum officinale* Baill by high-speed counter-current chromatography using pH-modulated stepwise elution. *J Chromatogr A.* 1999;858(1):103–107.

27. Sydiskis RJ, Owen DG, Lohr JL, Rosler KH, Blomster RN. Inactivation of enveloped viruses by anthraquinones extracted from plants. *Antimicrob Agents Chemother.* 1991;35(12):2463–2466.

28. Semple SJ, Pyke SM, Reynolds GD, Flower RL. *In vitro* antiviral activity of the anthraquinone chrysophanic acid against poliovirus. *Antiviral Res.* 2001;49(3):169–178.

29. The Rhubarb Compendium. http://www.rhubarbinfo.com/botanical. Accessed June 16, 2011.

30. Brown JP. A review of the genetic effects of naturally occurring flavonoids, anthraquinones and related compounds. *Mutat Res-Rev Genet.* 1980; 75(3):243–277.

31. Institute of Medicine. *Dietary Reference Intakes for Thiamin, Riboflavin, Niacin, Vitamin B6, Folate, Vitamin B12,Pantothenic Acid, Biotin and Choline.* Washington DC: National Academy Press; 1998.

32. Jacques PF, Taylor A, Moeller S, Hankinson SE, Rogers G, Tung W, Ludovico J, Willett WC, Chylack LT Jr. Long-term nutrient intake and 5-year change in nuclear lens opacities. *Arch Ophthalmol.* 2005;123(4):517–526.

R

33. Nabavi SF, Tenore GC, Daglia M, Tundis R, Loizzo MR, Nabavi SM. The cellular protective effects of rosmarinic acid: From bench to bedside. *Curr Neurovasc Res.* 2015;12(1):98–105.
34. Melo GA, Grespan R, Fonseca JP, Farinha TO, Silva EL, Romero AL, Bersani-Amado CA, Cuman RKN. *Rosmarinus officinalis* L. essential oil inhibits in vivo and in vitro leukocyte migration. *J Med Food.* 2011;14(9):944–946. Epub 2011 June 11.
35. Takaki I, Bersani-Amado LE, Vendruscolo A, Sartoretto SM, Diniz SP, Bersani-Amado CA, Cuman RK. Anti-inflammatory and antinociceptive effects of *Rosmarinus officinalis* L. essential oil in experimental animal models. *J Med Food.* 2008;11(4):741–746.
36. Antonious GF, Bomford M, Vincelli P. Screening *Brassica* species for glucosinolate content. *J Environ Sci Health B.* 2009;44(3):311–316.
37. Gorovic N, Afzal S, Tjønneland A, Overvad K, Vogel U, Albrechtsen C, Poulsen HE. Genetic variation in the hTAS2R38 taste receptor and brassica vegetable intake. *Scand J Clin Lab Invest.* 2011;71(4):274–249.
38. Mullin WJ, Sahas-Rabudhe MR. Glucosinolate content of cruciferous vegetable crops. *Can J Plant Sci.* 1977;57(4):1227–1230.

R

S

Sage (Salvia officinalis, Salvia lavandulaefolia)

definition

Earthy-flavored herb used fresh or dried to flavor meats, fish, and stews. Sage, in small quantities normally consumed as an herb, is not an appreciable source of nutrients. Its phytochemical constituents include phenolic compounds, catechin, chlorogenic acid, vanillic acid, caffeic acid, and epicatechin.[1] In traditional medicine, sage was boiled and drunk as a tea to treat dyspepsia, mouth and throat inflammation, excessive sweating, and minor skin inflammations.[2] Ancient Greek physicians used a solution of sage and water to stop wounds from bleeding and to clean sores and ulcers.[3]

scientific findings

S. officinalis has exhibited antioxidant and anti-inflammatory properties in experimental research.[4,5] Estrogenic flavonoids, compounds that exert anti-hot-flash (also called hot flush) activity, have been isolated in S. officinalis.[6] In laboratory research, S. lavandulaefolia (Spanish sage) extracts and constituents have demonstrated anticholinesterase, antioxidant, anti-inflammatory, estrogenic, and central nervous system depressant (sedative) effects.[7] There is insufficient scientific evidence to support its use as a treatment for sore throat.[3] Two small studies suggest that sage may improve mood and mental performance in healthy young people and memory and attention in older adults.[3] Findings of another small clinical trial found sage extract to be better than placebo to enhance thinking and learning in older adults with mild-to-moderate Alzheimer disease,[3,8] an explanation for which, according to researchers, could be related to sage's cholinergic binding properties, which have been demonstrated *in vitro*.[8]

bioactive dose

Not known.

S

safety

Sage contains the neurotoxin thujone, a monoterpene; however, when sage is used in normal dietary quantities, thujone poses little risk.[2] Thujone can have menstrual stimulant and abortifacient effects and is thought to reduce the mother's milk supply.[9] Taking large amounts of sage leaf or oil may result in restlessness, vomiting, vertigo, rapid heart rate, tremors, seizures, and kidney damage, and may lead to wheezing.[9] Twelve or more of drops of sage essential oil is considered a toxic dose.[9]

Saponin

definition

Glycoside compound found in a wide variety of plants, such as soybeans, chickpeas, peanuts, spinach, quinoa, and beer, but few used as food.[10] When fruits and vegetables are cut or otherwise processed, saponin produces a soapy foam.[10]

scientific findings

Dietary saponins, either isolated or as saponin-containing food plants, have reduced plasma cholesterol levels in animal studies.[10] Experimental data show saponins to be one of many bioactive ingredients in foods that has exhibited blood-pressure-lowering effects.[11]

bioactive dose

Not known.

safety

Presumed safe when consumed in normal dietary quantities by non-allergic individuals.

Selenium

definition

Trace mineral found in meat, especially organ meats, seafood, and certain plant foods, such as nuts. Brazil nuts, which supply 290 μg of selenium per one nut[12] (more than three times the Daily Reference Value of 70 μg or 415%DV), are an excellent source of the mineral. Selenium is an antioxidant that seems to inhibit cell proliferation[13]; it is also necessary for thyroid function,[14] immune function, and normal testicular development, spermatogenesis, and spermatozoa motility and function in males[15]; and it exhibits insulin-mimetic properties.[16]

scientific findings

Consuming one Brazil nut daily for 8 weeks improved selenium status, erythrocyte glutathione peroxidase activity, and measures of atherogenic risk, such as HDL cholesterol, in a small clinical trial (n = 38 selenium deficient, severely obese women).[12] The association between selenium status and cancer risk is being investigated. A meta-analysis of cancer studies examining the relationship between dietary selenium intake and cancers that included 49 prospective observational studies and 6 randomized controlled trials, concluded: "No reliable conclusions can be drawn regarding a causal relationship between low selenium exposure and an increased risk of cancer."[17] An analysis of toenail selenium was conducted in the Netherlands Cohort Study (n = 58,279 men aged 55–69 years at baseline) from a random subcohort of 898 advanced prostate cancer subjects and 1176 subcohort subjects. Incident advanced prostate cancer case subjects from the entire cohort were identified during 17.3 years of follow-up. The study found that "toenail selenium was associated with a substantial decrease in risk of advanced prostate cancer."[18] If there is a benefit of selenium on prostate cancer risk, it appears to be limited to patients who are selenium deficient.[19] In an observational study (n = 5587 participants in the 2007–2008 National Health and Nutrition Examination Survey) evaluating associations between self-reported sleep duration and intake of various dietary components, normal sleep duration was associated with the greatest food variety, and nutrients consumed less by short sleepers (<5 h per night) included selenium.[20] A selenium review found that low selenium levels or selenium deficiency may reduce the conversion of thyroxine (T4) to triiodothyronine (T3).[9] Another review stated that selenium status appears to have an impact on the development of thyroid pathologies.[21] Patients with newly diagnosed Graves Disease (n = 97) and/or autoimmune overt hypothyroidism (n = 96) had significantly lower serum selenium compared with random controls (n = 830), suggesting a link between inadequate selenium status and overt autoimmune thyroid disease, especially Graves Disease.[22]

bioactive dose

The RDA for adults aged 19–50 is 55 μg/day.

safety

The UL for adults aged 19–50 is 400 µg/day. "Signs and symptoms of selenosis (selenium toxicity) include pruritis, nail changes, brittle hair and nails, and garlic breath, and have been reported at serum selenium levels >1000 ng/mL corresponding to daily intakes >910 µg."[19]

Shallot (Allium cepa L. var. aggregatum)

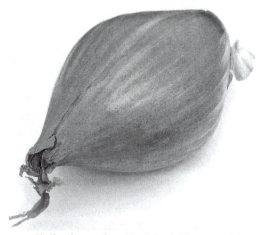

Shallot. (Image from NeydtStock/Shutterstock.)

definition

Miniature purple onion that contains allyl sulfides and flavonol glycosides, including quercetin.[23] Used for their strong, characteristically burning flavor in salads and salad dressings.

S

scientific findings

See *Allium* vegetables.

bioactive dose

Not known.

safety

Presumed safe when consumed in normal dietary quantities by non-allergic individuals.

Snap pea (Pisum sativum)

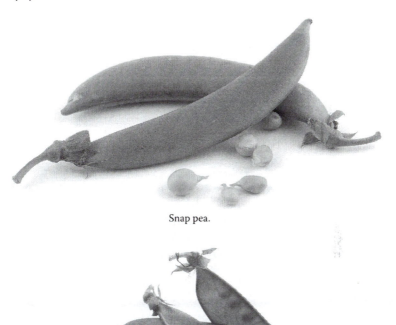

Snap pea.

Snow pea.

definition

Fabaceae green pod vegetable containing several edible peas. Snap peas are generally cooked or stir-fried; they are also sold as a freeze-dried, salted, ready-to-eat snack. Fresh shoots of the snap pea are used as micro-greens (sprouts from seeds) in salads or as a garnish. The snow pea (also called sugar snap pea) has a flat pod, while the snap pea pod is plump with tougher skin. Excellent source of vitamin C[24]; contains phenolic compounds.[25]

scientific findings

In an animal study, diets containing *P. sativum* reduced serum total cholesterol possibly due in part to an increased fecal bile acid output.[26]

S

bioactive dose

Not known.

safety

Presumed safe when consumed in normal dietary quantities by non-allergic individuals.

Soybean (Glycine max)

definition

Fabaceae vegetable that is a good source of protein and fiber and supplies isoflavones. Edamame are immature, raw soybeans, and tofu, tempeh, miso, and soy milk, in addition to soymilk-based infant formula, are products made from soybean. Soybean oil is a source of omega-3 fatty acid and a good source of vitamin E (6% DV) and vitamin K (31% DV).[27]

scientific findings

The physiological effects of consuming soy foods are as follows: (1) Eating modest amounts of soy foods during childhood and/or adolescence modestly reduces the risk of developing breast cancer.[9] More evidence is needed to determine the effect of soy foods on patients with existing breast cancer[28]; (2) Consuming soy protein seems to modestly reduce total and LDL cholesterol.[9] Soy foods lower the risk of coronary heart disease[28]; (3) Consuming soy protein isoflavones modestly decreases hot flashes in some menopausal women[9,28]; (4) Soy protein, according to most, but not all, evidence can increase bone mineral density or slow its loss and improve biochemical markers of bone turnover in peri- and postmenopausal women.[9,29] A review of 13 studies found unclear and conflicting evidence on the effect of increased soy food intake and blood pressure.[30]

bioactive dose

Not known. The dose of soy protein needed to achieve significant decreases in total or LDL cholesterol or triglycerides has not been established,[31] but a dose of 20–50 g of soy protein daily has been used for hyperlipidemia.[9]

safety

Presumed safe when consumed in normal dietary quantities by non-allergic individuals. Allergies to soybean have been reported. Soy protein products in doses up to 60 g/day have been safely used in studies lasting up to 16 weeks.[9]

Spinach (Spinacia oleracea)

definition

Dark green leaf vegetable that is a good source of folate and an excellent source of vitamins A and K.[32] Supplies lutein,[33] saponin, and oxalate, the latter of which gives raw spinach a distinctive mouth feel described as a film in one's mouth. Unlike many other dark green vegetables, spinach is a poor calcium source, providing only 30 mg per 1 cup (3%DV), and, despite its reputation to the contrary, spinach is not a good source of iron, providing only 0.8 mg of nonheme iron per 1 cup (4% DV).[34] The bioavailability of nonheme iron is poor compared to the bioavailability of heme iron. Baby spinach is a popular salad ingredient, and spinach is used in many casserole and pasta recipes, in addition to being a main ingredient in the Greek dish spanakopita (literally meaning "spinach with bread") that consists of cooked spinach layered with phyllo dough and feta cheese.

scientific findings

Consumption of green leafy vegetables is associated with a reduced risk of several types of cancer, such as pancreatic cancer, and cardiovascular disease.[35,36] A high intake of green leafy vegetables was linked to a reduced risk of non-Hodgkin's lymphoma in a population-based case–control study (n = 348 cases and 470 controls) that compared dietary intake of cases to controls.[37]

bioactive dose

Not known.

safety

Presumed safe when consumed in normal dietary quantities by non-allergic individuals.

Squash (Curcubita pepo)

definition

Winter squash is the hard-shelled, orange- or yellow-fleshed variety of squash such as spaghetti, acorn, butternut, or Hubbard, while summer squash has an edible, thin skin and white flesh, for example, zucchini.

Winter squash's hard skin serves to increase its storage life. It can be stored for up to 3 months in cool temperatures. Winter squash is prepared by baking in the shell or by removing the hard outer skin and then baking and mashing the flesh. Many winter squash varieties are rich in starch and, therefore, are counted as starchy vegetables for purposes of carbohydrate counting in diabetes. Winter squash per 1/2 cup supplies 4.5 grams of fiber and 400 IU of vitamin A,[38] making it a good source of both.[39] Certain summer squashes are good sources of vitamin A, for example, zucchini per 1/2 cup, supplies 1300 IU of vitamin A.[40]

scientific findings

The vitamin A activity of squash is due to its provitamin A carotenoid, β-carotene. β-carotene becomes active vitamin A if necessary, or remains in its antioxidant form. Since β-carotene from food has no potential for toxicity, it is a safe form of vitamin A, which has an upper limit of safety of ≥10,000 IU, and which may be important, for example, during pregnancy.[41]

bioactive dose

Not known. Adult women and men aged 19–50 require 2.5 cups or 3 cups of vegetables, per day, respectively, ideally including all subgroups, including "red and orange" vegetables to which winter squash belongs, and "other vegetables" to which zucchini belongs.

safety

Presumed safe when consumed in normal dietary quantities by non-allergic individuals.

Stanols, sterols

definition

Steroid compounds, such as sitostanol, campestanol, sitosterol, campesterol, and stigmasterol, that have chemical structures similar to cholesterol.[42] Found naturally in fruits, grains, vegetables and vegetable oils, nuts and seeds, wheat germ and wheat bran; peanuts; corn, sesame, canola, and olive oil; almonds; and brussels sprouts.[43] These compounds are under consumed. Normal dietary intake of plant sterols is 200–400 mg/day, a level that would not significantly affect cholesterol absorption, but when consumed at levels 5–10 times higher than normal, they have been shown to reduce total and LDL cholesterol.[44] Vegetable oil spreads, mayonnaise, yogurt, milk, orange juice, cereals, and snack bars that have been fortified with plant sterols and stanols are commonly available in grocery stores.[43]

scientific findings

Plant sterols and stanols in the diet help to lower blood total and LDL cholesterol levels.[45]

bioactive dose

The National Heart Lung and Blood Institute's National Cholesterol Education Program Therapeutic Lifestyle Changes recommends that individuals with elevated LDL cholesterol consume 2 g of plant sterols/stanols per day.[46] "A reduction of up to 10% total cholesterol is observed when 2–3 g of plant stanol/sterol esters are consumed daily."[44]

safety

An intake of 2–3 g of plant sterols and stanols per day generally appears to be safe.[47]

"It is unclear whether there are unintended AEs when consuming sterols. Some studies have detected no significant changes in the plasma concentrations of α-carotene, lycopene, and vitamins A, D, and E; however, other studies have found that the plasma concentrations of α-tocopherol and α- and β-carotene decrease after the consumption of sterols and stanols."[48]

Starchy vegetables

definition

S

Vegetables that generally have a higher carbohydrate content (~15 g of carbohydrate per 1/2–1 cup serving) than nonstarchy vegetables, such as lettuce and tomatoes (~5 g of carbohydrate per 1/2–1 cup serving), and therefore, are considered to be equivalent to grains for diet planning purposes.[49] Examples of starchy vegetables, according to The American Diabetes Association (ADA), include parsnips, winter squash, white potatoes, sweet potatoes, and yams. Examples of starchy vegetables according to ChooseMyPlate.gov differ from that of ADA, for example, ChooseMyPlate.gov classifies winter squash as an Orange and Red Vegetable, not a starchy vegetable, which should be noted in patients who are required to control their carbohydrate intake. The flesh and/or skin of many starchy vegetables can be rich sources of fiber.

scientific findings

Starch is a major glycemic carbohydrate in foods. Starchy vegetables may increase dietary glycemic load and raise blood glucose appreciably.[50] Some starchy vegetables contain resistant starches and fibers that either reduce or have no effect upon glycemic load in addition to having other health benefits.[51]

bioactive dose

Not applicable.

safety

Presumed safe when consumed in normal dietary quantities by non-allergic individuals.

Strawberry (Fragaria × ananassa)

definition

Popular snack fruit that is an excellent source of vitamin C and folate[52] and a source of flavonoids. Eaten fresh, frozen, dried, as juices, or added to cereals, desserts, or baked products.

scientific findings

Strawberry constituents ameliorated allergy symptoms in a laboratory study.[53] A laboratory study demonstrated synergism and antagonism among the seven phenolic compounds in strawberries, including p-coumaric acid, cyanidin, catechin, quercetin-3-glucoside, kaempferol, and ellagic acid,[54] illustrating the unique interactions that occur among phytochemicals within the complex food matrix using strawberry as a model. Strawberry phenolics are known for their antioxidant and anti-inflammatory action, and possess direct and indirect antimicrobial, anti-allergy and anti-hypertensive properties based on laboratory research.[55] They also inhibit the activities of some physiological enzymes and receptor properties which may have various disease-preventative implications.[55]

bioactive dose

Not known.

safety

Presumed safe when consumed in normal dietary quantities by non-allergic individuals. Allergy to strawberries have been reported.

Sulforaphane

definition

Isothiocyanate found in broccoli, broccoli sprouts, and other *Brassica* vegetables.

scientific findings

Sulforaphane exhibited chemoprotective properties in experimental research; it may prompt the body to make higher levels of chemoprotective enzymes.[56] In a small clinical trial (n = 20 men with recurrent prostate cancer), treatment with 200 µmoles/day of sulforaphane-rich broccoli sprout extract did not decrease prostate-specific antigen in the majority of patients.[57]

bioactive dose

Not known.

safety

Presumed safe when consumed in normal dietary quantities by non-allergic individuals.

Syringic acid

definition

A phenolic acid found in plants, such as sage and wheat.

scientific findings

In animal research, syringic acid exhibited hepatoprotective properties.[58]

bioactive dose

Not known.

S

safety

Presumed safe when consumed in normal dietary quantities by non-allergic individuals.

References

1. Rababah TM, Ereifej KI, Esoh RB, Al-U'datt MH, Alrababah MA, Yang W. Antioxidant activities, total phenolics and HPLC analyses of the phenolic compounds of extracts from common Mediterranean plants. *Nat Prod Res.* 2011;25(6):596–605.
2. Walch SG, Tinzoh LN, Zimmermann BF, Stühlinger W, Lachenmeier DW. Antioxidant capacity and polyphenolic composition as quality indicators for aqueous infusions of *Salvia officinalis* L. (sage tea). *Front Pharmacol.* 2011;2:79. Epub 2011 December 19.
3. National Institutes of Health. National Center for Complementary and Alternative Medicine. Herbs at a Glance. Sage. https://nccih.nih.gov/health/sage. Accessed March 17, 2015.
4. Wang M, Shao Y, Li J, Zhu N, Rangarajan M, LaVoie EJ, Ho CT. Antioxidative phenolic glycosides from sage (*Salvia officinalis*). *J Nat Prod.* 1999;62(3):454–456.
5. Oniga I, Pârvu AE, Toiu A, Benedec D. Effects of *Salvia officinalis* L. extract on experimental acute inflammation. *Rev Med Chir Soc Med Nat Iasi.* 2007;111(1):290–294.
6. Rahte S, Evans R, Eugster PJ, Marcourt L, Wolfender JL, Kortenkamp A, Tasdemir D. *Salvia officinalis* for hot flushes: Towards determination of mechanism of activity and active principles. *Planta Med.* 2013;79(9):753–760. doi: 10.1055/s-0032-1328552. Epub 2013 May 13.
7. Perry NS, Bollen C, Perry EK, Ballard C. Salvia for dementia therapy: Review of pharmacological activity and pilot tolerability clinical trial. *Pharmacol Biochem Behav.* 2003;75(3):651–659.
8. Akhondzadeh S, Noroozian M, Mohammadi M, Ohadinia S, Jamshidi AH, Khani M. *Salvia officinalis* extract in the treatment of patients with mild to moderate Alzheimer's disease: A double blind, randomized and placebo-controlled trial. *J Clin Pharm Ther.* 2003;28(1):53–59.
9. Jellin JM, Gregory PJ. *Natural Medicine Comprehensive Database.* Therapeutic Research Faculty. 2013. http://www.naturaldatabase.com. Accessed July 11, 2012.
10. Oakenfull, D. Saponins in food—A review. *Food Chem.* 1981;7(1):19–40.
11. Huang WY, Davidge ST, Wu J. Bioactive natural constituents from food sources-potential use in hypertension prevention and treatment. *Crit Rev Food Sci Nutr.* 2013;53(6):615–630. doi: 10.1080/10408398.2010.550071.
12. Cominetti C, de Bortoli MC, Garrido AB Jr, Cozzolino SM. Brazilian nut consumption improves selenium status and glutathione peroxidase activity and reduces atherogenic risk in obese women. *Nutr Res.* 2012;32(6):403–407. doi: 10.1016/j.nutres.2012.05.005. Epub 2012 June 12.
13. National Institutes of Health. Medline Plus. Selenium-Antioxidant. http://www.nlm.nih.gov/medlineplus/ency/imagepages/19304.htm. Accessed March 22, 2015.

14. National Institutes of Health. Office of Dietary Supplements. Dietary Supplement Fact Sheet. Selenium. http://ods.od.nih.gov/pdf/factsheets/selenium.pdf. Accessed June 16, 2011.
15. Moslemi MK, Tavanbakhsh S. Selenium-vitamin E supplementation in infertile men: Effects on semen parameters and pregnancy rate. *Int J Gen Med.* 2011;23(4):99–104.
16. Koyama H, Mutakin, Abdulah R, Yamazaki C, Kameo S. Selenium supplementation trials for cancer prevention and the subsequent risk of type 2 diabetes mellitus. *Nihon Eiseigaku Zasshi.* 2013;68(1):1–10.
17. Dennert G, Zwahlen M, Brinkman M, Vinceti M, Zeegers MP, Horneber M. Selenium for preventing cancer. *Cochrane Database Syst Rev.* 2011; May 11(5):CD005195. doi: 10.1002/14651858.CD005195.pub2.
18. Geybels MS, Verhage BA, van Schooten FJ, Goldbohm RA, van den Brandt PA. Advanced prostate cancer risk in relation to toenail selenium levels. *J Natl Cancer Inst.* 2013;105(18):1394–1401. Epub 2013 July 22. [Epub ahead of print.]
19. Fritz H, Kennedy D, Fergusson D, Fernandes R, Cooley K, Seely A, Sagar S, Wong R, Seely D. Selenium and lung cancer: A systematic review and meta analysis. *PLoS One.* 2011;6(11):e26259. doi: 10.1371/journal.pone.0026259.
20. Grandner MA, Jackson N, Gerstner JR, Knutson KL. Dietary nutrients associated with short and long sleep duration. Data from a nationally representative sample. *Appetite.* 2013;64:71–80. doi: 10.1016/j.appet.2013.01.004. Epub 2013 January 20.
21. Drutel A, Archambeaud F, Caron P. Selenium and the thyroid gland: More good news for clinicians. *Clin Endocrinol (Oxford).* 2013;78(2):155–64. doi: 10.1111/cen.12066.
22. Pedersen IB, Knudsen N, Carlé A, Schomburg L, Köhrle J, Jørgensen T, Rasmussen LB, Ovesen L, Laurberg P. Serum selenium is low in newly diagnosed Graves' disease: A population-based study. *Clin Endocrinol (Oxford).* 2013;79(4):584–590. Epub 2013 February 28. doi: 10.1111/cen.12185. [Epub ahead of print].
23. Price KR, Rhodes MJC. Analysis of the major flavonol glycosides present in four varieties of onion (*Allium cepa*) and changes in composition resulting from autolysis. *J Sci Food Agric.* 1997;74(3):331–339.
24. US Department of Agriculture. Agricultural Research Service. National Nutrient Database. Peas, raw. http://ndb.nal.usda.gov/ndb/foods/show/30 83?man=&lfacet=&count=&max=35&qlookup=snap+pea&offset=&sort=& format=Abridged&reportfmt=other&rptfrm=&ndbno=&nutrient1=&nut rient2=&nutrient3=&subset=&totCount=&measureby=&_action_show= Apply+Changes&Qv=1&Q5877=1&Q5878=0.5&Q5879=10.0. Accessed March 21, 2015.
25. Troszyńska A, Estrella I, Luisa López-Amóres M, Hernández T. Antioxidant activity of pea (*Pisum sativum* L.) seed coat acetone extract. *LWT—Food Sci Technol.* 2002;35(2):158–164.
26. Martins JM, Riottot M, de Abreu MC, Lanc MJ, Viegas-Crespo AM, Almeida JA, Freire JB, Bento OP. Dietary raw peas (*Pisum sativum* L.) reduce plasma total and LDL cholesterol and hepatic esterified cholesterol in intact and ileorectal anastomosed pigs fed cholesterol-rich diets. *J Nutr.* 2004;134:3305–3312.

S

27. US Department of Agriculture. National Nutrient Database. Soybean oil. http://ndb.nal.usda.gov/ndb/foods/show/635?fgcd=&manu=&lfacet=&format=&count=&max=35&offset=&sort=&qlookup=soybean+oil. April 15, 2015.

28. Messina M. Insights gained from 20 years of soy research. *J Nutr.* 2010; 140(12):2289S–2295S.

29. Lagari VS, Levis S. Phytoestrogens and bone health. *Curr Opin Endocrinol Diabetes Obes.* 2010;17(6):546–553. doi: 10.1097/MED.0b013e32833f4867.

30. Academy of Nutrition and Dietetics. Evidence Analysis Library. What evidence suggests a relationship between soy food intake and blood pressure in healthy and hypertensive adults? http://andevidencelibrary.com/conclusion.cfm?conclusion_statement_id=250680. Accessed July 29, 2013.

31. Academy of Nutrition and Dietetics. Evidence Analysis Library. Is there a dose–response relationship of the soy protein and/or isoflavone effects on cholesterol levels? http://andevidencelibrary.com/conclusion.cfm?conclusion_statement_id=95. Accessed July 29, 2013.

32. US Department of Agriculture. Agricultural Research Service. Nutrient Data Laboratory. Spinach, raw. http://ndb.nal.usda.gov/ndb/foods/show/3151?fg=&man=&lfacet=&format=&count=&max=25&offset=&sort=&qlookup=spinach%2C+raw. Accessed July 30, 2013.

33. Włodarek D, Głabska D. Influence of the lutein-rich products consumption on its supply in diet of individuals with age-related macular degeneration (AMD). *Klin Oczna.* 2011;113(1–3):42–46.

34. US Department of Agriculture. National Nutrient Database. Spinach, raw. http://ndb.nal.usda.gov/ndb/foods/show/3202?man=&lfacet=&count=&max=35&qlookup=spinach&offset=&sort=&format=Abridged&reportfmt=other&rptfrm=&ndbno=&nutrient1=&nutrient2=&nutrient3-=&subset=&totCount=&measureby=&_action_show=Apply + Changes&Qv=1&Q6075=1&Q6076=1&Q6077=1&Q6078=1. Accessed April 15, 2015.

35. Jin J, Koroleva OA, Gibson T, Swanston J, Magan J, Zhang Y, Rowland IR, Wagstaff C. Analysis of phytochemical composition and chemoprotective capacity of rocket (*Eruca sativa* and *Diplotaxis tenuifolia*) leafy salad following cultivation in different environments. *J Agric Food Chem.* 2009;57(12):5227–5234.

36. Jansen RJ, Robinson DP, Stolzenberg-Solomon RZ, Bamlet WR, de Andrade M, Oberg AL, Hammer TJ et al. Fruit and vegetable consumption is inversely associated with having pancreatic cancer. *Cancer Causes Control.* 2011;22(12):1613–1625. Epub 2011 September 14.

37. Chiu BC, Kwon S, Evens AM, Surawicz T, Smith SM, Weisenburger DD. Dietary intake of fruit and vegetables and risk of non-Hodgkin lymphoma. *Cancer Causes Control.* 2011;22(8):1183–1195. Epub 2011 June 22.

38. National Institutes of Health Centers for Disease Control. Fruit and veggies matter. Squash. http://www.fruitsandveggiesmatter.gov/month/winter_squash.html. Accessed June 25, 2011.

39. US Department of Agriculture. Agricultural Research Service. Nutrient Data Laboratory. Squash, winter, butternut, cooked. http://ndb.nal.usda.gov/ndb/foods/show/3173?fg=&man=&lfacet=&count=&max=25&qlookup=cooked+squash&offset=&sort=&format=Abridged&_action_show=Apply+Changes&Qv=1&Q5895=0.5. Accessed August 1, 2013.

40. US Department of Agriculture. Agricultural Research Service. Nutrient Data Laboratory. Squash, zucchini. http://ndb.nal.usda.gov/ndb/foods/sho w/3215?fg=&man=&lfacet=&count=&max=25&qlookup=zucchini&offset= &sort=&format=Abridged&reportfmt=other&rptfrm=&ndbno=&nutrien t1=&nutrient2=&nutrient3=&subset=&totCount=&measureby=&_action_ show=Apply+Changes&Qv=1&Q6099=0.5&Q6100=1&Q6101=1&Q6102=1& Q6103=1&Q6104=1. Accessed January 22, 2015.

41. Strobel M, Tinz J, Biesalski HK. The importance of beta-carotene as a source of vitamin A with special regard to pregnant and breastfeeding women. *Eur J Nutr.* 2007;46(Suppl 1):I1–20.

42. Talati R, Sobieraj DM, Makanji SS, Phung OJ, Coleman CI. The comparative efficacy of plant sterols and stanols on serum lipids: A systematic review and meta-analysis. *J Am Diet Assoc.* 2010;110(5):719–726.

43. Joslin Diabetes Center. Lower Your Cholesterol with Sterols and Stanols. http://www.joslin.org/info/lower-cholesterol-with-plant-sterols-and-stanols.html. Accessed August 1, 2013.

44. The American Dietetic Association Evidence Analysis Library. Diseases/ Health Conditions. Disorders of Lipid Metabolism. 2005. Plant Sterols/ Stanols Sterols and Stanols. http://www.adaevidencelibrary.com/ conclusion.cfm?conclusion_statement_id=47. Accessed January 10, 2012.

45. US Food and Drug Administration. Health claims: Plant sterol/stanol esters and risk of coronary heart disease (CHD). *CFR—Code of Federal Regulations Title* 21 Sec. 101.83.http://www.accessdata.fda.gov/scripts/cdrh/cfdocs/cfcfr/ CFRSearch.cfm?fr=101.83. Accessed April 14, 2015.

46. The National Institutes of Health. National Cholesterol Education Program Slideshow. *Therapeutic Lifestyle Changes Adult Treatment Panel III Guidelines.* http://hp2010.nhlbihin.net/ncep_slds/menu.htm#2. Accessed January 25, 2012.

47. The American Dietetic Association Evidence Analysis Library. Diseases/ Health Conditions. Disorders of Lipid Metabolism. 2005. Plant Sterols/ Stanols Sterols and Stanols. What does the research indicate about the safety of stanol and sterol intake? Accessed January 10, 2012.

48. The American Dietetic Association Evidence Analysis Library. Diseases/ Health Conditions. Disorders of Lipid Metabolism. 2005. Plant Sterols/ Stanols Sterols and Stanols. 2005. Are there any unintended adverse effects when consuming stanols and sterols? http://andevidencelibrary.com/con-clusion.cfm?conclusion_statement_id=52. Accessed August 1, 2013.

49. The American Diabetes Association. Whole Grain Foods. http://www. diabetes.org/food-and-fitness/food/what-can-i-eat/grains-and-starchy-vegetables.html. Accessed August 1, 2013.

50. Dauchet L, Amouyel P, Dallongeville J. Fruit and vegetable consumption and risk of stroke: A meta-analysis of cohort studies. *Neurology.* 2005;65(8):1193–1197.

51. Grabitske HA, Slavin JL. Gastrointestinal effects of low-digestible carbohy-drates. *Crit Rev Food Sci Nutr.* 2009;49(4):327–360.

52. US Department of Agriculture. Agricultural Research Service. Nutrient Data Laboratory. Strawberries, raw. http://ndb.nal.usda.gov/ndb/foods/sho w/2401?fg=&man=&lfacet=&count=&max=25&qlookup=strawberry&offset =&sort=&format=Abridged&_action_show=Apply + Changes&Qv=1&Q44 84=1.0&Q4485=0.5&Q4486=1.0&Q4487=1.0&Q4488=1.0&Q4489=1.0&Q4490 =1.0&Q4491=1.0&Q4492=1.0&Q4493=1.0. Accessed July 29, 2013.

S

53. Itoh T, Ninomiya M, Yasuda M, Koshikawa K, Deyashiki Y, Nozawa Y, Akao Y, Koketsu M. Inhibitory effects of flavonoids isolated from *Fragaria ananassa* Duch on IgE-mediated degranulation in rat basophilic leukemia RBL-2H3. *Bioorg Med Chem.* 2009;17(15):5374–5379.

54. Reber JD, Eggett DL, Parker TL. Antioxidant capacity interactions and a chemical/structural model of phenolic compounds found in strawberries. *Int J Food Sci Nutr.* 2011;62(5):445–452.

55. Giampieri F, Alvarez-Suarez JM, Mazzoni L, Romandini S, Bompadre S, Diamanti J, Capocasa F et al. The potential impact of strawberry on human health. *Nat Prod Res.* 2013;27(4–5):448–455. doi: 10.1080/14786419.2012.706294. Epub 2012 July 13.

56. American Cancer Society. Broccoli. http://www.cancer.org/Treatment/ TreatmentsandSideEffects/ComplementaryandAlternativeMedicine/ DietandNutrition/broccoli. Accessed January 25, 2012.

57. Alumkal JJ, Slottke R, Schwartzman J, Cherala G, Munar M, Graff JN, Beer TM et al. A phase II study of sulforaphane-rich broccoli sprout extracts in men with recurrent prostate cancer. *Invest New Drugs.* 2015;33(2):480–489. Epub 2014 November 29.

58. Itoh A, Isoda K, Kondoh M, Kawase M, Kobayashi M, Tamesada M. Yagi Hepatoprotective effect of syringic acid and vanillic acid on concanavalin a-induced liver injury. *Biol Pharm Bull.* 2009;32(7):1215–1219.

S

T

Tamarind (Tamarindus indica)

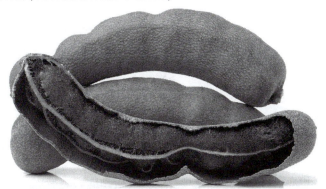

Tamarind. (Image from Jiang Hongyan/Shutterstock.)

definition

Pod-shaped fruit indigenous to tropical Africa[1] that is grown in Florida.[2] Tamarind is a good source of potassium[3] and contains tartaric acid.[4] Tamarind is used to make a sweet sauce that is used in Asian and Indian cooking.[4] The fruit is used in traditional medicine as a laxative, for abdominal pain, to treat diarrhea and dysentery, to treat helminthes infections, for wound healing, and to treat malaria, fever, constipation, inflammation, cell cytotoxicity, gonorrhea, and eye diseases.[5,6]

scientific findings

T. indica seeds exhibited antioxidant properties, and T. indica extract exhibited antidiabetic properties in experimental research.[7,8]

bioactive dose

Not known.

safety

Presumed safe when consumed in normal dietary quantities by non-allergic individuals.

Tangerine (Citrus reticulata)

definition

Small dark orange citrus fruit that is an excellent source of vitamin C and a source of the flavanones hesperetin and naringenin.[9] Its juice is a source of flavones, flavonols, and flavanones, such as kaempferol and quercetin. Tangerines are commonly eaten fresh and added to salads.

scientific findings

See *citrus*.

bioactive dose

Not known.

safety

Presumed safe when consumed in normal dietary quantities by non-allergic individuals.

Tannin

definition

Polyphenol found in black-eyed peas, grapes, lentils, persimmon, black and green teas, and red and white wines, in addition to many other foods.[10,11]

scientific findings

Tannins exhibited chemoprotective properties[10] and bound bile acids in experimental research.[11] Tannin inhibits nonheme iron absorption[12] and can have a significant impact on adult iron status.[13] Tea should be avoided during meals and for at least 1 h after meals to prevent its impairment of nonheme iron absorption.[13]

bioactive dose

Not known.

safety

Presumed safe when consumed in normal dietary quantities by non-allergic individuals.

Tarragon (Artemisia dracunculus)

definition

Culinary herb used fresh or dried. Tarragon pairs well with chicken and fish, including salmon, and can be used to flavor salad dressing. It has a licorice-like flavor. Tarragon is used orally as an antiepileptic remedy in middle Eastern folkloric medicine.[14]

scientific findings

In vitro, tarragon exhibited antioxidant properties.[15] Tarragon exhibited anticonvulsant and sedative effects that were attributed to its monoterpenoids content in experimental research.[14]

bioactive dose

Not known.

safety

Presumed safe when consumed in normal dietary quantities by non-allergic individuals.

Tartaric acid

definition

Organic plant acid found naturally in foods such as grapes raisins, and tamarind.[16,17] Tartaric acid is used in manufacturing sour-flavored confections; for leavening when used in combination with baking soda, in baked goods, and as a food preservative to maintain the quality of processed foods.[18]

T

scientific findings

Tartaric acids in dried fruits, along with other naturally occurring compounds, such as sugar alcohols and fiber, may positively affect bowel regularity.[17]

bioactive dose

Not known.

safety

Presumed safe when consumed in normal dietary quantities by non-allergic individuals.

Tea (Camellia sinensis)

definition

Beverage prepared with leaves that have undergone varying degrees of fermentation corresponding to color differences, such as green (without fermentation), red (lightly fermented), oolong (medium fermentation), and black (fermented). All teas contain caffeine and are traditionally consumed for their mild central nervous system stimulating effects. In addition, all types of tea provide between 100 and 300 mg of flavonoids, such as flavon-3-ol, per serving.[19] Tea is consumed hot, iced, and sweetened or unsweetened. It may also be added to recipes as a marinade.

scientific findings

Epidemiological studies support the potential health-protective effects of flavan-3-ols and their derived compounds upon chronic diseases.[20] The flavonoid catechin is found to a great degree within green tea as compared to black and oolong tea because the latter are processed by fermenting, which destroys catechins. Epidemiologic studies suggest that green tea consumption is associated with cardiovascular benefits and that it may possess antioxidative, antihypertensive, anti-inflammatory, antiproliferative, antithrombogenic, and lipid-lowering properties.[21-23] Epidemiologic studies examining the association between tea consumption and cancer risk have been inconclusive.[13] A number of human observational studies found that tea catechins were associated with a reduced risk of stroke[24]; however, a large observational study in elderly men found no association between tea and stroke, but did find a reduced risk of ischemic heart disease.[25]

bioactive dose

Not known.

safety

Presumed safe when consumed in normal dietary quantities by non-allergic individuals. See also tannin.

Terpenoids

definition

Group of phytochemicals whose main subclasses are monoterpenes (including limonene, carvone, and carveol); diterpenes (including the retinoids); and tetraterpenes (including α- and β-carotene, lutein, lycopene, xeaxanthin, and cryptoxanthin). Terpenoids occur in nearly every natural food,[26] and, along with other phytochemical constituents in foods, impart sensory qualities, for example, the characteristic "'green,' 'woody,' 'earthy,' 'fruity,' 'floral,' 'sweet,' and 'musty'" flavors of plant foods.[27] Foods that contain terpenoids include citrus fruits, coriander, lemon grass, caraway, peppermint, rosemary, sage, and thyme.[28]

scientific findings

Terpenoids exhibited antimicrobial effects in a laboratory study.[26] Cancer-prevention advice to eat at least 2.5 cups of vegetables and fruits each day is based on plant foods' "numerous potentially beneficial bioactive substances, such as terpenes ... that may help prevent cancer."[29]

bioactive dose

Not known.

safety

Presumed safe when consumed in normal dietary quantities by non-allergic individuals.

Thiamin (Vitamin B1)

definition

Water-soluble vitamin required for carbohydrate and ethanol metabolism. It is found in whole, fortified, and enriched grains, legumes, and pork products. The average U.S. diet maintains an adequate thiamin status.[30] However, thiamin status may be reduced if sufficient thiamin is not ingested (for example, due to poor diet or dietary intake < RDA during conditions of heightened requirement, such as pregnancy or hyperthyroidism[31]). Thiamin can also increase (due to alcoholism), or losses can occur (due to malabsorptive disorders). Clinical signs of thiamin deficiency include anorexia, weight loss, mental changes, apathy, decreases in short-term memory, confusion, irritability, muscle weakness, and cardiovascular abnormalities,[30] the latter of which is characterized by symptoms ranging from pedal edema and anasarca to severe cardiac abnormalities.[32] Dry beriberi is characterized by peripheral neuropathy[33] and mental status changes,[34] which may clinically manifest as Wernicke encephalopathy, Wernicke–Korsakoff syndrome, and structural and functional brain injury.[35]

scientific findings

A high dietary intake of thiamin was associated with a reduced risk of lens opacification in a 5-year study (n = 408 women from the Nurses' Health Study aged 52–74 years at baseline) evaluating nutrition and vision.[36] Higher intake of thiamin was associated with reduced prevalence of nuclear cataract in a population-based study (2900 healthy people aged 49–97 years).[37]

bioactive dose

The RDA is 1.2 mg for men aged 19–50 and 1.1 mg for women aged 19–50.

safety

No UL has been established for thiamin. Thiamin is generally considered nontoxic, though rare hypersensitivity reactions have been reported.[31]

Thiols

definition

Sulfur compounds that impart characteristic aromas to foods found in fruits, such as grapefruit, vegetables, beer, and wine.[38–40]

scientific findings

In vitro, thiols exhibited antioxidant properties.[41]

bioactive dose

Not known.

safety

Presumed safe when consumed in normal dietary quantities by non-allergic individuals.

Thyme (Thymus vulgaris)

definition

Culinary herb that contains phenolics, flavonoids, and terpenoids.[42] Used fresh or dried to flavor meats, and tomato-based soups such as seafood chowder.

scientific findings

Phenolic compounds have exerted antioxidant, anti-inflammatory, and antimicrobial effects in laboratory studies.[43-45] Thyme exerted DNA-protective activity in a laboratory study.[46]

bioactive dose

Not known.

safety

Presumed safe when consumed in normal dietary quantities by non-allergic individuals.

Tofu

definition

White gelatin-like curd formed when soybean protein is precipitated. Its firmness is determined by the amount of liquid it contains. Silken tofu contains a high amount of liquid, whereas firm tofu contains less liquid. Tofu is a rich source of soy protein and can be a good source of calcium, depending on whether the soybean is precipitated with a calcium compound, such as calcium chloride; it is not a source of vitamin B12 (unless it has been fortified with vitamin B12 which would be stated on the ingredients label). Tofu is used raw or cooked in Asian-inspired cooking as a meat substitute.

T

scientific findings

Research suggests that a daily intake of soy protein has a mild LDL-lowering effect,[47] especially when soy protein is substituted for animal protein.[48] A population study found Western-culture women who ate tofu once weekly, compared to women who did not, reduce their risk of premenopausal bilateral breast cancer.[31]

bioactive dose

Not known.

safety

Presumed safe when consumed in normal dietary quantities by non-allergic individuals.

Tomato (Lycopersicon esculentum)

definition

Popular culinary vegetable that is botanically classified as a fruit. A good source of vitamin C and a source of many phytochemicals including lycopene, a carotenoid, the parent compound of which is a terpenoid.

scientific findings

Consuming ≥10 servings/week of tomato-based foods as compared to consuming <1.5 servings/week, significantly, but only modestly, improved total cholesterol, total cholesterol:HDL ratio, and hemoglobin A1C in an observational trial of women.[49] Eating a tomato-rich diet is associated in epidemiology with a decreased risk of prostate cancer,[50] but "there is insufficient evidence to either support, or refute, the use of lycopene for the prevention of prostate cancer," according to a recent meta-analysis and review.[51] Some epidemiological studies suggest that the risk of prostate cancer is decreased modestly in men who consume tomato products, including tomatoes, tomato sauce, pizza, or tomato juice, one time or more per week, according to a review, which also found that other epidemiological evidence suggests that tomato consumption is not associated with a reduced risk of prostate cancer.[31] For preventing prostate cancer, four or more servings of tomato products per week (equivalent to a dietary lycopene intake greater than 6 mg daily) have been used.[31]

bioactive dose

Not known.

safety

Presumed safe when consumed in normal dietary quantities by non-allergic individuals.

Tomatillo (Physalis philadelphica)

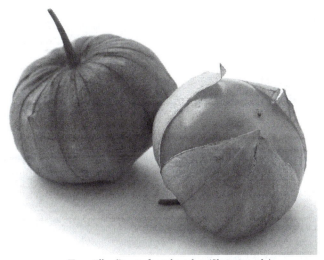

Tomatillo. (Image from bonchan/Shutterstock.)

definition

Small, green tomato-like vegetable used to make salsa verde (green salsa). A small, 34-g tomatillo contains 10 cal, 1 g of fiber, 6% DV for vitamin C, 2% DV for iron, and is a source of phytochemicals including lutein, β-carotene, and ixocarpalactone A.[52,53]

scientific findings

Ixocarpalactone A has been shown to be a cancer chemopreventive agent cytotoxic against human cancer cell lines in laboratory studies.[52,54]

bioactive dose

Not known.

T

safety

Presumed safe when consumed in normal dietary quantities by non-allergic individuals.

Turmeric (Curcuma longa)

definition

Herb member of the ginger family known for its golden color that is used to prepare curry powder and yellow mustard. Traditional use of turmeric to aid in digestion and liver function, relieve arthritis pain, and regulate menstruation involves drying the rhizome (underground stem) and taking turmeric powder in capsules, teas, or liquid extracts.[55] However, few clinical trials have been conducted to evaluate these effects in humans.[31] A biologically effective dose of curcumin in humans has not been reported;[56] however, a dose of 500 mg of turmeric four times daily has been used for dyspepsia,[31] and a dose of 500 mg of turmeric extract four times daily has been used for osteoarthritis.[31]

scientific findings

Curcumin, a vanilloid compound in turmeric, exhibited apoptotic, anti-inflammatory, chemoprotective, antitumor, antioxidant, antiarthritic, antiamyloid, anti-ischemic, anti-inflammatory, and bone-protective effects.[57–61] Some clinical research shows that taking turmeric orally can relieve symptoms of dyspepsia,[31] but turmeric has not been adequately studied for effectiveness in humans for any health condition.[55]

bioactive dose

Not known.

safety

Presumed safe when consumed in normal dietary quantities by nonallergic individuals. High doses or long-term use of turmeric may cause indigestion, nausea, or diarrhea.[55] People with gallbladder disease should avoid using turmeric as a dietary supplement, as it may worsen the condition.[55]

Turnip (Brassica rapa)

definition

White or white-and-purple Brassica root vegetable about the size of a small onion that has been used as a vegetable for human consumption in Europe since prehistoric times.[62] One cup of raw turnip is low in calories, supplying 36 cal, 8 g of carbohydrates, 2 g of fiber, and 250 mg of potassium, and 38 mg of vitamin C, making it an excellent source of vitamin C.[66] Its greens, commonly boiled or cooked with ingredients such as meats, onions, and garlic, are a source of vitamins C and K, magnesium, potassium, phenolics and glucosinolates[64]; canned turnip greens contain more iron than fresh turnip greens.[65]

scientific findings

See *Brassica vegetables*.

bioactive dose

Not known.

safety

Presumed safe when consumed in normal dietary quantities by non-allergic individuals.

References

1. Tamarind. Purdue University. http://www.hort.purdue.edu/newcrop/morton/tamarind.html. Accessed August 3, 2013.
2. US Department of Agriculture. Natural Resources Conservation Service. *Tamarindus indica* L. Plants Profile. http://plants.usda.gov/java/county?state_name=Florida&statefips=12&symbol=TAIN2. Accessed August 3, 2013.
3. US Department of Agriculture. Agricultural Research Service. Nutrient Data Laboratory. Tamarind, raw. http://ndb.nal.usda.gov/ndb/foods/show/2407?fg=&man=&lfacet=&count=&max=25&qlookup=tamarind&offset=&sort=&format=Abridged&_action_show=Apply+Changes&Qv=1&Q4505=0.5&Q4506=1.0. Accessed August 3, 2013.
4. Pugalenthi M, Vadivel V, Gurumoorthi P, Janardhanan K. Comparative nutritional evaluation of little known legumes, *Tamarindus indica, Erythrina indica*, and *Sesbania bispinosa. Trop Subtrop Agroecosyst*. 2004;4(3):107–123.
5. Havinga RM, Hart A, Putscher J, Prehsler S, Buchmann C, Vogl CR. *Tamarindus indica* L. (Fabaceae): Patterns of use in traditional African medicine. *J Ethnopharmacol*. 2010;127(3):573–588. doi: 10.1016/j.jep.2009.11.028. Epub 2009 December 4.
6. Bhadoriya SS, Ganeshpurkar A, Narwaria J, Rai G, Jain AP. *Tamarindus indica*: Extent of explored potential. *Pharmacogn Rev*. 2011;5(9):73–81. doi: 10.4103/0973-7847.79102.
7. Siddhuraju P. Antioxidant activity of polyphenolic compounds extracted from defatted raw and dry heated *Tamarindus indica* seed coat. *Food Sci Technol-LEB*. 2007;40(6):982–990.

T

8. Mairi R, Jana D, Das UK, Ghosh D. Antidiabetic effect of aqueous extract of seed of *Tamarindus indica* in streptozotocin-induced diabetic rats. *J Ethnopharmacol.* 2004;92(1):85–91.

9. US Department of Agriculture. Agricultural Research Service. Nutrient Data Laboratory. USDA Database for the Flavonoid Content of Selected Foods— 2003. http://www.ars.usda.gov/Services/docs.htm?docid=6231. Accessed August 2, 2013.

10. Whitney ER, Rolfes SR. *Understanding Nutrition*, 12th edn. Belmont, CA: Wadsworth Cengage; 2011.

11. Takekawa K, Matsumoto K. Water-insoluble condensed tannins content of young persimmon fruits-derived crude fibre relates to its bile acid-binding ability. *Nat Prod Res.* 2012;26(23):2255–2258. Epub 2012 January 18.

12. Harkness R, Bratman S. *Mosby's Handbook of Drug-Herb and Drug-Supplement Interactions*. St. Louis, MO: Mosby; 2003.

13. National Institutes of Health. National Cancer Institute. Tea and Cancer Prevention: Strengths and Limits of the Evidence http://www.cancer.gov/cancertopics/factsheet/prevention/tea. Accessed January 2, 2011.

14. Kamalinejad M, Nadjafria L, Sayyah M. Anticonvulsant activity and chemical composition of *Artemisia dracunculus* L. essential oil. *J Ethnopharmacol.* 2004;94(2–3):283–287.

15. Plumb GW, Chambers SJ, Lambert N, Bartolome B, Heaney RK, Wantigatunga SU, Aruoma OL, Halliwell B, Williamson G. Antioxidant actions of fruit, herb and spice extracts. *J Food Lipids.* 1996;3(3):171–188.

16. Mudhavi DL, Deshpande DS, Salunkhe DK. *Food Antioxidants Technological, Toxicological and Health Aspects*. New York, NY: Marcel Dekker; 1996.

17. Alasalvar C, Shahidi F. Composition, phytochemicals, and beneficial health effects of dried fruits: An overview. In: *Phytochemicals and Health Effects*. Ames, Iowa: John Wiley & Sons, Inc.; 2013:12.

18. Over KF, Hettiarachchy NS, Perumalla AV, Johnson MG, Meullenet JF, Dickson JS, Holtzbauer MJ, Niebuhr SE, Davis B. Antilisterial activity and consumer acceptance of irradiated chicken breast meat vacuum-infused with grape seed and green tea extracts and tartaric acid. *J Food Sci.* 2010;75(7):M455–M461.

19. Webb D. Hot & cold—Despite tea's popularity worldwide, research on its health benefits remains inconsistent. *Today's Diet.* 2011;13(1):32.

20. Knaze V, Zamora-Ros R, Luján-Barroso L, Romieu I, Scalbert A, Slimani N, Riboli E et al. Intake estimation of total and individual flavan-3-ols, proanthocyanidins and theaflavins, their food sources and determinants in the European Prospective Investigation into Cancer and Nutrition (EPIC) study. *Br J Nutr.* 2012;108(6):1095–1108. Epub 2011:1–14.

21. Babu PV, Liu D. Green tea catechins and cardiovascular health: An update. *Curr Med Chem.* 2008;15(18):1840–1850.

22. Suzuki J, Isobe M, Morishita R, Nagai R. Tea polyphenols regulate key mediators on inflammatory cardiovascular diseases. *Mediators Inflammation.* 2009;2009:1–5.

23. Chow HH, Hakim IA, Vining DR, Crowell JA, Ranger-Moore J, Chew WM, Celaya CA, Rodney SR, Hara Y, Alberts DS. Effects of dosing condition on the oral bioavailability of green tea catechins after single-dose administration of polyphenon E in healthy individuals. *Clin Cancer Res.* 2005;11(12):4627–4633.

24. Arab L, Liebeskind DS. Tea, flavonoids and stroke in man and mouse. *Arch Biochem Biophys*. 2010;501(1):31–36.

25. Arts IC, Hollman PC, Feskens EJ, Bueno de Mesquita HB, Kromhout D. Catechin intake might explain the inverse relation between tea consumption and ischemic heart disease: The Zutphen Elderly Study. *Am J Clin Nutr*. 2001;74(2):227–232.

26. Wagner K-H, Elmadfa I. Biological relevance of terpenoids. *Ann Nutr Metab*. 2003;47(3–4):95–106.

27. Mayuoni-Kirshinbaum L, Porat R. The flavor of pomegranate fruit: A review. *J Sci Food Agric*. 2014;94(1):21–27. Epub 2013 July 23. doi: 10.1002/jsfa.6311. [Epub ahead of print]

28. Breitmaier E. Terpenes: Importance, general structure, and biosynthesis. In: Bretimaier E, ed. *Terpenes*. Weinheim, Germany: Wiley VCH Verlag; 2006, 1–9.

29. Kushi LH, Doyle C, McCullough M, Rock CL, Demark-Wahnefried W, Bandera EV, Gapstur S, Patel AV, Andrews K, Gansler T. The American Cancer Society 2010. Nutrition and Physical Activity Guidelines Advisory Committee. American Cancer Society guidelines on nutrition and physical activity for cancer prevention: Reducing the risk of cancer with healthy food choices and physical activity. *CA Cancer J Clin*. 2012;62(1):30–67.

30. Institute of Medicine. *Dietary Reference Intakes for Thiamin, Riboflavin, Niacin, Vitamin B6, Folate, Vitamin B12, Pantothenic Acid, Biotin, and Choline*. Washington, DC: National Academy Press; 1998.

31. Jellin JM, Gregory PJ. *Natural Medicines Comprehensive Database*. Therapeutic Research Faculty. 2013. www.naturaldatabase.com. Accessed 07/11/2012.

32. Rao SN, Chandak GR. Cardiac beriberi: Often a missed diagnosis. *J Trop Pediatr*. 2010;56(4):284–285. doi: 10.1093/tropej/fmp108. Epub 2009 November 24.

33. Imai N, Kubota M, Saitou M, Yagi N, Serizawa M, Kobari M. Increase of serum vascular endothelial growth factors in wet beriberi: Two case reports. *Intern Med*. 2012;51(8):929–932. Epub 2012 April 15.

34. Becker DA, Ingala EE, Martinez-Lage M, Price RS, Galetta SL. Dry Beriberi and Wernicke's encephalopathy following gastric lap band surgery. *J Clin Neurosci*. 2012;19(7):1050–1052. doi: 10.1016/j.jocn.2011.11.006. Epub 2012 April 22.

35. Osiezagha K, Ali S, Freeman C, Barker NC, Jabeen S, Maitra S, Olagbemiro Y, Richie W, Bailey RK. Thiamine deficiency and delirium. *Innovations Clin Neurosci*. 2013;10(4):26–32.

36. Jacques PF, Taylor A, Moeller S, Hankinson SE, Rogers G, Tung W, Ludovico J, Willett WC, Chylack LT Jr. Long-term nutrient intake and 5-year change in nuclear lens opacities. *Arch Ophthalmol*. 2005;123(4):517–526.

37. Cumming RG, Mitchell P, Smith W. Diet and cataract: The Blue Mountains Eye Study. *Ophthalmology*. 2000;107(3):450–456.

38. Demirkol O, Adams C, Ercal N. Biologically important thiols in various vegetables and fruits. *J Agric Food Chem*. 2004;52:8151–8154.

39. Swiegers JH, Kievit RL, Siebert T, Lattey KA, Bramley BR, Francis IL, King ES, Pretorius IS. The influence of yeast on the aroma of Sauvignon Blanc wine. *Food Microbiol*. 2009;26(2):204–211. Epub 2008 November 5.

T

40. Takoi K, Degueil M, Shinkaruk S, Thibon C, Maeda K, Ito K, Bennetau B, Dubourdieu D, Tominaga T. Identification and characteristics of new volatile thiols derived from the hop (*Humulus lupulus* L.) cultivar Nelson Sauvin (dagger). *J Agric Food Chem*. 2009;25:57(6):2493–502.
41. Packer L, Cadenas E. *Biothiols in Health and Disease*. New York, NY: Marcel Dekker, Inc.; 1995.
42. USDA Agricultural Research Service. Medicinal Plants and Herbs. Thyme. http://www.pl.barc.usda.gov/usda_plant/plant_home.cfm. Accessed June 19, 2011.
43. Martínez-Valverde I, Periago MJ, Ros G. Nutritional importance of phenolic compounds in the diet. *Arch Latinoam Nutr*. 2000;50(1):5–18.
44. Abidi W, Jiménez S, Moreno MÁ, Gogorcena Y. Evaluation of antioxidant compounds and total sugar content in a nectarine [*Prunus persica* (L.) Batsch] progeny. *Int J Mol Sci*. 2011;12(10):6919–6935. Epub 2011 October 19.
45. Crozier A, Jaganath IB, Clifford MN. Dietary phenolics: Chemistry, bioavailability and effects on health. *Nat Prod Rep*. 2009;26(8):1001–1043. Epub 2009 May 13.
46. Kozics K, Klusová V, Srančíková A, Mučaji P, Slameňová D, Hunáková L, Kusznierewicz B, Horváthová E. Effects of Salvia officinalis and *Thymus vulgaris* on oxidant-induced DNA damage and antioxidant status in HepG2 cells. *Food Chem*. 2013;141(3):2198–2206. doi: 10.1016/j.foodchem.2013.04.089. Epub 2013 May 9.
47. National Institutes of Health National Center for Complementary and Alternative Medicine. Herbs at a glance. Soy. http://nccam.nih.gov/health/soy/ataglance.htm. Accessed January 25, 2012.
48. Academy of Nutrition and Dietetics Evidence Analysis Library. *Critical Illness Nutrition Practice Guideline*. http://www.adaevidencelibrary.com/topic.cfm?cat = 2799&library = EBG. Accessed March 10, 2011.
49. Sesso HD, Wang L, Ridker PM, Buring JE. Tomato-based food products are related to clinically modest improvements in selected coronary biomarkers in women. *J Nutr*. 2012;142(2):326–333. Epub 2012 January 5.
50. Giovannucci E, Liu Y, Platz EA, Stampfer MJ, Willett WC. Risk factors for prostate cancer incidence and progression in the health professionals follow-up study. *Int J Cancer*. 2007;121(7):1571–1578.
51. Ilic D, Forbes KM, Hassed C. Lycopene for the prevention of prostate cancer. *Cochrane Database Syst Rev*. 2011;11:CD008007.
52. Elizalde-González MP, Hernández-Ogarcía SG. Effect of cooking processes on the contents of two bioactive carotenoids in *Solanum lycopersicum* tomatoes and *Physalis ixocarpa* and *Physalis philadelphica* tomatillos. *Molecules*. 2007;12(8):1829–1835.
53. US Department of Agriculture. SNAP-Ed Connection. Tomatillos. http://snap.nal.usda.gov/nutrition-through-seasons/seasonal-produce/tomatillos. Accessed March 24, 2015.
54. Maldonado E, Pérez-Castorena AL, Garcés C, Martínez M. Philadelphicalactones C and D and other cytotoxic compounds from *Physalis philadelphica*. *Steroids*. 2011;76(7):724–728.
55. National Institutes of Health. National Center for Complementary and Integrative Health. Turmeric. https://nccih.nih.gov/health/turmeric/ataglance.htm. Accessed April 8, 2015.

56. Cheng AL, Hsu CH, Lin JK, Hsu MM, Ho YF, Shen TS, Ko JY et al. Phase I clinical trial of curcumin, a chemopreventive agent, in patients with high-risk or pre-malignant lesions. *Anticancer Res.* 2001;21(4B):2895–2900.

57. Shukla PK, Khanna VK, Ali MM, Khan MY, Srimal RC. Anti-ischemic effect of curcumin in rat brain. *Neurochem Res.* 2008;33(6):1036–1043.

58. Stix G. Spice Healer. Scientific American (February 2007). http://www.scientificamerican.com/article.cfm?id=spice-healer. Accessed August 3, 2013.

59. Aggarwal BB, Shishodia S. Molecular targets of dietary agents for prevention and therapy of cancer. *Biochem Pharmacol.* 2006;71(10):1397–1421.

60. Choi H, Chun YS, Kim SW, Kim MS, Park JW. Curcumin inhibits hypoxia-inducible factor-1 by degrading aryl hydrocarbon receptor nuclear translocator: A mechanism of tumor growth inhibition. *Mol Pharmacol (Am Soc Pharmacol Exp Ther).* 2006;70(5):1664–1671.

61. Wright LE, Frye JB, Timmermann BN. Protection of trabecular bone in ovariectomized rats by turmeric *Curcuma longa* L. is dependent on extract composition. *J Agric Food Chem.* 2010;58(17):9498–9504.

62. Undersander DJ, Kaminski AR, Oakley EA, Smith LH, Doll JD, Schulte EE, Plunger ES. *Turnip. Alternative Field Crops Manual.* University of Wisconsin-Extension, Cooperative Extension, University of Minnesota. http://www.hort.purdue.edu/newcrop/afcm/turnip.html. Accessed March 24, 2015.

63. US Department of Agriculture. Agricultural Research Service. Nutrient Data Lab. Turnip raw. http://ndb.nal.usda.gov/ndb/foods/show/3274?fgcd=&manu=&lfacet=&format=&count=&max=35&offset=&sort=&qlookup=turnip. Accessed March 25, 2015.

64. Francisco M, Crate ME, Songs P, Velasco P. Effect of genotype and environmental conditions on health-promoting compounds in Brassica rape. *J Agric Food Chem.* 2011;59(6):2421–2431.

65. US Department of Agriculture. Agricultural Research Service. Nutrient Data Laboratory. Turnip greens cooked, boiled, drained; turnip greens, canned. http://ndb.nal.usda.gov/ndb/foods/list. Accessed January 26, 2012.

T

U

Ugli fruit (Citrus paradisi × reticulata)

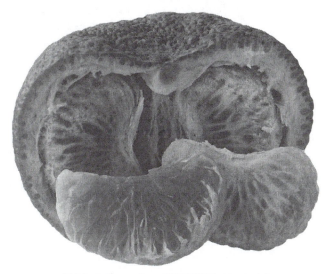

Ugli fruit. (Image from 75857518/Shutterstock.)

definition

Also known as unique fruit and ugli tangelo. Hybrid of a mandarin and a grapefruit[1] that is native to Jamaica.[2] Larger than an orange with yellow–green, easily peeled skin, ugli fruit eaten fresh is an excellent source of vitamin C (70% DV) and a good source of fiber (% DV).[2]

scientific findings

See *citrus fruits.*

bioactive dose

Not known.

safety

Presumed safe when consumed in normal dietary quantities by non-allergic individuals.

References

1. Purdue University. Tangelo *Citrus paradisi x Citrus reticulata*. http://www.hort.purdue.edu/newcrop/morton/tangelo.html. Accessed April 14, 2015.
2. Produce for Better Health Foundation. Ugli fruit. http://www.fruitsandveggiesmorematters.org/ugli-fruit-nutrition-selection-storage. Accessed April 2, 2015.

U

V

Vanilloid

definition

Phytochemical family that includes capsaicin in *Capsicum frutescens* (chili pepper),[1] curcumin in the spice turmeric,[2] and gingerol in ginger.[3]

scientific findings

In laboratory studies, vanilloids exhibited hepatoprotective,[4] anti-inflammatory,[5] and antioxidative properties.[3]

bioactive dose

Not known.

safety

Presumed safe when used in normal dietary quantities in foods by non-allergic individuals.

Vegetable Foods Group

definition

Underconsumed food group[6] that is a source of folate, β-carotene, vitamin C, vitamin K, vitamin E, magnesium, potassium, and fiber[7] which has been divided into five subgroups by color: dark green (e.g., broccoli), starchy (e.g., potatoes), beans and peas (e.g. lentils), red and orange (e.g. tomatoes and carrots), and other (e.g. artichokes, mushrooms, wax beans, zucchini etc.). Dark green vegetables are particularly rich in folate, vitamin K, and magnesium and chlorophyll, and likewise, other subgroups contribute unique nutrients and phytochemicals. Naturally low in fat, calories, and cholesterol, the low-energy density of vegetables makes them good food choices to include for weight reduction; due to their fiber content, vegetables can help to promote a feeling of fullness as well.[8] It is

V

estimated that there could be more than 100 different phytochemicals in just a single serving of vegetables.[9]

scientific findings

Reduced vegetable consumption is a factor, along with reduced fruit consumption, that is linked to poor health and increased risk of noncommunicable diseases.[10] A diet rich in vegetables, as part of an overall healthy diet, may reduce the risk of heart disease, including heart attack and stroke; certain types of cancer; obesity; type 2 diabetes; blood pressure; kidney stones; and bone loss.[11] Biologic mechanisms, whereby vegetables exert healthful effects, are likely to be multiple and are likely to include both nutrients and phytochemicals.[12] People whose diets are rich in vegetables (and fruits) have a lower risk of developing cancers of the mouth, pharynx, larynx, esophagus, stomach, and lung; and some evidence suggests this dietary pattern also lowers the risk of cancers of the colon, pancreas, and prostate, in addition to lowering the risk of developing diabetes, heart disease, hypertension, and overweight.[13] Consuming a diet containing high amounts of vegetables (and fruits) is associated with fewer age-related diseases such as Alzheimer disease.[14]

bioactive dose

The daily vegetable recommendation for general health for 19-to-50-year-old women is 2.5 cups and for 19-to-50-year-old men is 3 cups.[8] Cancer preventative recommendations for men and women are similar: to consume approximately 1.25–4 cups/day emphasizing dark green and orange vegetables and legumes.[13]

safety

Presumed safe when consumed in normal dietary quantities by non-allergic individuals.

Vitamin A

definition

Fat-soluble vitamin whose roles include (1) vision because it converts light energy into nerve impulses that enable vision and because it maintains the cornea; (2) bone growth; (3) maintaining the integrity of epithelial cells, which occur in the eye, respiratory tract, genitourinary tract, and intestinal tract; (4) reproduction; (5) gene expression; (6) immunity;

(7) embryonic development; and (8) cell differentiation, in addition to other functions.[15,16] Preformed, active vitamin A (e.g., retinol) is found in animal foods, such as fortified milk, fish oils, and liver. Provitamin A carotenoids, such as β-carotene, α-carotene, and β-cryptoxanthin,[15] are found in dark green, orange, and yellow fruits and vegetables, such as spinach, apricots, squash, and pumpkin. The median intake of vitamin A in the United States is higher than the RDA for vitamin A.[15] Vitamin A deficiency is characterized by eye and visual changes, such as drying and hardening of the cornea and night blindness, progressing to blindness, skin keratinization, susceptibility of the salivary glands and other mucous membranes to infection, general body-wide susceptibility to infection, and impaired digestion and absorption.[17] "Vitamin A deficiency can occur due to abnormal storage and transport of vitamin A in people with abetalipoproteinemia, protein deficiency, diabetes mellitus, hyperthyroidism, fever, liver disease, and cystic fibrosis."[18] To assess vitamin A status, plasma retinol and carotenoid levels are typically measured; however, these values have limited utility in assessing marginal vitamin A status, because they do not decline until vitamin A levels in the liver are almost depleted.[15,19]

scientific findings

Epidemiological evidence suggests that high intake of vitamin A from foods is associated with a reduced risk of breast cancer among premenopausal women with a positive family history of breast cancer; it is not known whether supplemental vitamin A has a similar benefit.[18] High dietary intake of vitamin A was associated with a reduced risk of cataracts.[18]

bioactive dose

The RDA for adult men aged 19–50 is 900 µg/day Retinol Activity Equivalents (RAE)[19] (approximately 3000 IU)* and for adult women aged 19–50 is 700 µg/day RAE[19] (approximately 2333 IU).†

safety

The vitamin A UL is 3000 µg[16] (approximately 10,000 IU).‡ Either short-term, massive intakes or chronic intakes of high amounts of vitamin A can

---

* Conversion from mcg to IU by Diane Kraft: 900 µg/0.3 = 3000 IU.
† Conversion from mcg to IU by Diane Kraft: 700 µg/0.3 = 2333 IU.
‡ Conversion from mcg to IU by Diane Kraft: 3000 µg/0.3 = 10,000 IU.

V

cause tissue levels of vitamin A to rise and hypervitaminosis A to occur, as characterized by increased intracranial pressure, headache, dizziness, nausea, skin irritation, pain in joints and bones, coma, liver damage, and even death. Tissue levels take a long time to fall after high doses, and the resulting liver damage may or may not be reversible after discontinuing the vitamin A.[15,19] Exceeding the UL during pregnancy is teratogenic and has been associated with development of fetal orofacial malformations, such as cleft palate.[20]

Vitamin B6 (B6)

definition

Water-soluble vitamin also called pyridoxine that is required for protein, fat, and carbohydrate metabolism.[21] Sources include fortified, ready-to-eat cereals; meats, fish, and poultry; white potatoes and starchy vegetables; and noncitrus fruits, including bananas and watermelon.[21] Vitamin B6 (B6) can also be synthesized in the lower gut. Median B6 intake of adults is higher than the B6 RDA.[21] Deficiency of B6 is characterized by depression, confusion, seborrheic dermatitis, microcytic anemia, convulsions,[21] poor growth, and decreased immune function.[21] B6 status is measured by using plasma 5′-pyridoxal phosphate; a value of 20 nmol/L or higher is adequate.[21]

scientific findings

Low B6 status was associated with increased pro-inflammatory markers.[22] Epidemiological research suggests that male smokers with higher serum levels of pyridoxine have a lower risk of lung cancer.[18] Deficiency of vitamin B6 increases blood homocysteine,[18] a marker for cardiovascular disease that also has been suggested as a cause or mechanism in the development of Alzheimer's disease and other forms of dementia.[23]

bioactive dose

The RDA is 1.3 mg/day for adults aged 19–50.

safety

The tolerable UL for adults is 100 mg of B6 per day, an amount that is likelier to be reached from taking dietary supplements of B6 rather than from foods.

Vitamin B12 (B12)

definition

Also called cobalamin and cyanocobalamin. Water-soluble vitamin found naturally in animal foods, such as meat, poultry, fish and shellfish, eggs, and dairy products, but generally not in plant foods except for scant amounts in mushrooms and nori (seaweed),[24] hence, the rule of thumb: "Nothing that grows out of the ground contains vitamin B12."[25] Soy milk, cereal, and vegetarian meat substitutes may be fortified with crystalline B12, which is also used in dietary supplements. Crystalline B12 is absorbed better than naturally occurring B12 in food.[26] B12 is necessary for folate metabolism, DNA synthesis, red blood cell formation, to convert homocysteine to methionine, and to synthesize the myelin sheath of nerves.[27] Absorption of B12 is unique. In the stomach, gastric acid and pepsin separate B12 from the protein to which it is bound in food.[25] Free B12 attaches to intrinsic factor, a gastric secretion, forming an intrinsic factor (IF)-B12 complex that is absorbed in the small intestine.[25] A small amount of B12 not bound to IF can be absorbed by passive diffusion.[25] B12 is stored in the liver.[25]

scientific findings

The elderly are considered to be at high-risk for B12 deficiency because they have a higher incidence of gastric mucosa atrophy, altered production of intrinsic factor, and altered gastric acid secretion.[26] Approximately, 10%–30% of people over the age of 50 do not absorb food-bound B12 efficiently, and therefore, should meet their RDA mainly by consuming foods fortified with B12 or a B12 supplement,[28] rather than attempting to get B12 strictly from dietary sources.[24] Low serum vitamin B12 concentrations are found in more than 10% of older adults.[29] Average age of onset of B12 deficiency in the elderly has been estimated to be between 60 and 70 years.[30] Other groups at risk for B12 deficiency include those who eat a vegan diet,[26] cannot produce intrinsic factor, and/or have pernicious anemia, and/or malabsorption, such as from celiac disease or gastrectomy; use proton pump inhibitor drugs or metformin on a prolonged basis[24]; have thyrotoxicosis, hemolytic anemia, hemorrhage, malignancy, hepatic disease, renal disease, myeloproliferative disorders, or who are pregnant.[18,30,32] Individuals at high risk of B12 deficiency should consume B12-fortified food and/or take dietary supplements of B12 to help them meet the RDA.[24] Diagnosis of B12 deficiency requires a complete blood count and measurement of serum B12,[24] but measurement of serum homocysteine and methylmalonic acid should be used to confirm deficiency in asymptomatic high-risk patients with low-normal levels of B12.[24] Serum holotranscobalamin has been proposed as a better marker for assessing initial vitamin B12 status, to replace serum vitamin B12, and to accompany

V

serum methylmalonic acid and serum homocysteine levels.[30] Serum vitamin B12 is neither sensitive nor specific for vitamin B12 deficiency, which might explain why many deficient subjects would be overlooked by utilizing it as a status marker, whereas, serum holotranscobalamin is an earlier marker that becomes decreased before serum vitamin B12.[33] B12 deficiency is characterized by megaloblastic anemia, low or low-normal serum B12, elevated homocysteine, elevated methylmalonic acid, and low serum holotranscobalamin; in addition, neuropathy, and a variety of neuropsychiatric symptoms, such as paresthesia, loss of sensation and strength in the limbs, ataxia, slowed or increased reflexes, and vibration and position sensitivity, irritability, memory loss, and dementia,[18,24,30,34,35] may be present though patients with the disorder may not exhibit all of the symptoms because B12 deficiency symptoms span a continuum.[31]

bioactive dose

The RDA is 2.4 µg/day for adults aged 19–50. Further research is required to determine appropriate levels of B12 for deficient older adults; however, it is recommended that individuals aged 50 and older consume vitamin B12 in its crystalline form, available in fortified foods and supplements, to assure absorption.[36,37]

safety

No UL has been established for vitamin B12. "No adverse effects have been associated with excess B12 intake from food or supplements in healthy individuals."[30]

Vitamin C

definition

Also called ascorbic acid and ascorbate. Water-soluble antioxidant vitamin that reduces cellular oxidative stress, scavenges free radicals, and inhibits peroxidation of membrane phospholipids. It is necessary for immunity and the synthesis of amino acids, collagen, carnitine, cholesterol, hormones, and neurotransmitters.[38–40] Vitamin C increases the intestinal absorption of nonheme iron[41] either by reducing iron from the ferrous ionic state to the ferric state (in its capacity as an electron donor) or by forming a soluble complex with the iron in the alkaline pH of the small intestine.[42] Vitamin C deficiency, which causes scurvy, might affect up to 30% of the population, including those of low socioeconomic status or who suffer from alcoholism, severe psychiatric illness leading to poor nutrition, and other critical illness.[43] Perhaps the most recognizable symptoms of scurvy are those involving decreased collagen synthesis, such as impaired wound healing, petechiae, bleeding gums, and loose teeth, but rheumatologic and other symptoms can occur, and include synovitis with effusion, anemia, markedly elevated erythrocyte sedimentation rate and C-reactive protein levels, pulmonary hypertension, purpuric rash, and hemarthrosis.[44]

scientific findings

Vitamin C has been shown to affect immune function.[45] Vitamin C depletion has been correlated with histaminemia, but its role in allergy is not well understood.[46] Vitamin C deficiency has been associated with the development of age-related macular degeneration according to a review citing "clinical and laboratory studies",[47] but increasing dietary vitamin C does not appear to significantly reduce the risk of developing age-related macular degeneration.[43] Plasma ascorbic acid concentration was inversely related to mortality from all causes, including cardiovascular disease and ischemic heart disease in men and women, and to cancer mortality in men but not women, in a prospective observational study (n = 19,496 men and women aged 45–79 years), that concluded eating the equivalent of a 50-g serving (one typical serving) of fruit or vegetables daily increased plasma ascorbate levels to cancer-protective levels.[45] Some research suggests that dietary vitamin C reduces breast cancer risk, while other research suggests no association between vitamin C intake and breast cancer risk.[43] Overall, dietary vitamin C appears to slow progression of atherosclerosis, and decrease the risk of atherosclerosis and peripheral arterial disease.[43] Dietary restriction of vitamin C is associated with increases in both diastolic and systolic blood pressure.[43] Consuming vitamin C from dietary sources seems to reduce blood concentrations of lead.[43]

bioactive dose

The RDA is 75 and 90 mg/daily for nonsmoking women and men, respectively, aged 19–50.

safety

The UL is 2000 mg for adults aged 19–50.

Vitamin D

definition

Fat-soluble vitamin found naturally in beef, egg yolk, fatty fish, and mushrooms, and added to vitamin-D-fortified milk (and milk alternates, such as vitamin-D-fortified soy milk), margarine, and vitamin-D-fortified ready-to-eat breakfast cereals. One 8-oz glass of milk supplies approximately 100 IU of vitamin D, which meets 1/6 of the adult RDA (of 600 IU). Dairy products other than milk are generally not fortified with vitamin D. Vitamin D_2 (ergocalciferol) and vitamin D_3 (cholecalciferol) are the two major, naturally occurring forms.[48] Both are found in dietary supplements, but some evidence indicates that ergocalciferol (D_2) is less potent than cholecalciferol (D_3).[48] D_2 is found in mushrooms.[18] D_3 is found in animal foods; it is used to fortify milk and cereal; in addition, provitamin D_3 in skin is converted into vitamin D_3 by exposure to ultra violet B (UVB) radiation.[49] Vitamin D is classified as a nonessential nutrient because it can be synthesized by exposure of skin to sun. Both D_2 and D_3 require hydroxylation by the kidney and liver to be converted into active vitamin D, 1,25-dihydroxyvitamin D ($1,25(OH)_2D$), also called calcitriol.[48,50] Blood level of 25-hydroxyvitamin D ($25(OH)D$) is used to measure body status of vitamin D, and it reflects dietary and cutaneously synthesized vitamin D.[51] A blood value of 25–80 ng/mL has been described as the target range for $25(OH)D$.[48] Vitamin D promotes intestinal calcium and phosphorus absorption, regulating bone metabolism, and controlling parathyroid hormone secretion.[48] Every tissue and cell has a vitamin D receptor,[53] and vitamin D performs diverse roles body-wide including that it regulates arterial blood pressure; modulates immunological responses, regulates insulin production,[49] modulates male and female reproductive processes,[52] and it is necessary for neuromuscular function.[53] It has been estimated that 25%–50% or more of patients encountered in clinical practice are vitamin D deficient.[48] The Centers for Disease Control and Prevention have reported that 30% of whites and 5% of blacks have sufficient vitamin D levels, using 25-hydroxyvitamin D of ≥ 30 ng/mL as a marker of vitamin D adequacy.[45] Symptoms of hypovitaminosis D include bone pain, myalgias, and generalized weakness, and laboratory values will include $25(OH)D$ <25 ng/mL, normal calcium and phosphorus blood levels, elevated or high-normal levels of PTH, normal to elevated levels of alkaline phosphatase, and a low 24-h urine calcium excretion rate.[45] Common risk factors for vitamin D deficiency include decreased intake, GI malabsorption, hepatic or renal disease, use of certain medications that suppress vitamin D absorption, obesity, and decreased skin synthesis of vitamin D caused by older age, low sun exposure (indoor occupation, time of day, season, latitude), use of sunscreens, and ethnicity (other than Caucasian).[45,47]

scientific findings

Vitamin D deficiency has been linked to an increased risk of autoimmune diseases.[47,48] Bone manifestations of vitamin D deficiency include osteomalacia in adults and rickets in children,[45] increasing risk of fracture.[53] Vitamin D deficiency in athletes has been linked to decreased physical performance and a predisposition to stress fractures.[54] A study that searched the literature for evidence of a cancer–vitamin D relationship yielded 63 observational studies of vitamin D status in relation to cancer risk, including 30 of colon, 13 of breast, 26 of prostate, and 7 of ovarian cancer, and several that assessed the association of vitamin D receptor genotype with cancer risk. The majority of studies found a protective relationship between sufficient vitamin D status and lower risk of cancer.[55] The greatest risk for cancer appears to be associated with 25(OH)D levels below 20 ng/mL.[56] Vitamin D intake may play a key role in the prevention of cardiovascular disease.[57] Vitamin D deficiency is often present in patients with chronic obstructive pulmonary disease and evidence suggests that vitamin D plays a role in the lung pathology of patients with chronic obstructive pulmonary disease.[58] The relation between Vitamin D deficiency with depressive and fatigue symptoms in healthy populations and patients with multiple sclerosis have been reported.[59] Poor vitamin D status was significantly associated with increased depression symptoms in a study (n = 178) of pregnant African-American women.[60]

Chronic vitamin D deficiency is associated with an increased risk of type 1 and type 2 diabetes.[53] Vitamin D deficiency has been associated with decreased spermatogenesis and decreased male fertility,[61] while vitamin D is positively associated with semen quality and androgen status.[52]

Vitamin D might influence steroidogenesis of the sex hormones estradiol and progesterone in healthy women and high 25(OH)D levels might be associated with endometriosis.[52] Population research suggests that lower 25(OH)D levels are associated with a higher risk of developing hypertension compared to people with higher vitamin D levels.[51] Hypovitaminosis D is considered to be an important environmental factor associated in the etiology of multiple sclerosis according to physiological, experimental, epidemiological, immunological, and biological studies.[59] Vitamin D plays a role in skeletal muscle health and function; and vitamin D deficiency is characterized by myopathy; muscle weakness and atrophy.[56] Vitamin D deficiency in athletes has been linked to decreased physical performance.[54] Adequate vitamin D intake in pregnancy is optimal for maternal, fetal, and child health. Adverse health outcomes of low vitamin D status during pregnancy include preeclampsia; gestational diabetes mellitus, and caesarean section, while consequences to newborns include increased risk of low birth weight, neonatal rickets, neonatal hypocalcaemia, asthma, and/or type 1 diabetes.[62] Population research suggests that low vitamin D levels are associated with increased risk of upper respiratory infection in children.[53]

V

bioactive dose

The RDA for adults aged 19–50, who are vitamin-D-adequate, is 600 IU.[63] Eight ounces of vitamin-D fortified milk (note not all dairy products are fortified with vitamin D) supplies approximately 100 IU. The vitamin D RDA was based upon the amount of vitamin D needed to maintain adequate bone mineral density not on the extra-skeletal roles of vitamin D.[51] Hypovitaminosis D (25(OH)D <10 ng/mL) has been treated with 50,000 IU of vitamin D orally once weekly for 2–3 months or three times weekly for 1 month, though the practice has not been validated in clinical trials.[48]

safety

A UL of 4000 IU/day has been established for adults aged 19–50. Vitamin D toxicity is "extremely rare and generally only occurs after ingestion of large doses of vitamin D (>10,000 IU) for prolonged periods in patients with normal gut function or in patients who may be concurrently ingesting generous if not excessive amounts of calcium."[48] Most patients with vitamin D toxicity have levels of 25(OH)D > 150 ng/mL, hypercalcemia, and usually, but not always, hypercalciuria and hyperphosphatemia.[48]

Vitamin E

definition

Fat-soluble antioxidant vitamin of which there are more than eight naturally occurring forms; γ-tocopherol is the predominate form in foods[64] though α-tocopherol and other tocopherols are also found in foods.[65] In addition to vegetable oils and products made from them, such as salad dressing, nuts, seeds, whole grains, and certain fruits and vegetables are sources of vitamin E. Vitamin E serves as an antioxidant, and is involved in immune function, cell signaling, regulation of gene expression, various metabolic processes, and inhibits platelet aggregation.[66] Consuming salad and salad dressing promoted adequate vitamin E intake in a dietary examination study (n = 9466 women and 8282 men).[45] Vitamin E deficiency is rare and most commonly occurs in people with malabsorption disorders such as abetalipoproteinemia; cystic fibrosis; gastrectomy; hepatitic-biliary tract disease including chronic cholestasis, hepatic cirrhosis, biliary atresia, and obstructive jaundice; in infants receiving formula with insufficient vitamin E; and in intestinal disease, such as celiac disease and regional enteritis.[18]

scientific findings

γ-tocopherol, but not α-tocopherol, inhibits cyclooxygenase activity and, thus, possesses anti-inflammatory properties.[64] Some human and animal studies indicate that plasma concentrations of γ-tocopherol are inversely associated with the incidence of cardiovascular disease and prostate cancer.[64] Different forms of vitamin E appear to exert different effects on prostate cancer, with α-tocopherol potentially increasing and γ-tocopherol potentially decreasing risk of the disease.[67] Extensive evidence has demonstrated that many antioxidants, such as vitamin E, have protective effects in preventing cardiovascular disease.[68] Some population study data suggest that increasing dietary vitamin E from food is associated with a reduced risk of prostate cancer, but other population study data suggest that increasing food vitamin E is not associated with prostate cancer risk.[18]

bioactive dose

The RDA is 15 mg/day of α-tocopherol for adults aged 19–50. This is equivalent to 22 IU of natural vitamin E or 33 IU of synthetic vitamin E.[18]

safety

A UL of 1000 mg for adults aged 19–50 (approximately equivalent to 1100 IU of synthetic vitamin E or 1500 IU of natural vitamin E[69]) has been established.

Vitamin K (Phylloquinone)

definition

Fat-soluble vitamin that functions as a coenzyme in the synthesis of proteins involved in blood coagulation and bone metabolism.[16] Vitamin K occurs as phylloquinone, also called vitamin K1, and menaquinone, also referred to as vitamin K2. Phylloquinone is concentrated in dark green, chlorophyll-rich leafy vegetables, such as collards and spinach; in addition, certain plant oils including soybean, canola, cottonseed, and olive, and products made from them, such as margarine and salad dressings, are important dietary sources of phylloquinone.[70] Menaquinone is primarily the product of bacterial production or conversion from dietary phylloquinone or is consumed as menaquinone-4 found in kidney, milk, butter, and cheese.[70] The vitamin gets its name for the Danish word "koagulation."

V

scientific findings

Low circulating vitamin K levels have been observed in subjects with reduced bone mineral density in two of three observational studies.[16] Vitamin K intakes were inversely associated with the risk of hip fracture in a large observational study (n = 71,327 women aged 38 to 63).[16] Vitamin K deficiency increases prothrombin time.[16] Evidence from randomized controlled trials (n = 32 subjects) on the benefits of routine vitamin K supplementation for people with cystic fibrosis is weak and limited to two studies of limited duration.[71]

bioactive dose

The AI is 90 µg for women and 120 µg for men aged 19–50. Vitamin K1 (phytonadione) 2.5–25 mg is administered to newborns to prevent hypoprothrombinemia and hemorrheage.[18]

safety

No UL has been established for vitamin K.

References

1. Arpad Szallasi A, Blumber PM. Vanilloid (Capsaicin) receptors and mechanisms. *Pharmacol Rev.* 1999;51(2):159–212.
2. National Institutes of Health. National Center for Complementary and Integrative Health. Turmeric. https://nccih.nih.gov/health/turmeric/ataglance.htm. Accessed April 8, 2015.
3. Ray A. Cancer preventive role of selected dietary factors. *Indian J Cancer.* 2005;42(1):15–24.
4. Itoh A, Isoda K, Kondoh M, Kawase M, Kobayashi M, Tamesada M, Yagi. Hepatoprotective effect of syringic acid and vanillic acid on concanavalin A-induced liver injury. *K Biol Pharm Bull.* 2009;32(7):1215–1219.
5. Lee E, Surh YJ. Induction of apoptosis in HL-60 cells by pungent vanilloids, [6]-gingerol and [6]-paradol. *Cancer Lett.* 1998;134(2):163–168.
6. Nicklas TA, Jahns L, Bogle ML, Chester DN, Giovanni M, Klurfeld DM, Laugero K, Liu Y, Lopez S, Tucker KL. Barriers and facilitators for consumer adherence to the dietary guidelines for Americans: The HEALTH Study. *J Acad Nutr Diet.* 2013;113(10):1317–1331. Epub 2013 July 16. doi: 10.1016/j.jand.2013.05.004. [Epub ahead of print]
7. Whitney ER, Rolfes SR. *Understanding Nutrition*, 12th edn. Belmont, CA: Wadsworth Cengage; 2011.
8. National Institutes of Health. National Heart, Lung and Blood Institute. Aim for a Healthy Weight. http://www.nhlbi.nih.gov/health/public/heart/obesity/aim_hwt.pdf. Accessed June 4, 2011.
9. Surh Y-J. Cancer chemoprevention with dietary phytochemicals. *Nature Rev.* 2003;3:768–779.

V

10. World Health Organization. e-Library of Evidence for Nutrition Actions. Increasing fruit and vegetable consumption to reduce the risk of noncommunicable diseases. http://www.who.int/elena/titles/fruit_vegetables_ncds/en/. Accessed April 9, 2015.

11. US Department of Agriculture. Choose MyPlate.gov. Vegetables. Why is it important to eat vegetables? http://www.choosemyplate.gov/food-groups/vegetables-why.html. Accessed January 28, 2012.

12. Bazzano LA, Serdula MK, Liu S. Dietary intake of fruits and vegetables and risk of cardiovascular disease. *Curr Atheroscler Rep.* 2003;5(6):492–499.

13. National Cancer Institute. Cancer Progress Trends Report. http://progress-report.cancer.gov/prevention/fruit_vegetable. Accessed February 6, 2015.

14. Joseph JA, Shukitt-Hale B, Willis LM. Grape juice, berries, and walnuts affect brain aging and behavior. *J Nutr.* 2009;139(9):1813S–1817S.

15. National Institutes of Health. Office of Dietary Supplements. Dietary Supplement Fact Sheet: Vitamin A and Carotenoids. http://ods.od.nih.gov/factsheets/VitaminA-HealthProfessional/. Accessed June 23, 2011.

16. Institute of Medicine. *Dietary Reference Intakes for Vitamin A, Vitamin K, Arsenic, Boron, Chromium, Copper, Iodine, Iron, Manganese, Molybdenum, Nickel, Silicon, Vanadium and Zinc.* Washington, DC: National Academy Press; 2001.

17. Whitney ER, DeBruyne LK, Pinna K, Rolfes SR. *Nutrition for Health and Health Care,* 4th edn. Belmont, CA: Cengage; 2011.

18. Jellin JM, Gregory PJ. *Natural Medicine Comprehensive Database.* Therapeutic Research Faculty. 2013. http://www.naturaldatabase.com. Accessed July 11, 2012.

19. National Institutes of Health Office of Dietary Supplements. Vitamin A—Health Professional Fact Sheet. http://ods.od.nih.gov/factsheets/VitaminA-HealthProfessional/. Accessed August 5, 2013.

20. Rothman KH, Moore LL, Singer MR, Nguyen T-SDT, Mannino S, Milunsky A. Teratogenicity of high vitamin A intake. *N Engl J Med.* 1995;333(21):1369–1373.

21. Institute of Medicine. *Dietary Reference Intakes for Thiamin, Riboflavin, Niacin, Vitamin B6, Folate, Vitamin B12, Pantothenic Acid, Biotin and Choline.* Washington DC: National Academy Press; 1998.

22. Friso S, Jacques PF, Wilson PWF, Rosenberg IH, Selhub J. Low circulating vitamin B6 is associated with elevation of the inflammation marker C-Reactive protein independently of plasma homocysteine levels. *Circulation.* 2001;103:2788–2791.

23. Malouf R, Grimley Evans J. The effect of vitamin B6 on cognition. *Cochrane Database Syst Rev.* 2003;(4):CD004393.

24. Watanabe F, Yabuta Y, Tanioka Y, Bito T. Biologically active vitamin B12 compounds in foods for preventing deficiency among vegetarians and elderly subjects. *J Agric Food Chem.* 2013;61(28):6769–6775. doi: 10.1021/jf401545z. Epub 2013 July 2.

25. Herbert V, Subak-Sharpe GJ. *The Mount Sinai School of Medicine Complete Book of Nutrition.* New York: St. Martin's Press; 1990.

26. Langan RC, Zawistoski KJ. Update on vitamin B12 deficiency. *Am Fam Physician.* 2011;83(12):1425–1430.

27. Brito A, Hertrampf E, Olivares M, Gaitán D, Sánchez H, Allen LH, Uauy R. Folate, vitamin B12 and human health. *Rev Med Chile.* 2012;140(11):1464–75. doi: 10.1590/S0034-98872012001100014.

V

28. Institute of Medicine. *Dietary Reference Intakes for Thiamin, Riboflavin, Niacin, Vitamin B6, Folate, Vitamin B12, Pantothenic Acid, Biotin and Choline.* Washington DC: National Academy Press; 1998.

29. Malouf R, Areosa Sastre A. Vitamin B12 for cognition. *Cochrane Database Syst Rev.* 2003;(3):CD004326.

30. Martinez Estrada KM, Cadabal Rodriguez T, Miguens Blanco I, García Méndez L. Neurological signs due to isolated vitamin B12 deficiency. *Semergen.* 2013;39(5):e8–e11. doi: 10.1016/j.semerg.2012.06.006. Epub 2012 August 11.

31. Robert Langan MD. (B12 Expert) in discussion with Diane Kraft, September 3, 2015.

32. Cinemre H, Serinkan Cinemre BF, Çekdemir D, Aydemir B, Tamer A, Yazar H. Diagnosis of vitamin B12 deficiency in patients with myeloproliferative disorders. *J Invest Med.* 2015;63(4):636–40. doi: 10.1097/JIM.0000000000000187.

33. Herrmann W, Obeid R. Cobalamin deficiency. *Subcell Biochem.* 2012;56:301–22. doi: 10.1007/978-94-007-2199-9_16.

34. Dangour AD, Allen E, Clarke R, Elbourne D, Fasey N, Fletcher AE, Letley L et al. A randomised controlled trial investigating the effect of vitamin B12 supplementation on neurological function in healthy older people: The Older People and Enhanced Neurological function (OPEN) study protocol [ISRCTN54195799]. *Nutr J.* 2011;10:22. doi: 10.1186/1475-2891-10-22. http://www.ncbi.nlm.nih.gov/pmc/articles/PMC3062585/

35. Neumann WL, Coss E, Rugge M, Genta RM. Autoimmune atrophic gastritis-pathogenesis, pathology and management. *Nat Rev Gastroenterol Hepatol.* 2013;10(9):529–541. Epub 2013 June 18. doi: 10.1038/nrgastro.2013.101. [Epub ahead of print]

36. US Department of Agriculture. US Department of Health and Human Services. *Dietary Guidelines for Americans,* 2010, 7th edn. Washington, DC: U.S. Government Printing Office, December 2010.

37. Academy of Nutrition and Dietetics Evidence Analysis Library. What is the evidence regarding the effect of oral vitamin B12 supplementation and/or fortification on serum cobalamin levels in deficient older adults? http://www.andeal.org/topic.cfm?menu=3580&cat=3768. Accessed April 6, 2015.

38. Shaik-Dasthagirisaheb YB, Varvara G, Murmura G, Saggini A, Caraffa A, Antinolfi P, Tete' S et al. Role of vitamins D, E and C in immunity and inflammation. *J Biol Regul Homeost Agents.* 2013;27(2):291–295.

39. Institute of Medicine. *Dietary Reference Intakes for Vitamin C, Vitamin E, Selenium and Carotenoids.* Washington, DC: National Academy Press; 2000.

40. Grosso G, Bei R, Mistretta A, Marventano S, Calabrese G, Masuelli L, Giganti MG, Modesti A, Galvano F, Gazzolo D. Effects of vitamin C on health: A review of evidence. *Front Biosci (Landmark Ed).* 2013;18:1017–1029.

41. Wolber FM, Beck KL, Conlon CA, Kruger MC. Kiwifruit and mineral nutrition. *Adv Food Nutr Res.* 2013;68:233–256. doi: 10.1016/B978-0-12-394294-4.00013-4.

42. Gropper SS, Smith JL, Groff JL. *Advanced Nutrition and Human Metabolism,* 4th edn. Belmont CA: Wadsworth Cengage Learning; 2005.

43. Doll S, Ricou B. Severe vitamin C deficiency in a critically ill adult: A case report. *Eur J Clin Nutr.* 2013;67(8):881–882. doi: 10.1038/ejcn.2013.42. Epub 2013 April 3.

44. Mertens MT, Gertner E. Rheumatic manifestations of scurvy: A report of three recent cases in a major urban center and a review. *Semin Arthritis Rheum.* 2011; 41(2):286–290. doi: 10.1016/j.semarthrit.2010.10.005. Epub 2010 December 23.

45. Institute of Medicine. *Dietary Reference Intakes for Vitamins C, E, Selenium, and Carotenoids.* Washington DC: National Academy Press; 2000.
46. Khaw KT, Bingham S, Welch A, Luben R, Wareham N, Oakes S, Day N. Relation between plasma ascorbic acid and mortality in men and women in EPIC-Norfolk prospective study: A prospective population study. European Prospective Investigation into Cancer and Nutrition. *Lancet.* 2001;357(9257):657–663.
47. Tso MO. Pathogenetic factors of aging macular degeneration. *Ophthalmology.* 1985;92(5):628–635.
48. Kennel KA, Drake MT, Hurley DL. Vitamin D deficiency in adults: When to test and how to treat. *Mayo Clin Proc.* 2010; 85(8):753–758.
49. Jäpelt RB, Jakobsen J. Vitamin D in plants: A review of occurrence, analysis, and biosynthesis. *Front Plant Sci.* 2013;4:136. doi: 10.3389/fpls.2013.00136. eCollection 2013.
50. Neve A, Corrado A, Cantatore FP. Immunomodulatory effects of vitamin D in peripheral blood monocyte-derived macrophages from patients with rheumatoid arthritis. *Clin Exp Med.* 2014;14(3):275–283. Epub 2013 July 4.
51. Institute of Medicine. Dietary Reference Intakes for Calcium and Vitamin D. http://books.nap.edu/openbook.php?record_id=13050&page=8. Accessed August 13, 2013.
52. Lerchbaum E, Obermayer-Pietsch B. Vitamin D and fertility: A systematic review. *Eur J Endocrinol.* 2012;166(5):765–778. doi: 10.1530/EJE-11-0984. Epub 2012 January 24. Epub 2012 January 24.
53. Holick MF. Vitamin D: A d-lightful solution for health. *J Invest Med.* 2011;59(6):872–880. doi: 10.231/JIM.0b013e318214ea2d.
54. Watkins CM, Lively MW. A review of vitamin D and its effects on athletes. *Phys Sportsmed.* 2012;40(3):26–31. doi: 10.3810/psm.2012.09.1977.
55. Garland CF, Garland FC, Gorham ED, Lipkin M, Newmark H, Mohr SB, Holick MF. The role of vitamin D in cancer prevention. *Am J Public Health.* 2006;96(2):252–261.
56. Bouillon R, Van Schoor NM, Gielen E, Boonen S, Mathieu C, Vanderschueren D, Lips P. Optimal vitamin D status: A critical analysis on the basis of evidence-based medicine. *J Clin Endocrinol Metab.* 2013;98(8):E1283–304.
57. Fung GJ, Steffen LM, Zhou X, Harnack L, Tang W, Lutsey PL, Loria CM, Reis JP, Van Horn LV. Vitamin D intake is inversely related to risk of developing metabolic syndrome in African American and white men and women over 20 y: The Coronary Artery Risk Development in Young Adults study. *Am J Clin Nutr.* 2012;96(1):24–29. Epub 2012 May 30.
58. Christakos S, Hewison M, Gardner DG, Wagner CL, Sergeev IN, Rutten E, Pittas AG, Boland R, Ferrucci L, Bikle DD. Vitamin D: Beyond bone. *Ann N Y Acad Sci.* 2013;1287:45–58. Epub 2013 May 17.
59. Ashtari F, Ajalli M, Shaygannejad V, Akbari M, Hovsepian S. The relation between Vitamin D status with fatigue and depressive symptoms of multiple sclerosis. *J Res Med Sci.* 2013;18(3):193–197.
60. Cassidy-Bushrow AE, Peters RM, Johnson DA, Li J, Rao DS. Vitamin D nutritional status and antenatal depressive symptoms in African American women. *J Women's Health (Larchmt).* 2012;21(11):1189–1195. Epub 2012 July 23.
61. Jensen MB, Nielsen JE, Jorgensen A, Rajpert-De Meyts E, Møbjerg Kristensen D, Jørgensen N, Skakkebaek NE, Juul A, Leffers H. Vitamin D receptor and

V

vitamin D metabolizing enzymes are expressed in the human male reproductive tract. *Hum Reprod.* 2010;25(5):1303–1311.

62. Kaushal M, Magon N. Vitamin D in pregnancy: A metabolic outlook. *Indian J Endocrinol Metab.* 2013;17(1):76–82.

63. National Institutes of Health. Office of Dietary Supplements. Dietary Supplement Fact Sheet: Vitamin D. http://ods.od.nih.gov/factsheets/VitaminD-HealthProfessional/. Accessed August 5, 2013.

64. Jiang Q, Christen S, Shigenaga MK, Ames BN. Gamma-tocopherol, the major form of vitamin E in the US diet, deserves more attention. *Am J Clin Nutr.* 2001;74(6):714–722.

65. US Department of Agriculture. National Nutrient Database. Nutrient List for Alpha-, Beta-, and Gamma-Tocopherol. http://ndb.nal.usda.gov/ndb/nutrients/index. Accessed April 9, 2015.

66. National Institutes of Health. Office of Dietary Supplements. Vitamin E Fact Sheet for Health Professionals. http://ods.od.nih.gov/factsheets/VitaminE-HealthProfessional/. Accessed April 4, 2015.

67. Vance TM, Su J, Fontham ET, Koo SI, Chun OK. Dietary antioxidants and prostate cancer: A review. *Nutr Cancer.* 2013;65(6):793–801.

68. Wang Y, Chun OK, Song WO. Plasma and dietary antioxidant status as cardiovascular disease risk factors: A review of human studies. *Nutrients.* 2013;5(8):2969–3004.

69. Regulatory Affairs Vitamin Converter. http://www.robert-forbes.com/public_html/index.php?option=com_content&view=article&id=61&Itemid=90. Accessed January 5, 2015.

70. Booth SL. Vitamin K: Food composition and dietary intakes. *Food Nutr Res.* 2012;56. Epub 2012 April 2.

71. Jagannath VA, Fedorowicz Z, Thaker V, Chang AB. Vitamin K supplementation for cystic fibrosis. *Cochrane Database Syst Rev.* 2015;18;1:CD008482. doi: 10.1002/14651858.CD008482.pub4.

V

W

Walnut (Juglans regia L.)

definition

Also called English walnut. Common tree nut that is a source of protein, monounsaturated fatty acids, polyunsaturated fatty acids, including omega-3 fatty acid, carotenoids, phytosterols, flavonoids, proanthocyanidins, phytates, and lignans.[1]

scientific findings

A small, randomized clinical trial (n = 18 healthy men) found that replacing 20% of calories from high-fat foods in the diet with walnuts within a cholesterol-lowering diet for 4 weeks decreased serum levels of total cholesterol.[2] Some research suggests that people who increase consumption of walnuts and other nuts might have a lower risk of coronary heart disease and death due to coronary events, and that substituting walnuts for other dietary fats may improve HDL and cholesterol-to-total-cholesterol ratios in patients with type 2 diabetes.[3]

bioactive dose

Not known. "For lowering cholesterol, approximately 30–56 grams English walnuts (about 1/4 to 1/2 cup or 8 to 11 nuts) has been substituted for other dietary fats."[3]

safety

Presumed safe when consumed in normal dietary quantities by non-allergic individuals. Allergic and fatal anaphylactic reactions to walnuts have been reported.[4]

W

Wasabi (Wasabia japonica)

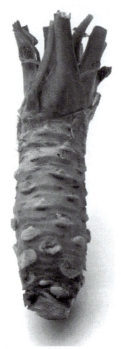

Wasabi. (Image from matin/Shutterstock.)

definition

Also known as Japanese radish, a pine-cone-shaped *Brassica* vegetable that is ground into a pungent sushi condiment. It contains isothiocyanates.[5]

scientific findings

In laboratory studies, *Wasabia japonica* killed *Helicobacter pylori*,[6] exhibited detoxification, anti-inflammation, cancer cell apoptosis, and colon cancer cell apoptosis.[7]

bioactive dose

Not known.

W

safety

Presumed safe when consumed in normal dietary quantities by non-allergic individuals, except for the adverse effects of extreme burning sensations.

Water

definition

Essential nutrient necessary for many functions, including hydration and maintenance of adequate blood volume and blood pressure, regulation of body temperature, and transporting nutrients, oxygen, and other substances in blood. Total water intake includes drinking water, water in nonalcoholic beverages, and water (moisture) in foods. There are no uniform standards for water purity. Collecting urine for 24 h to measure the volume of urine produced is a proxy of water intake.[8] The normal range for 24-h urine volume is 800–2000 mL/day (with a normal fluid intake of about 2 L/day).[9] Hydration status is assessed by several methods, the primary indicator being plasma or serum osmolality[8] that measures the concentration of chemical particles found in the fluid part of blood (and normal values range from 275 to 295 milliosmoles/kilogram).[10]

scientific findings

Hard water is a source of magnesium and calcium, which are associated with the maintenance of normal blood pressure, while soft water is higher in sodium and can aggravate high blood pressure and heart disease.[11,12] Effects of dehydration include metabolic and functional abnormalities, and low intake of water is associated with some chronic diseases.[8]

bioactive dose

The AI for total water is 2.7 L/day for women and 3.7 L/day for men aged 19–50 years, which is met by drinking water and nonalcoholic beverages and eating fruits, vegetables, and other foods[8]; however, water needs are highly variable based on size, body composition, physical activity level, climate, and other factors,[13] and therefore water intake exceeding the AI is required for individuals, including athletes.

W

safety

Although no UL has been established for water, excessive water intake, without concomitant electrolyte consumption, can cause water intoxication and hyponatremia that is potentially life-threatening.

Watercress (Nasturtium officinale)

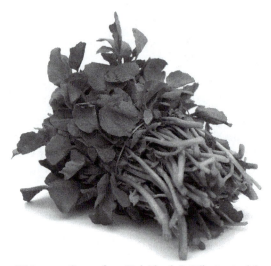

Watercress. (Image from Binh Thanh Bui/Shutterstock.)

definition

Dark green *Brassica* salad vegetable whose small leaves and soft stems have a radish-like flavor. Watercress is a good source of calcium[14] and is also a source of lutein and carotenes.[15] Watercress has been traditionally used as an antioxidant, anti-inflammatory, hypolipidemic, and cardioprotective agent.[15]

scientific findings

In an experimental study in animals, watercress juice protected cells and did not damage DNA.[16] In a single-blind, randomized, crossover study (n = 30 smokers and 30 nonsmoking men and women, mean age 33 years), subjects were fed 85 g raw watercress daily for 8 weeks in addition to their usual diet. The effect of watercress supplementation was measured on a range of end points, including DNA damage in lymphocytes, activity of detoxifying enzymes (glutathione peroxidase and superoxide dismutase) in erythrocytes, plasma antioxidants (retinol, ascorbic acid, α-tocopherol,

W

lutein, and β-carotene), plasma total antioxidant status, and plasma lipid profile. Watercress supplementation in the treated group compared to the control group was associated with beneficial reductions in markers of DNA damage, and plasma lutein and β-carotene increased significantly, with beneficial changes being more significant in smokers than in non-smokers after watercress supplementation.[15]

bioactive dose

Not known.

safety

Presumed safe when consumed in normal dietary quantities by non-allergic individuals.

Watermelon (Citrullis lanatus)

definition

Member of the cucumber and squash family that includes fruits of different sizes, shapes, rind patterns, and flesh colors.[17] Watermelon contains a relatively high sugar content, consisting of sucrose, fructose, and glucose,[18] and is a source of lycopene.[19] Eaten fresh, alone, or in fruit salads; its pickled rind is eaten in certain cultures.

scientific findings

A case–control study (n = 438 Chinese women age matched to n = 438 controls) that examined dietary intake and breast cancer risk found consumption of the "watermelon/papaya/cantaloupe" fruit group was significantly inversely associated with breast cancer risk.[20]

bioactive dose

Not known.

safety

Presumed safe when consumed in normal dietary quantities by non-allergic individuals.

W

Wheat germ

definition

Wheat grain embryo that contains high concentrations of unsaturated fats, protein, and vitamin E, it is removed from the grain to reduce grain perishability when whole grains are refined. Eaten by the spoonful or sprinkled onto other foods.

scientific findings

In animal studies, wheat germ improved markers of antioxidant status in animal tissues.[21]

bioactive dose

Not known.

safety

Presumed safe when consumed in normal dietary quantities by non-allergic individuals.

Whey

definition

Complete protein found within the watery portion of milk. Whey comprises 20% of milk protein, while casein makes up 80%.[22] Cheese is a source of whey, and whey is filtered from milk to make cheese. Greek-style yogurt has most of the water and whey strained out, whereas thin-style (non-Greek) yogurt contains whey. Whey contains lactose and provides more than 20% of the DV for calcium per cup.[23]

scientific findings

Whey has exerted chemoprotective, anti-HIV effects, and reduced body weight gain relative to red meat consumption in laboratory animals.[24–26] In healthy and type 2 diabetes subjects, whey protein has exerted insulinotropic and glucose-lowering properties, according to a review that theorized whey protein may generate bioactive products during digestion that stimulate the release of gut hormones that in turn regulate food intake or potentiate insulin secretion.[22]

bioactive dose

Not known.

safety

Presumed safe when consumed in normal dietary quantities by non-allergic individuals.

References

1. Bolling BW, Chen CY, McKay DL, Blumberg JB. Tree nut phytochemicals: Composition, antioxidant capacity, bioactivity, impact factors. A systematic review of almonds, Brazils, cashews, hazelnuts, macadamias, pecans, pine nuts, pistachios and walnuts. *Nutr Res Rev.* 2011;24(2):244–275. doi: 10.1017/S095442241100014X. Epub 2011 December 12.

2. Sabate J, Fraser GE, Burke K, Knutsen SF, Bennett H, Lindsted KD. Effects of walnuts on serum lipid levels and blood pressure in normal men. *N Engl J Med.* 1993;328:603–607.

3. Jellin JM, Gregory PJ. Natural Medicines Comprehensive Database. http://www.naturaldatabase.com. Accessed July 11, 2012. Therapeutic Research Faculty; 2013.

4. DerMarderosian A, Beutler JA. *Review of Natural Products*, 5th edn. St. Louis, MO: Wolters Kluwer; 2008.

5. Nakamura T, Kitamoto N, Osawa T, Kato Y. Immunochemical detection of food-derived isothiocyanate as a lysine conjugate. *Biosci Biotechnol Biochem.* 2010;74(3):536–540. Epub 2010 March 7.

6. Shin IS, Masuda H, Naohide K. Bactericidal activity of wasabi (*Wasabia japonica*) against *Helicobacter pylori*. *Int J Food Microbiol.* 2004; 94(3):255–261.

7. Hsuan SW, Chyau CC, Hung HY, Chen JH, Chou FP. The induction of apoptosis and autophagy by *Wasabia japonica* extract in colon cancer. *Eur J Nutr.* 2015 February 27. [Epub ahead of print].

8. Institute of Medicine. *Dietary Reference Intakes for Water, Potassium, Sodium, Chloride and Sulfate*, Washington, DC: National Academy Press; 2005.

9. National Institutes of Health Medline Plus. Urine 24 Hour Volume. http://www.nlm.nih.gov/medlineplus/ency/article/003425.htm. Accessed March 8, 2015.

10. National Institutes of Health Medline Plus. Osmolality-blood test. http://www.nlm.nih.gov/medlineplus/ency/article/003463.htm. Accessed March 8, 2015.

11. Blaszczyk U, Duda-Chodak A. Magnesium: Its role in nutrition and carcinogenesis. *Rocz Panstw Zakl Hig.* 2013;64(3):165–171.

12. Whitney E, Rolfes SR. *Understanding Nutrition*, 11th edn. Belmont, CA: Cengage, Thomson Wadsworth; 2008.

13. Hedrick Fink H, Mikesky AE, Burgoon LA. *Practical Applications in Sports Nutrition*, 3rd edn. Burlington, MA: Jones & Bartlett Learning; 2012.

14. Whitney ER, Rolfes SR. *Understanding Nutrition*, 12th edn. Belmont, CA: Wadsworth Cengage; 2011.

15. Gill CI, Haldar S, Boyd LA, Bennett R, Whiteford J, Butler M, Pearson JR, Bradbury I, Rowland IR. Watercress supplementation in diet reduces lymphocyte DNA damage and alters blood antioxidant status in healthy adults. *Am J Clin Nutr.* 2007;85(2):504–510.

16. Casanova NA, Ariagno JI, López Nigro MM, Mendeluk GR, Gette Mde L, Petenatti E, Palaoro LA, Carballo MA. *In vivo* antigenotoxic activity of watercress juice (*Nasturtium officinale*) against induced DNA damage. *J Appl Toxicol.* 2013;33(9):880–885. doi: 10.1002/jat.2746. Epub 2012 April 4.

17. Gusmini G, Wehner TC. Qualitative inheritance of rind pattern and flesh color in watermelon. *J Hered.* 2006;97(2):177–185. Epub 2006 February 17.

W

18. Yativ M, Harary I, Wolf SJ. Sucrose accumulation in watermelon fruits: Genetic variation and biochemical analysis. *Plant Physiol.* 2010; 167(8):589–596. Epub 2009 December 29.

19. Tarazona-Díaz MP, Aguayo E. Influence of acidification, pasteurization, centrifugation, time and storage temperature on watermelon juice quality. *J Sci Food Agric.* 2013;93(15):3863–3869. Epub 2013 July 31. doi: 10.1002/jsfa.6332. [Epub ahead of print.]

20. Zhang CX, Ho SC, Chen YM, Fu JH, Cheng SZ, Lin FY. Greater vegetable and fruit intake is associated with a lower risk of breast cancer among Chinese women. *Int J Cancer.* 2009;125(1):181–188.

21. Leenhardt F, Fardet A, Lyan B, Gueux E, Rock E, Mazur A, Chanliaud E, Demigné C, Rémésy C. Wheat germ supplementation of a low vitamin E diet in rats affords effective antioxidant protection in tissues. *J Am Coll Nutr.* 2008;27(2):222–228.

22. Jakubowicz D, Froy O. Biochemical and metabolic mechanisms by which dietary whey protein may combat obesity and type 2 diabetes. *J Nutr Biochem.* 2013;24(1):1–5. doi: 10.1016/j.jnutbio.2012.07.008. Epub 2012 September 17.

23. US Department of Agriculture. Agricultural Research Service. Nutrient Data Laboratory. Whey protein. http://ndb.nal.usda.gov/ndb/foods/show/100. Accessed January 31, 2012.

24. Belobrajdic DP, McIntosh GH, Owens JA. A high-whey-protein diet reduces body weight gain and alters insulin sensitivity relative to red meat in Wistar rats. *J Nutr.* 2004;134:1454–1458.

25. Baruchel S, Olivier R, Wainberg M. Anti-HIV and anti-apoptotic activity of the whey protein concentrate. *Immunocal Int Conf AIDS.* 1994;10:32 (abstract # 421A).

26. Bounous G, Batist G, Gold P. Whey proteins in cancer prevention. *Cancer Lett.* 1991;7:91–94.

W

X

Xeaxanthin

definition

Also spelled *zeaxanthin*. Xanthophyll carotenoid that occurs commonly with lutein in foods. Rich sources of xeaxanthin include egg yolk, dark green leafy vegetables, orange bell pepper, kiwi fruit, grapes, spinach, zucchini, corn, and squash.[1,2]

scientific findings

The macular region of the retina is yellow owing to the presence of macular pigment, consisting largely of lutein and xeaxanthin.[2] The amount of macular pigment correlates with dietary intake of lutein and xeaxanthin and other factors,[3] and may be protective against age-related macular degeneration according to epidemiological evidence.[2] Laboratory data suggest inverse correlations between plasma xanthophyll carotenoids and oxidative damage in DNA and lipids.[4]

bioactive dose

Not known.

safety

Presumed safe when consumed in normal dietary quantities by non-allergic individuals.

References

1. Sommerburg O, Keunen JE, Bird AC, van Kuijk FJ. Fruits and vegetables that are sources for lutein and xeaxanthin: The macular pigment in human eyes. *Br J Ophthalmic*. 1998;82(8):907–910.
2. Krinsky NI, Landrum JT, Bone RA. Biologic mechanisms of the protective role of lutein and xeaxanthin in the eye. *Annu Rev Nutr*. 2003;23:171–201.

X

3. Curran-Celentano J, Hammond Jr. BR, Ciulla TA, Cooper DA, Pratt LM, Danis RB. Relation between dietary intake, serum concentrations, and retinal concentrations of lutein and xeaxanthin in adults in a Midwest population. *Am J Clin Nutr.* 2001;74(6):796–802.
4. Haegele AD, Gillette C, O'Neill C, Wolfe P, Heimendinger J, Sedlacek S, Thompson HJ. Plasma xanthophyll carotenoids correlate inversely with indices of oxidative DNA damage and lipid peroxidation. *Cancer Epidemiol Biomarkers Prev.* 2000;9:421–425.

X

Y

Yam (Dioscorea rotundata)

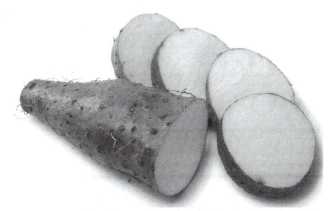

Yam. (Image from jiangdi/Shutterstock.)

definition

Tuber root vegetable that is long and cylindrical whose flesh, depending on species, can range from off-white to yellow or pink or purple, with skin that is off-white to dark brown.[1] Yam differs from the darker orange sweet potato, *Ipomoea batatas*, which is classified under a different botanical family, and because yams are not dark orange in color, their vitamin A content is much lower than sweet potatoes. Approximately 150 different species of yam are commercially cultivated, and white yam (*D. rotundata*) is the most predominant yam species produced worldwide.[2] In traditional folk medicine, yams have been used to treat menopausal symptoms. Yam contains natural steroid precursors but does not have oral contraceptive properties, contrary to popular belief that the phytochemical diosgenin found in wild yam is used to manufacture human steroidal hormones, such as dehydroepiandrosterone, though "taking wild yam extract will not increase dehydroepiandrosterone levels in humans."[3] Yams are baked, boiled, or fried. They are a good source of fiber and an excellent source of vitamin C, folate, and potassium.[4]

Y

scientific findings

In a clinical trial (n = 24 postmenopausal women), replacing a staple food with 390 g of the *Dioscorea alata* species of yam per day for 30 days increased serum levels of sex hormones (estrone, sex hormone binding globulin, and estradiol) compared to a control group (n = 19 healthy postmenopausal women) fed 240 g of sweet potato for 41 days who had no change in serum levels of hormones.[5] A laboratory study found yam extract to protect against cancer proliferation in human breast cancer cells.[6]

bioactive dose

Not known.

safety

Presumed safe when consumed in normal dietary quantities by non-allergic individuals.

References

1. University of California. Agriculture & Natural Resources. Sweet potato or yam? http://cesolano.ucdavis.edu/files/59967.pdf. Accessed March 25, 2015.
2. Dania VO, Fadina OO, Ayodele M, Kumar PL. Efficacy of *Oryza sativa* husk and *Quercus phillyraeoides* extracts for the *in vitro* and *in vivo* control of fungal rot disease of white yam (*Dioscorea rotundata* Poir). *SpringerPlus*. 2014;3:711.
3. Jellin JM, Gregory PJ. Natural Medicine Comprehensive Database. Therapeutic Research Faculty. 2013. http://www.naturaldatabase.com. Accessed July 11, 2012.
4. USDA Agricultural Research Service National Nutrient Database. Yam. http://ndb.nal.usda.gov/ndb/search/list. Accessed March 2, 2012.
5. Wu WH, Liu LY, Chung CJ, Jou HJ, Wang TA. Estrogenic effect of yam ingestion in healthy postmenopausal women. *J Am Coll Nutr.* 2005;24(4):235–243.
6. Park MK, Kwon HY, Ahn WS, Bae S, Rhyu MR, Lee Y. Estrogen activities and the cellular effects of natural progesterone from wild yam extract in MCF-7 human breast cancer cells. *Am J Chin Med.* 2009;37(1):159–167.

Y

Z

Zinc

definition

Trace mineral necessary for immune function, growth, protein and DNA synthesis, wound healing, and taste and sense perception.[1,2] Rich sources of zinc include red meat, seafood, such as oysters, crab and lobster, whole grains, and zinc-fortified breakfast cereals.[3] The median intake of zinc for adults exceeds the zinc RDA (median intake for women is 9 mg/day and for men is 13 mg/day[3]).

scientific findings

Certain individuals may be at risk for zinc deficiency, including vegetarians and vegans who ingest insufficient amounts; people who have severe diarrhea or malabsorption syndromes (e.g., due to weight loss surgery, or digestive disorders, such as ulcerative colitis or Crohn's disease); liver cirrhosis; after major surgery; during long-term administration of total parenteral nutrition; older infants who are breastfed because breast milk does not have enough zinc for infants over 6 months of age; alcoholics due to their limited, unvaried diet, and because alcohol decreases zinc absorption and increases urinary zinc excretion; and possibly people with sickle cell anemia.[1,4] Zinc deficiency symptoms include slowed growth in children, delayed sexual development in adolescents, impotence in men, hair loss, diarrhea, eye and skin sores, a loss of appetite, impaired immune function, decreased taste sensation, weight loss, delayed wound healing, and reduced mental alertness.[3] Zinc deficiency decreases spermatogenesis and impairs male fertility.[5] Zinc adequacy is necessary for male fertility for testicular development, sperm maturation, and testosterone synthesis; and for female fertility because it plays a role in female sexual development, ovulation, and the menstrual cycle.[6]

bioactive dose

The RDA for adult women (aged 19–50 years) is 8 mg/day and for adult men (aged 19–50 years) is 11 mg/day.

safety

An UL of 40 mg/day has been established for adult men and women aged 19–50 years.

Zucchini (Cucurbita pepo)

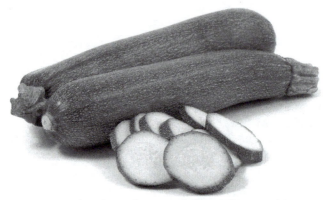

Zucchini. (Image from unverdorben jr/Shutterstock.)

definition

Mild-flavored, white-fleshed vegetable that resembles a cucumber in its cylindrical shape and green skin. It supplies >1000 IU of vitamin A per 1/2 cup cooked, in addition to cucurbitosides, flavonoids, triterpenes, sterols, lutein, and xeaxanthin.[7,8] Zucchini is commonly stir-fried, used in casseroles, or cooked with tomato as an ingredient in ratatouille; zucchini may be cut into ribbons and substituted for fettucini.[9]

scientific findings

Zucchini contains substantial amounts of lutein and xeaxanthin whose intake is associated with a decreased risk of age-related macular degeneration.[10]

bioactive dose

Not known.

safety

Presumed safe when consumed in normal dietary quantities by non-allergic individuals.

Z

References

1. National Institute of Health. Office of Dietary Supplements. Dietary Supplement Fact Sheet: Zinc. http://ods.od.nih.gov/factsheets/Zinc-QuickFacts/. Accessed June 13, 2011.
2. Ibs K-H, Rink R. Zinc-altered immune function. *J Nutr*. 2003;133(5):1452S–1456S.
3. Institute of Medicine. *Dietary References Intakes for Vitamin A, Vitamin K, Arsenic, Boron, Chromium, Copper, Iodine, Iron, Manganese, Molybdenum, Nickel, Silicon, Vanadium, and Zinc*. Washington DC: National Academy Press; 2002.
4. Temiye EO, Duke ES, Owolabi MA, Renner JK. Relationship between painful crisis and serum zinc level in children with sickle cell anaemia. *Anemia*. 2014;2011:1-7. doi:10.1155/2011/698586
5. Wong WY, Thomas CMG, Merkus JMWM, Zielhuis GA, Steegers-Theunissen RPM. Male factor subfertility: Possible causes and the impact of nutritional factors. *Fertil Steril*. 2000;73(3):435–442.
6. Ebisch IM, Thomas CM, Peters WH, Braat DD, Steegers-Theunissen RP. The importance of folate, zinc and antioxidants in the pathogenesis and prevention of subfertility. *Hum Reprod Update*. 2007;13(2):163–174. Epub 2006 November 11.
7. US Department of Agriculture. Agricultural Research Service. Phytochemical Database. *Cucurbita pepo*. http://www.pl.barc.usda.gov/usda_plant/plant. Accessed June 2, 2011.
8. US Department of Agriculture. Agricultural Research Service. Nutrient Data Laboratory. Zucchini, cooked, mashed. http://ndb.nal.usda.gov/ndb/foods/show/3247. Accessed January 28, 2012.
9. The New York Times. Health. Zucchini pasta. http://www.nytimes.com/2008/08/23/health/22recipehealth.html. Accessed January 28, 2012.
10. Sommerburg O, Keunen JE, Bird AC, van Kuijk FJ. Fruits and vegetables that are sources for lutein and xeaxanthin: The macular pigment in human eyes. *Br J Ophthalmol*. 1998;82(8):907–910.

Z

Appendix

Table A1 Major phytochemical groups and specific phytochemicals
addressed in this guide

Major phytochemical category	Specific phytochemicals in foods addressed in this guide
Dietary fiber	Insoluble fiber • Cellulose • Lignin Soluble fiber • Beta-glucan • Fructooligosaccharide • Pectin
Fatty acids	Monounsaturated fatty acids Polyunsaturated fatty acids • Linoleic acid (omega-6-fatty acid) • Linolenic acid (omega-6 fatty acid)
Glucosinolates	Aglycones Indoles • Piperine Isothiocyanates • Sulforaphane Organosulfur compounds, also called sulfur compounds or sulfides • Allyl sulfides • Thiols
Phenolic compounds	Aromatic acids • Phenolic acids (chlorogenic acid, ferulic acid, syringic acid, vanillic acid) • Hydroxycinnaminic acids (caffeic acid, chlorogenic acid, ferulic acid, gingerol)

(Continued)

Table A1 (Continued) Major phytochemical groups and specific
phytochemicals addressed in this guide

Major phytochemical category	Specific phytochemicals in foods addressed in this guide
	Capsaicin
	Polyphenols
	• Curcuminoids (curcumin)
	• Flavonoids (anthocyanins, catechins, chalcones, flavanols, flavones, flavonols, flavanones, glycosides, glycoalkaloids)
	• Isoflavonoids (isoflavones)
	• Lignans (lignan)
	• Stilbenoids (resveratrol, stilbene)
	• Tannin
Terpenoids	Monoterpenes
	• Limonene
	Diterpenes
	• Retinol
	Tetraterpenes
	• Carotenoids (carotenes, xanthophylls)
	Triterpenoids
	• Glycosides
	Steroids
	• Stanols
	• Sterols
	• Tocopherol

Index